FIRST AID®
CASES
FOR THE
USMLE
STEP 1

Third Edition

TAO LE, MD, MHS
Associate Clinical Professor of Medicine and Pediatrics
Chief, Section of Allergy and Immunology
Department of Medicine
University of Louisville

JAMES S. YEH, MD
Resident Physician
Clinical Fellow in Medicine
Cambridge Health Alliance
Harvard Medical School

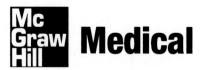
Medical

New York / Chicago / San Francisco / Lisbon / London / Madrid / Mexico City
Milan / New Delhi / San Juan / Seoul / Singapore / Sydney / Toronto

The McGraw·Hill Companies

First Aid® Cases for the USMLE Step 1, Third Edition

1 2 3 4 5 6 7 8 9 0   QDB/QDB   14 13 12

ISBN 978-0-07-174397-6
MHID 0-07-174397-9
ISSN 1559-5757

Notice

Medicine is an ever-changing science. As new research and clinical experience broaden our knowledge, changes in treatment and drug therapy are required. The authors and the publisher of this work have checked with sources believed to be reliable in their efforts to provide information that is complete and generally in accord with the standards accepted at the time of publication. However, in view of the possibility of human error or changes in medical sciences, neither the authors nor the publisher nor any other party who has been involved in the preparation or publication of this work warrants that the information contained herein is in every respect accurate or complete, and they disclaim all responsibility for any errors or omissions or for the results obtained from use of the information contained in this work. Readers are encouraged to confirm the information contained herein with other sources. For example and in particular, readers are advised to check the product information sheet included in the package of each drug they plan to administer to be certain that the information contained in this work is accurate and that changes have not been made in the recommended dose or in the contraindications for administration. This recommendation is of particular importance in connection with new or infrequently used drugs.

This book was set in Avenir by Rainbow Graphics.
The editors were Catherine A. Johnson and Cindy Yoo.
The production supervisor was Jeffrey Herzich.
Project management was provided by Rainbow Graphics.
The designer was Mary McKeon.
Quad/Graphics was printer and binder.

This book is printed on acid-free paper.

DEDICATION

To the contributors of this and future editions, who took time to share their knowledge, insight, and humor for the benefit of students.

and

To our families, friends, and loved ones, who supported us in the task of assembling this guide.

CONTENTS

SECTION I   GENERAL PRINCIPLES

SECTION II   ORGAN SYSTEMS

CONTRIBUTING AUTHORS

Eike Blohm
Johns Hopkins University School of Medicine
Class of 2012

Vivek Buch
Warren Alpert Medical School of Brown University
Class of 2013

Phil Eye
Boston University School of Medicine
Class of 2012

John Hegde
Harvard Medical School
Class of 2013

Kimberly Kallianos, MD
Harvard Medical School
Class of 2011

Donnie Matsuda, MD
Stanford University School of Medicine
Class of 2010

Bethany L. Strong
Harvard Medical School
Class of 2012

Daniel Verdini, MD
Internal Medicine-Preliminary
University of Nevada School of Medicine

FACULTY REVIEWERS

Mark J. Albanese, MD
Assistant Clinical Professor of Psychiatry
Department of Psychiatry
Cambridge Health Alliance
Harvard Medical School

David H. Bor, MD
Charles S. Davidson Associate Professor of Medicine
Chief of Medicine
Department of Medicine, Infectious Diseases
Cambridge Health Alliance
Harvard Medical School

Erica Childs, MD
Instructor in Medicine
Department of Medicine
Cambridge Health Alliance
Harvard Medical School

Pieter A. Cohen, MD
Assistant Professor of Medicine
Department of Medicine
Cambridge Health Alliance
Harvard Medical School

Malgorzata Dawiskiba, MD
Clinical Fellow in Medicine
Department of Medicine
Cambridge Health Alliance
Harvard Medical School

Michael A. Gillette, MD, PhD
Instructor in Medicine
Department of Medicine, Pulmonary/Critical Care
Broad Institute
Cambridge Health Alliance
Dana-Farber Cancer Institute
Massachusetts General Hospital
Harvard Medical School

Eirini Iliaki, MD, MPH
Clinical Fellow in Medicine
Department of Medicine
Cambridge Health Alliance
Harvard Medical School

Melisa W. Lai Becker, MD
Chief, Department of Emergency Medicine
Instructor in Medicine, Department of Emergency Medicine
Director, Division of Medical Toxicology
Beth Israel Deaconness Medical Center
Cambridge Health Alliance
Children's Hospital, Boston
Harvard Medical School

Maria Livshin, MD
Instructor in Medicine
Department of Medicine, Gastroenterology
Cambridge Health Alliance
Harvard Medical School

Omar H. Maarouf, MD
Clinical Fellow in Medicine
Department of Medicine, Nephrology
Brigham and Women's Hospital
Massachusetts General Hospital
Harvard Medical School

Paul G. Mathew, MD
Instructor in Neurology
Division of Neurology
Director of Headache Medicine
Brigham and Women's Hospital
Cambridge Health Alliance
Harvard Medical School

Rachel Nardin, MD
Assistant Professor of Neurology
Chief of Neurology
Division of Neurology
Cambridge Health Alliance
Harvard Medical School

Eva D. Patalas, MD
Instructor in Pathology
Department of Pathology
Cambridge Health Alliance
Massachusetts General Hospital
Harvard Medical School

Richard J. Pels, MD
Assistant Professor of Medicine
Associate Chief of Medicine
Department of Medicine
Director, Graduate Medical Education
Cambridge Health Alliance
Harvard Medical School

Lisa B. Weissmann, MD
Assistant Professor of Medicine
Department of Medicine, Hematology/Oncology
Cambridge Health Alliance
Mount Auburn Hospital
Harvard Medical School

PREFACE

With *First Aid Cases for the USMLE Step 1*, 3rd edition, we continue our commitment to providing students with the most useful and up-to-date preparation guides for the USMLE Step 1. This edition represents an outstanding effort by a talented group of authors and includes the following:

- An all-new, two-color tabular design for efficient and effective study.
- Updated USMLE-style cases with expanded differentials and commonly asked question stems seen on the USMLE Step 1.
- Concise yet complete with relevant pathophysiology explanations.
- New high-yield figures and tables complement the questions and answers.
- Organized as a perfect supplement to *First Aid for the USMLE Step 1*.

We invite you to share your thoughts and ideas to help us improve *First Aid Cases for the USMLE Step 1*. See "How to Contribute," on p. xxiii.

Louisville	Tao Le
Cambridge	James S. Yeh

ACKNOWLEDGMENTS

We gratefully acknowledge the thoughtful comments, corrections, and advice of the many medical students, international medical graduates, and faculty who have supported the authors in the development of *First Aid® Cases for the USMLE Step 1,* 3rd edition.

For support and encouragement throughout the process, we are grateful to Thao Pham, Selina Franklin, and Louise Petersen.

Thanks to our publisher, McGraw-Hill, for the valuable assistance of their staff. For enthusiasm, support, and commitment to this challenging project, thanks to our editor, Catherine A. Johnson. For outstanding editorial work, we thank Emma D. Underdown, Isabel Nogueira, and Carol Ayres. A special thanks to Rainbow Graphics for remarkable production work.

Louisville	Tao Le
Cambridge	James S. Yeh

HOW TO CONTRIBUTE

To continue to produce a high-yield review source for the USMLE Step 1 you are invited to submit any suggestions or corrections. We also offer paid internships in medical education and publishing ranging from three months to one year (see below for details). Please send us your suggestions for:

- New facts, mnemonics, diagrams, and illustrations
- High-yield topics that may reappear on future Step 1 examinations
- Corrections and other suggestions

For each entry incorporated into the next edition, you will receive a $10 gift certificate, as well as personal acknowledgment in the next edition. Diagrams, tables, partial entries, updates, corrections, and study hints are also appreciated, and significant contributions will be compensated at the discretion of the authors. Also let us know about material in this edition that you feel is low yield and should be deleted.

The preferred way to submit entries, suggestions, or corrections is via our blog:

www.firstaidteam.com.

Otherwise, you can e-mail us directly at:

firstaidteam@yahoo.com

NOTE TO CONTRIBUTORS

All entries become property of the authors and are subject to editing and reviewing. Please verify all data and spellings carefully. In the event that similar or duplicate entries are received, only the first entry received will be used. Include a reference to a standard textbook to facilitate verification of the fact. Please follow the style, punctuation, and format of this edition, if possible.

AUTHOR OPPORTUNITIES

The author team is pleased to offer opportunities in medical education and publishing to motivated medical students and physicians. Projects may range from three months (eg, a summer) up to a full year. Participants will have an opportunity to author, edit, and earn academic credit on a wide variety of projects, including the popular First Aid series. English writing/editing experience, familiarity with Microsoft Word, and Internet access are required. Go to our blog **www.firstaidteam.com** to apply for an internship. A sample of your work or a proposal of a specific project is helpful.

Behavioral Science

■ CASE 1

A 44-year-old man is brought to the emergency department by paramedics after he was found stumbling and confused at home. On physical examination, the patient appears slightly sedated and admits to recent heavy drinking but says his last drink was 34 hours ago. He also says he vomited three times earlier that morning. He denies chest and abdominal pain. He has a 15-year history of heavy alcohol abuse and usually drinks six to seven beers a day. CT scan of the head is negative for mass lesions or bleeding. Relevant laboratory findings are as follows:

Aspartate aminotransferase: 57 U/L
Alanine aminotransferase: 18 U/L
Lactate dehydrogenase: 398 U/L

What is the most likely diagnosis?
Alcohol withdrawal.

What is the pathophysiology of this condition?
Alcohol is a central nervous system depressant that causes neuronal changes, including stimulation of the γ-aminobutyric acid (GABA)$_A$ receptor. Repeated consumption of alcohol desensitizes GABA$_A$ receptors, resulting in tolerance and physical dependence. When a person suddenly stops consuming alcohol, the nervous system is hyperaroused and synapses fire uncontrollably; the result is the symptoms seen in alcohol withdrawal. Increased serum norepinephrine and altered serotonin levels have also been implicated in both alcohol craving and tolerance.

What are the symptoms of this condition?
Minor symptoms (occurring 6–36 hours after the last drink) include: diaphoresis, GI upset, headache, nausea and vomiting, palpitations, and tremulousness. Seizures can occur within 6–48 hours of the last drink. Visual (or less commonly, tactile or auditory) hallucinations can occur within 12–48 hours of the last drink, and delirium tremens may occur within 48–96 hours.

What is delirium tremens?
Delirium tremens is a collection of severe alcohol withdrawal symptoms that includes delirium, agitations, and autonomic instability such as tachycardia, hypertension, low-grade fever, and diaphoresis. Approximately 5% of patients with alcohol withdrawal symptoms develop delirium tremens.

What is the appropriate treatment for this condition?
Benzodiazepines, particularly lorazepam or diazepam, are the treatment of choice for all types of alcohol withdrawal symptoms.

■ CASE 2

A 24-year-old woman is brought to the emergency department with confusion, blurred vision, dizziness, and somnolence. Her friend states that the woman is generally healthy but is taking medication for occasional episodes of intense fear, sweating, nausea, and abdominal and chest pain. Physical examination reveals a respiratory rate of 8/min.

What is the most likely diagnosis?

Benzodiazepine toxicity, as characterized by respiratory depression, confusion, and other symptoms of central nervous system depression.

What class of drugs might be responsible for this patient's symptoms?

Her friend's description is consistent with a diagnosis of panic disorder. Benzodiazepines (such as clonazepam, lorazepam, and alprazolam) are commonly used in the short-term treatment of panic disorder.

What treatment was likely administered to this patient in the emergency department?

Flumazenil, a competitive antagonist at the γ-aminobutyric acid (GABA) receptor, is effective in reversing symptoms of benzodiazepine overdose.

How does the mechanism of action of benzodiazepines differ from that of barbiturates?

Normally, $GABA_A$ receptors respond to GABA binding by opening chloride channels, which raises the membrane potential of the neuron and inhibits neuronal firing. Benzodiazepines and barbiturates enhance the affinity of GABA for $GABA_A$ receptors. **Benzodiazepines** increase the **frequency** of chloride channel openings. **Barbiturates** increase the **duration** of chloride channel openings.

What are the advantages of treatment with benzodiazepines over barbiturates?

Benzodiazepines have a lower risk of dependence, P450 system involvement, respiratory depression, coma, and loss of rapid eye movement sleep. They are considered to be much safer than barbiturates in cases of overdose (specifically, barbiturates have a lower therapeutic index).

What drugs, when taken with benzodiazepines, increase the risk of toxicity?

- Acetaminophen
- Alcohol
- Cimetidine
- Disulfiram
- Isoniazid
- Valproic acid

▮ CASE 3

A 16-year-old girl is brought to the physician by her mother who is worried about her daughter's rapid weight loss and erratic behavior. The girl states she has been exercising frequently and has not had menses for several months. Upon further questioning, she reluctantly states that she is afraid of gaining weight and eats only cereal and vegetables. Her weight is 44.1 kg (97 lb) and her body mass index is 17 kg/m². She complains of right foot pain and an x-ray of her foot is taken (Figure 1-1). Relevant laboratory findings are as follows:

Hemoglobin: 10.8 g/dL
Hematocrit: 33.5%
Mean corpuscular volume (MCV): 78.5 fL

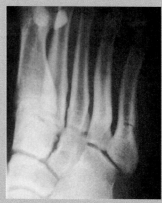

FIGURE 1-1. (Courtesy of Alan B. Storrow, MD, as published in Knoop KJ, Stack LB, Storrow AB. *Atlas of Emergency Medicine*, 2nd ed. New York: McGraw-Hill, 2002: 343.)

What is the most likely diagnosis?
Anorexia nervosa.

What other symptoms of this condition are common at presentation?

Patients typically present with severe weight loss (with body weight < 85% of ideal body weight) and clinical manifestations of multiple nutritional deficiencies. Despite being underweight, anorexic patients are obsessed with calories, preoccupied with dieting, and intensely fearful of gaining weight. Dental caries and erosions (Figure 1-2) may be present if patients are also inducing vomiting. Additional purging via laxative abuse may cause palpitations, lightheadedness, or chest pain due to electrolyte abnormalities.

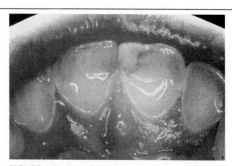

FIGURE 1-2. **Dental erosions in patients with vomiting.** (Courtesy of David P. Kretzschmar, DDS, MS, as published in Knoop KJ, Stack LB, Storrow AB. *Atlas of Emergency Medicine*, 2nd ed. New York: McGraw-Hill, 2002: 175.)

What is Russell's sign?
Russell's sign is scarring on the knuckles due to repeatedly sticking fingers down one's throat to induce vomiting.

What nutritional deficiency may contribute to the radiographic findings in Figure 1-1?
Fractures of the fifth metatarsal bone in anorexic patients are often related in part to osteopenia or osteoporosis secondary to vitamin D and calcium deficiency.

How is this condition differentiated from bulimia?
Bulimia nervosa can present with findings similar to anorexia. Its hallmark is uncontrollable binge eating followed by purging. Patients with bulimia usually have normal weight and irregular menses. Nutritional deficiencies, however, are uncommon.

What region of the brain regulates appetite and is thought to play a role in eating disorders?
The "feeding center" is located in the lateral nucleus of the hypothalamus. When stimulated, it promotes eating/appetite. The "satiety center" is located in the ventromedial nucleus. When stimulated, it signals the body to stop eating. Lesions to this area cause hyperphagia and obesity.

What kind of anemia does this patient likely have?
Low hematocrit and low MCV suggest **microcytic anemia**, most likely due to iron deficiency, a common feature in patients with anorexia. Inadequate vitamin B$_{12}$ and folate intake cause **macrocytic anemia**. Some patients may have overall **normocytic anemia** due to the combined microcytic and macrocytic anemias.

What is the treatment and prognosis of this condition?
A multidisciplinary treatment approach focuses on restoring the patient to a healthy weight and uses psychotherapy to correct the thoughts and behaviors that initially caused the disordered eating. Prognosis is variable, as one fifth of patients remain severely ill, one fifth recover fully, and three fifths have a fluctuating, chronic course.

▮ CASE 4

An overseer of clinical trials is given an application for the study of a new drug that is intended to independently reduce anxiety. The company seeking to test this drug wants to distribute it to volunteer members of local meditation groups for 3 weeks and then follow up with participants 3 months later.

In terms of study design, what is bias?

Bias refers to any source of error in the determination of association between the exposure (drug use, in this case) and outcome (reduction in anxiety, in this case).

What types of bias can be found in this study?

There are three types of bias in this drug company's proposal:

- **Sampling bias:** All the subjects are members of a meditation group and are therefore likely to have less anxiety than members of the general population. For this reason, the results of the trial cannot be generalized to the targeted population as a whole.
- **Selection bias:** All the subjects are able to choose whether they want to try the new drug. Because of this nonrandom assignment, there is no way to eliminate the placebo effects of the drug.
- **Recall bias:** The drug company plans to contact participants 3 months after the study is completed. Because they know what is expected of them, the subjects may be more likely to claim that they have less anxiety.

What is another important type of bias found in the research design of some studies?

Late-look bias, which pertains to information gathered at an inappropriate time, is another type of bias; an example would be following up on results after another intervention outside of the study has taken place.

What are some ways that bias can be reduced?

Bias can be reduced by using placebos, randomizing the subjects who are using the drug, designing a double-blind study, and employing a crossover study in which the subject acts as his or her own control.

What is blinding and what types of blinding are there?

Blinding is an aspect of study design that conceals information that could bias the results of the study from some or all of the persons involved in the study. Trials may be single-blind or double-blind. In single-blind trials, subjects do not know whether they have been assigned to the experimental or the control group. In double-blind trials, neither the subjects nor the researchers know who has been assigned to the experimental group and who has been assigned to the control group.

■ CASE 5

A 27-year-old woman comes to the emergency department with bruises on her wrists and forearms. X-ray of the chest shows three broken ribs. Upon questioning, the woman tells the physician that her boyfriend got upset with her because she overcooked his steak. She claims that she provoked the incident by not preparing his food correctly and asks the doctor not to tell the police or anyone else.

What should the physician do in this scenario?

Because the patient is not considered to be a minor or an elderly patient (defined as being older than 65 years of age), the patient's right to confidentiality must be respected. Although the physician should make all resources available to her, such as a battered women's home, the ethical principles of patient autonomy and privacy must be followed.

Should the physician contact members of the woman's family or close friends named in the social history?

No, the physician should not contact friends or relatives of the patient; doing so when clearly told not to by the patient would break the principle of autonomy. Also, the physician is bound by the privacy rule of the Health Insurance Portability and Accountability Act (HIPAA).

What are the exceptions to confidentiality?

There are a number of exceptions to confidentiality besides the age parameters that protect minors and the elderly. These exceptions rely on the physician's judgment. If the potential harm to self or others is great or serious, then confidentiality may be violated to preserve the principle of beneficence. It is the responsibility of the physician to take steps to prevent harm if there are no alternative means to protect those at risk.

What is the *Tarasoff* decision?

The *Tarasoff* decision is a law requiring a physician to *directly* inform and protect potential victims from harm. In this case, for example, if the woman told the physician that she had a gun and was going to go back home and kill her boyfriend for abusing her, the physician would have a duty to inform the boyfriend and detain the patient.

What is the physician's duty if a patient has a serious infectious disease and is putting others at risk?

Physicians have a duty to warn public officials and other identifiable persons at risk if a patient has certain infectious diseases. These diseases include hepatitis A and B, salmonella, shigella, syphilis, measles, mumps, AIDS, rubella, tuberculosis, chickenpox, and gonorrhea.

■ CASE 6

A 67-year-old man presents with a crushing, substernal chest pain that he claims used to occur only on exertion but now occurs randomly throughout the day. His wife is concerned and asks the attending physician what she thinks can be done. The attending physician meets with the patient and his wife and discusses the diagnosis of unstable angina and its association with myocardial infarction. The physician then explains the option of bypass surgery and asks the patient if he would like to have this surgery.

If the patient decides, with full mental capacity, that he does not want to have this surgery, what should the physician do?

Under the core ethical principle of **autonomy,** the physician has an obligation to respect and honor the medical care choices of the patient.

If the physician believes that not proceeding with this surgery is against the patient's best interest, what should the physician do?

The physician has a fiduciary duty to act in the patient's best interest under the ethical principle of **beneficence;** however, if the patient can make an **informed decision** (ie, is aware of the risks, benefits, and alternatives to surgery/treatment), he has the right to decide what type of treatment he will receive and the physician must respect that decision.

What ethical principle is violated in all surgeries?

Because the benefits of a surgical intervention often outweigh the risks, the principle of **nonmaleficence,** or "do no harm," is often broken as a means to a better end.

What is the fourth ethical principle that the physician must follow?

The last of the four core ethical principles is **justice,** which is to treat all persons fairly without exception.

If the patient decides he wants to proceed with the surgery, what should the physician do?

The physician must obtain **informed consent** from the patient. This is a process in which the physician discloses the risks and benefits of the procedure, the available alternatives, and the risks and benefits of refusing the procedure. As a result, the patient is able to make an informed decision about whether he will have the procedure.

CASE 7

A 65-year-old diabetic man is admitted to the hospital for repair of a hip fracture. On postoperative day 4, his wife reports that he is confused and cannot remember her name. Evaluation confirms that the patient is inattentive and confused. However, his nurse notes that he was fine both the day before and 3 hours earlier. The patient is taking morphine as well as previously prescribed β-blockers and angiotensin-converting enzyme inhibitors for hypertension. He is afebrile, and his blood pressure is 105/51 mm Hg. Relevant laboratory findings are as follows:

Sodium: 133 mEq/L	Phosphate: 3.0 mg/dL
Calcium: 8.9 mg/dL	Blood urea nitrogen: 18 mg/dL
Potassium: 3.9 mEq/L	Creatinine: 1.5 mg/dL
Chloride: 99 mEq/L	Glucose: 58 mg/dL
Magnesium: 1.9 mg/dL	Urinalysis: unremarkable
Bicarbonate: 25.1 mEq/L	

What is the most likely diagnosis?

Delirium. Key features include: acute onset, reduced attention, waxing and waning course, disorganized thinking, altered level of consciousness.

How is this condition distinguished from dementia?

Acute presentation and a waxing and waning course are found in delirium but not dementia whereas dementia is a chronic presentation. The ability to stay focused is significantly impaired in delirium, whereas patients with dementia generally remain alert.

What risk factors are associated with this condition?

Prolonged hospitalization, pain, dehydration, metabolic and electrolyte disturbances, medication-induced, infections, and postoperative state.

What drugs most commonly cause this condition?

Major classes of drugs that commonly cause delirium are opioids, anticholinergic agents, sedative-hypnotics, antihistamine agents, benzodiazepines, and corticosteroids.

What are the appropriate treatments for this condition?

The key is to treat the underlying etiology. The first step of the evaluation is a thorough review of the medication list and lab abnormalities that can contribute to delirium and to examine the patient for evidence of infection and pain control. The next step is reorient the patient.

CASE 8

A 19-year-old college student is brought to the emergency department by his roommate, who found him sitting outside their room breathing shallowly. The patient is difficult to understand because he is intoxicated, has slurred speech, and is drowsy. Physical examination reveals pinpoint pupils. The roommate admits they were both drinking at a party earlier in the evening, but he lost track of the patient and is not sure what else he could have ingested.

What drugs of abuse could be involved in this case?
- Alcohol
- Amphetamines
- Benzodiazepines or barbiturates
- Cocaine
- Heroin (opioids)
- Lysergic acid diethylamide (LSD)
- Phencyclidine (PCP)

What signs and symptoms are associated with alcohol intoxication and withdrawal?
- Intoxication: Slurred speech, incoordination, unsteady gait, nystagmus, impaired attention, stupor/coma.
- Withdrawal: Autonomic hyperactivity, tremor, insomnia, nausea, hallucinations, agitation, anxiety, seizures.

What signs and symptoms are associated with opioid intoxication and withdrawal?
- Intoxication: Intense euphoria, drowsiness, slurred speech, decreased memory, pupil constriction, decreased respirations.
- Withdrawal: Nausea, vomiting, pupil dilation, insomnia.

What signs and symptoms are associated with cocaine intoxication and withdrawal?
- Intoxication: Tachycardia, hallucinations, paranoid delusions, dilated pupils.
- Withdrawal: Increased appetite, irritability, depressed mood.

What signs and symptoms are associated with benzodiazepine or barbiturate intoxication and withdrawal?
- Intoxication: Respiratory and cardiac depression, disinhibition, unsteady gait.
- Withdrawal: Agitation, anxiety, depression, tremor, seizures, delirium.

What signs and symptoms are associated with PCP and LSD intoxication and withdrawal?
- PCP intoxication: Intense psychosis, violence, rhabdomyolysis, hyperthermia.
- PCP withdrawal: Anxiety, depression, irritable and angry mood.
- LSD intoxication: Increased sensation (colors richer, tastes heightened), visual hallucinations, dilated pupils.
- There are no withdrawal symptoms from LSD.

CASE 9

Scientists in Japan have devised a new HIV screening test and have administered it to 400 persons. Although 57 of the 400 persons are infected, this new test is positive in only 30 cases. Among uninfected persons, the test is negative in 300 cases (Table 1-1).

TABLE 1-1	Determining Diagnostic Test Data		
	PERSONS WITH INFECTION	PERSONS WITHOUT INFECTION	NUMBER OF PERSONS TESTED
Test positive	30	43	73
Test negative	27	300	327
Total	57	343	400

What is the sensitivity of this test?

Sensitivity is defined as the percentage of test subjects who have the infection and test positive for it. In other words, sensitivity = true positives/(true positives + false negatives). Therefore, the sensitivity of this test is 30/57, or 52.6%.

What is the specificity of this test?

Specificity is defined as the percentage of test subjects who do not have the infection and test negative for it. In other words, specificity = true negatives/(true negatives + false positives). Therefore, the specificity of this test is 300/343, or 87.5%.

What is the positive predictive value (PPV) of this test?

PPV is defined as the probability that a person with a positive test result is actually infected. Therefore, the PPV of this test is 30/73, or 41.1%. The PPV is directly proportional to the prevalence of the disease being tested; therefore, if the disease is prevalent, the PPV of the test will be high.

What is the negative predictive value (NPV) of this test?

NPV is defined as the probability that a person who is truly uninfected will have a negative test result. Therefore, the NPV of this test is 300/327, or 91.7%.

What is the prevalence of HIV in the population tested?

Prevalence is defined as the proportion of people who actually have the infection in relation to the total population at a point in time. Therefore, the prevalence of HIV in this population is 57/400, or 14.3%.

■ CASE 10

The mother of 15-month-old fraternal twin boys consults her pediatrician because she is concerned about the development of one twin. The older twin began to walk at approximately 12 months of age, but the younger twin is still unable to walk by himself. Physical examination reveals no significant issues.

Is it normal that the younger twin has not begun to walk?

Yes. The approximate age that children reach the motor milestone of walking is 15 months. Between 6 and 9 months of age, children should be able to sit without help.

By what age should the infant reflexes have disappeared?

Infant reflexes normally disappear within the first year. They include the Moro reflex (extension of limbs when startled), the rooting reflex (nipple seeking when cheek brushed), the palmar reflex (grasping of objects in palm), and the Babinski reflex (large toe dorsiflexion with plantar stimulation).

What cognitive/social milestones should these infants have reached?

Cognitive/social milestones reached by this age include social smile (3 mo), recognition of people (4–5 mo), stranger anxiety (7–9 mo), voice orientation (7–9 mo), and separation anxiety (15 mo).

What language milestones should these infants have reached?

Language milestones reached by this age include "cooing" (3 mo), babbling (6 mo), saying a couple of words like "mama" or "dada" (12 mo), and speaking a few words (15 mo).

What motor milestones should these infants have reached?

Motor milestones reached by this age include sitting without support (6–8 mo), cruising (12 mo), and walking independently (12–14 mo).

What is an APGAR score?

APGAR is an acronym for the scoring system that measures: **A**ppearance, **P**ulse, **G**rimace, **A**ctivity, and **R**espiration (Table 1-2). Each category is scored from 0–2 (Table 1-2); a total of 10 is a perfect score. Scoring is done at 1 and 5 minutes after birth. APGAR score is not a prognostic tool for future childhood developmental milestones.

TABLE 1-2	APGAR Scoring System		
CATEGORY	SCORE 0	SCORE 1	SCORE 2
Appearance (color)	Blue/pale	Trunk pink	All pink
Pulse	None	< 100/min	> 100/min
Grimace (reflex irritability)	None	Grimace	Grimace + cough
Activity (muscle tone)	Limp	Some	Active
Respiration (effort)	None	Irregular	Regular

What upcoming motor milestones should the mother expect to see?

Upcoming motor milestones include: climbing stairs (12–24 mo), stacking six blocks (18–24 mo), riding a tricycle (3 yrs), and hopping on one foot (4 yrs).

■ CASE 11

A 40-year-old woman in Miami consults a plastic surgeon for abdominal liposuction. After the surgeon fully explains the procedure and its possible complications, the woman agrees to have the operation and is scheduled for surgery the following week. Approximately 3 weeks after the liposuction, the woman's abdominal skin becomes dimpled in the area where the surgery was performed. Extremely upset with the outcome, she threatens to file a malpractice suit against the plastic surgeon if he does not repair it.

What is a malpractice suit, and what criteria justify it?

A malpractice suit is a civil suit under negligence that requires four fundamental criteria, also referred to as the "four Ds": **duty, dereliction, damage,** and **direct.** First, it must be understood that the physician had a **duty** or responsibility to the patient. Second, the physician must have breached that duty, which is called **dereliction.** Third, the patient must suffer harm or **damage.** Finally, the harm caused must be a **direct** cause of the dereliction.

In this case, if the physician decides not to perform a reparative procedure, are the grounds for malpractice justified?

It depends. Although the duty and damage are present in this case, it is unclear whether the physician was derelict in his duty and whether the patient's abdomen dimple is the result of dereliction. For example, if the patient did not follow postoperative instructions, even though she was told to do so to prevent complications, the physician's actions would not be the cause of the harm. But if the surgeon did not follow the standard of care in her treatment and this caused her complication, the woman would be justified in suing.

What is the difference between a criminal suit and a malpractice suit regarding the burden of proof?

In a criminal suit, the burden of proof must be "beyond a reasonable doubt"; in a malpractice suit, the burden of proof is more along the lines of "lack of reasonable and ordinary care or skill on the part of the physician."

What is the most common reason for litigation between a patient and a physician?

The number one factor leading to litigation is poor communication between the physician and the patient.

What action should the physician in this case take?

The physician should try to find the reason for the dimpling. If it is determined that he made an error in surgery, he should immediately apologize to the patient. Studies show that if a physician is honest and upfront about an error, he or she is less likely to be sued by the patient. Lastly, if miscommunication was the culprit, the physician should make every effort to prevent such miscommunication in the future.

■ CASE 12

A couple is eating dinner at home with their quiet 6-year-old son. The couple gets into an argument and the father starts to yell at his son, who begins to cry. The mother gives the child candy, which temporarily relieves the crying. Throughout the meal, she continues to give him candy every time he cries. The father then yells at the child and takes away the candy because children who cry should not be given candy. The child is upset that his candy has been taken away and begins to throw food across the dining room table.

What defense mechanism is the father using?

The father is using **displacement**, which is characterized by the transfer of feelings from one object or person to another. In this case, the father's anger at the mother is displaced onto the child.

What defense mechanism is the child using?

The child is **acting out**, which is characterized by the use of extreme behavior to express a thought or feeling. In this case, the child is so overcome with anger that he cannot simply state, "I'm angry with you"; instead, he acts out by throwing food across the table.

What type of reinforcement is the child using on the mother?

This is an example of **positive reinforcement**, in which the consequences of a response increase the likelihood that the response will recur. Specifically, the child cries because crying makes it more likely the mother will continue to give him candy.

How does negative reinforcement differ from punishment?

In **negative reinforcement**, a behavior is encouraged or reinforced by the removal of an aversive stimulus (eg, if a mother constantly yells at her child to pick up his toys, he will learn to pick up his toys to avoid mom's yelling). In **punishment**, behavior is discouraged and reduced by administration of an aversive stimulus (eg, the mother puts the boy in a "time out" because he did not pick up his toys).

Which method of conditioning is the father using by removing the reward?

The father is employing **extinction**, which is the elimination of a behavior by nonreinforcement. The child likely will stop crying after discovering that there is no reward for the behavior.

■ CASE 13

A newborn baby boy who was delivered at home is brought to the emergency department by his grandmother 30 minutes after birth. The grandmother says the baby "isn't acting right." He weighs 2700 g (approximately 6 lb) and was born at 35 weeks' gestation. He is limp and unresponsive and breathing infrequently, with bluish skin and pupils 2 mm in diameter. The infant is immediately resuscitated and stabilized for transfer to the neonatal intensive care unit. On day 3 of life, his nurse says he is vomiting, has diarrhea, and cries excessively. Physical examination reveals tachycardia, tachypnea, dilated pupils, diaphoresis, tremors, increased muscle tone, and piloerection.

What is the most likely diagnosis?

The infant most likely has **opioid intoxication**, heralded by the triad of (1) respiratory depression, (2) central nervous system depression, and (3) pinpoint pupils. Importantly, **pinpoint pupils** due to opioid intoxication will be present despite opioid tolerance. Other common findings in infants exposed to opioids include low birth weight, premature birth, and intrauterine growth retardation syndrome.

What pharmacologic agent should this patient receive in the emergency department?

Naloxone, an opioid antagonist, reverses the effects of opioid agonists by selectively binding to opioid receptors.

What is the most likely diagnosis on day 3 of life?

On day 3, the infant demonstrates symptoms of opiate withdrawal, also known as **neonatal abstinence syndrome.** Tachycardia, dilated pupils, diaphoresis, and other opiate withdrawal symptoms are related to sympathetic hyperactivity.

What is the Finnegan scale?

The Finnegan scale assesses 21 common signs and symptoms of neonatal drug withdrawal syndrome, including central nervous system, respiratory, metabolic, and gastrointestinal disturbances. The scale determines the severity of drug withdrawal symptoms in the neonate and assesses the resolution of symptoms after treatment has begun.

What is the appropriate long-term treatment for this patient?

An opioid agonist, such as methadone, relieves symptoms of acute opiate withdrawal. Methadone administration can be tapered as the baby is weaned.

Once the newborn is stabilized, what other issues need to be addressed?

The mother may need substance abuse treatment and counseling. Drug abuse during pregnancy is associated with medical and psychological problems that require evaluation and treatment. If she admits to IV drug use, she should be screened for infectious diseases, including HIV, hepatitis B, and hepatitis C. Also, it is important to arrange adequate follow-up care within the first few weeks of discharge.

CASE 14

A 21-year-old man and his mother visit the clinic because his daytime sleepiness is interfering with his studies. The man is slightly obese and has a history of pulmonary hypertension. His mother says that he has a medication "for sleep" but that he does not use it. On questioning, the man says he has a prescription for amphetamines and is taking sertraline. His mother also mentions that while they were in the waiting room, the man heard "bells ringing," which no one else heard. Shortly thereafter, the young man fell asleep during their conversation.

What is the diagnosis?

The hallucinations, sudden onset of sleep, and amphetamine treatment are consistent with a diagnosis of **narcolepsy.** This condition has a strong genetic component.

What kind of hallucinations is the patient having?

Hallucinations that occur before falling asleep are termed **hypnagogic hallucinations** ("gogic"—"go" to sleep). **Hypnopompic hallucinations,** which occur during waking, are also associated with narcolepsy.

What are the four classic signs and symptoms of this diagnosis?

The four classic signs and symptoms of narcolepsy are:

- Cataplexy: A sudden, transient loss of muscle tone ranging from mild weakness to full body collapse.
- Sleep paralysis: The inability to talk or move upon waking or falling asleep.
- Hypnagogic hallucinations.
- Excessive daytime sleepiness.

What sleep stage is the patient likely to enter immediately after falling asleep?

Narcolepsy is associated with rapid eye movement (**REM**) sleep within 10 minutes of falling asleep.

What behavioral and pharmacologic therapies can be used to treat this condition?

Central nervous system stimulants (eg, methylphenidate and amphetamine) are used to treat excessive daytime sleepiness, and tricyclic antidepressants (eg, clomipramine and imipramine) are used to treat cataplexy. Lifestyle changes, including reducing stress, increasing exercise, and taking frequent daytime naps, can also be therapeutic.

What other electroencephalographic (EEG) abnormalities might be expected in this patient?

Sertraline, a selective serotonin reuptake inhibitor, suggests depression. **Depression** is associated with decreased REM latency and decreased stage 4, slow-wave sleep. Effective treatment with antidepressants, however, usually reverses EEG abnormalities caused by major depression.

What other common sleep abnormality might account for poor quality of sleep?

Obesity and pulmonary hypertension are associated with **sleep apnea,** which can be disruptive and can lead to significant daytime fatigue. Arrhythmias and loud snoring are also associated with sleep apnea.

■ CASE 15

An 8-year-old boy who has been consistently incontinent at night is diagnosed with primary nocturnal enuresis. After several months of unsuccessful nonpharmacologic therapy, the family returns to the pediatrician. The boy is going to a 3-week summer camp in 1 month, and his parents are concerned about the social and psychological implications of his enuresis. They are interested in pharmacologic therapy to prevent enuresis while he is at camp.

In what stage of sleep is this patient's enuresis occurring?
Enuresis occurs during stage 4 sleep, which is the deepest non–rapid eye movement (non-REM) sleep (Table 1-3).

TABLE 1-3	Stages of Sleep	
STAGE (% OF SLEEP)	DESCRIPTION	EEG WAVEFORM
Awake	Active mentally, alert	Beta (highest frequency, lowest amplitude)
Awake/eyes closed		Alpha
Stage 1 (5%)	Light sleep	Theta
Stage 2 (45%)	Deeper sleep	Sleep spindles and K complexes
Stage 3–4 (25%)	Deepest non-REM sleep	Delta (lowest frequency, highest amplitude; slow-wave sleep)
REM (25%)	Dreaming, loss of motor tone	Beta

At what age is this condition considered a problem?
Most girls can stay dry at night by 6 years of age, and most boys stay dry at night by 7 years of age. Boys are more likely to wet their beds than girls.

What pharmacologic treatment is appropriate for this patient?
Imipramine is a tricyclic antidepressant used to treat primary nocturnal enuresis in children. It works by decreasing the duration of stage 4 sleep.

Which neurotransmitters influence sleep?
Serotonin (from the raphe nucleus) initiates sleep; acetylcholine promotes REM sleep; and, conversely, norepinephrine reduces REM sleep.

What physiologic changes occur in REM sleep?
During REM sleep, the pulse increases in rate and variability, REMs occur, blood pressure rises and has increased variability, and penile or clitoral tumescence occurs. The percentage of sleep spent in REM sleep decreases with age.

What are night terrors?
Night terrors are abrupt awakenings from sleep, often with gasping or screaming. Once the episode is over, the person goes back to sleep with no recollection of the event.

What class of drugs is used to treat night terrors?
Benzodiazepines are used for this purpose, as they shorten stage 4 sleep.

Biochemistry

▉ CASE 1

A 45-year-old man presents to his physician for chronic arthritis, which is worsening and affecting his lower back, hips, and knees. On physical examination, the patient's sclerae are noted to be brown-blue; however, his vision is unchanged from prior examinations. His ear cartilage is similarly discolored. An x-ray of the spine reveals disk degeneration and dense calcification that is most prominent in the lumbar region. Upon voiding for urinalysis, the man's urine is a normal color; however, after standing, the urine turns dark.

What is the most likely diagnosis?

Alkaptonuria (ochronosis).

What is the biochemical defect in this condition?

Alkaptonuria is characterized by the absence of **homogentisate oxidase,** an enzyme of tyrosine metabolism that catalyzes the conversion of homogentisate to maleylacetoacetate (Figure 2-1). The accumulation of homogentisate in cartilage leads to arthritis as well as to the discoloration of sclerae and other areas of the body.

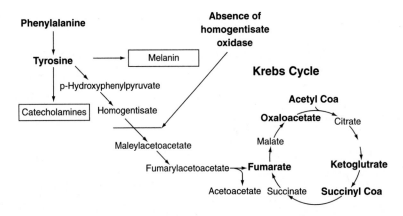

FIGURE 2-1. **Flow chart showing conversion of homogentisate to maleylacetoacetate in phenylalanine metabolism.**

The metabolite that accumulates in this condition is derived from an essential amino acid. Which amino acid is this?

Homogentisate is derived from phenylalanine. Homogentisate oxidase is necessary for the metabolism of this amino acid, which is both glucogenic and ketogenic. Homogentisate is normally metabolized to acetoacetate (a ketone) and fumarate (part of the tricarboxylic acid cycle).

Given the extent of joint disease in this patient, how might his mental functioning be affected?

Alkaptonuria has no effect on cognitive functioning. Aside from its effects on joints and discoloration of the sclerae and skin, the disease is benign.

What is the appropriate treatment for this condition?

There are no known ways to prevent the build-up of homogentisate. Dietary restriction of tyrosine and phenylalanine reduces the production of homogentisate, but this approach has demonstrated no benefit on the overall condition. Treating the symptoms of the patient's arthritis is the only recommended therapy in this case.

■ CASE 2

A 36-year-old chemist with a 15-year history of bipolar disorder is rushed to the emergency department by his wife, who found him lying unconscious in the living room of their home. The patient's wife reports that he is prescribed lithium but does not regularly take it. The man's skin is bright red, and he is breathing rapidly. Upon presentation, his breath smells like bitter almonds.

What is the most likely diagnosis?

This man has ingested cyanide (the "bitter almond" breath is pathognomonic). During a manic episode, patients with bipolar disorder are more likely to use illegal drugs and engage in self-injurious behavior so a toxicology screen is mandatory. Other causes of unconsciousness, including dehydration, metabolic acidosis, and diabetic ketoacidosis, should be investigated.

What biochemical process is disrupted in this condition?

Cyanide is a direct inhibitor of one step in the electron transport chain (Figure 2-2). Cyanide inhibits cytochrome oxidase.

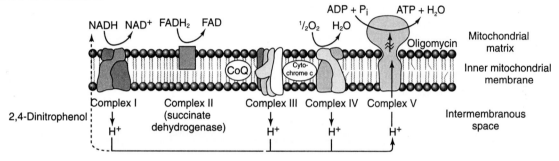

FIGURE 2-2. Cyanide inhibition of oxidative phosphorylation in the electron transport chain. ADP = adenosine diphosphate; ATP = adenosine triphosphate; FAD = oxidized flavin adenine dinucleotide; FADH$_2$ = reduced flavin adenine dinucleotide; NAD$^+$ = oxidized nicotinamide adenine dinucleotide phosphate; NADH = reduced nicotinamide adenine dinucleotide. (Reproduced, with permission, from Le T, et al. *First Aid for the USMLE Step 1: 2011*. New York: McGraw-Hill, 2011: 100.)

Does this patient have a greater-than-normal or lower-than-normal proton concentration in the intermembrane space of his mitochondria?

The man has a lower proton concentration. The electron transport chain fuels the transport of protons from the mitochondrial matrix to the intermembrane space. Because this patient ingested cyanide and thus inhibited this process, his proton gradient is weakened; therefore, he has a lower concentration of protons in the intermembrane spaces of his mitochondria.

What is the appropriate treatment for this condition?

Amyl nitrite is used to treat cyanide poisoning. Amyl nitrate oxidizes hemoglobin to methemoglobin. This is normally undesirable because this form of hemoglobin binds oxygen less avidly. However, methemoglobin strongly binds cyanide, preventing it from further disrupting electron transport.

What other substances inhibit the electron transport chain?

Amytal, rotenone, antimycin A, azide, and **carbon monoxide** also inhibit the electron transport chain.

What other substances act within the mitochondria and reduce adenosine triphosphate (ATP) synthesis?

- Oligomycin is an example of a chemical that can directly inhibit mitochondrial ATP synthase. Although the proton gradient forms, ATP is not produced. As a result, electron transport ceases.
- Uncoupling agents such as 2,4-dinitrophenol allow protons to cross the inner mitochondrial membrane. Electron transport is not disrupted, but protons are able to flow into the matrix from the intermembrane space. This reduces the proton gradient that drives ATP formation.

■ CASE 3

A 6-month-old boy with a history of frequent infections is brought to the emergency department because of stiff muscles and difficulty feeding. On examination he is found to have a carpopedal spasm, and tapping on his face in front of his ears leads to spasm of the facial muscle.

What is the most likely diagnosis?

This child has DiGeorge syndrome (22q11 syndrome), which is characterized by hypoparathyroidism and T-cell deficiency. Severe combined immunodeficiency may cause both B- and T-cell deficiencies or T-cell deficiency exclusively in a given host. Hyper-IgM syndrome, IgA deficiency, and Bruton agammaglobulinemia all primarily affect B cells.

What is the etiology of this condition?

DiGeorge syndrome is caused by a developmental defect involving the third and fourth pharyngeal pouches. It results in a hypoplastic thymus and parathyroid glands. Laboratory tests of this patient would show hypocalcemia and low T-cell count. The hypocalcemia causes tetany and carpopedal spasm. Chvostek sign involves tapping on the facial nerve in front of the ear and observing spasm of the facial muscle; it is another indication of hypocalcemia.

This patient is at risk for developing what type of infections?

Because of the aplastic thymus, patients with this disorder have ineffective T cells and are particularly susceptible to viral and fungal infections.

What abnormality may be observed on an x-ray of the chest in this patient?

An x-ray of the chest in a child with DiGeorge syndrome may show a reduced thymic shadow.

What other abnormalities are associated with this condition?

CATCH 22 is a mnemonic for the 22q11 syndrome, which involves a deletion in this region of chromosome 22. Clinical manifestations include Cardiac abnormalities, Abnormal facies, Thymic hypoplasia, Cleft palate, and Hypocalcemia. Velocardiofacial syndrome also arises from this gene and involves cardiac abnormalities, abnormal facies, and cleft palate.

▮ CASE 4

A 27-year-old man with little prior medical care was brought to the emergency department because of chest pain followed by sudden collapse. Resuscitation attempts were unsuccessful. On autopsy, he was found to have thick atherosclerotic plaques in his arteries, including the coronary arteries, aorta (Figure 2-3), and renal arteries. He also had small, raised yellow-brown lesions on the extensor surfaces of his arms.

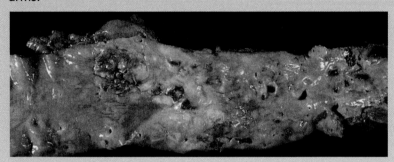

FIGURE 2-3. **Severe atherosclerosis of the aorta.** (Courtesy of the Centers for Disease Control and Prevention Public Health Image Library. http://phil.cdc.gov.)

What is the most likely diagnosis?

- This patient had familial hypercholesterolemia (FH), an inherited disorder characterized by extremely high serum cholesterol levels.
- Type I familial hyperlipidemia is caused by lipoprotein lipase deficiency and results in abdominal pain, xanthomas, and hepatosplenomegaly.
- Type III is caused by a defect in apolipoprotein E2 synthesis and results in palmar xanthomas and tuboeruptive xanthomas.
- Type IV is caused by increased very-low-density lipoprotein (VLDL) production and decreased elimination.

What is the genetic pattern of this condition?

FH is inherited in an autosomal manner. Heterozygotes typically have high cholesterol, approximately 370 mg/dL, and are at increased risk of myocardial infarctions. Homozygotes frequently have extremely high cholesterol levels, up to 1000 mg/dL, and frequently die before 30 years of age from cardiovascular disease. Normal total cholesterol is < 200 mg/dL, and levels > 240 mg/dL are considered elevated.

What is the molecular basis of this condition?

In FH there is a mutation in the LDL receptor gene. This results in a smaller number of functional LDL receptors. Normally, LDL circulates in the blood and binds to its receptor on hepatocyte membranes and is then taken up into the liver and metabolized. In FH patients, LDL is taken up by the hepatocytes less efficiently, leading to elevated LDL levels in the blood.

What would the microscopic examination of the lesions on this patient's arms show?

Cholesterol deposits in the skin, called xanthomas, form when there is a persistently elevated LDL level. They are composed largely of lipid-laden macrophages.

Statin drugs are frequently used to treat this condition. What is their mechanism of action?

Statins inhibit 3-hydroxy-3-methylglutaryl coenzyme A reductase, a hepatic enzyme that catalyzes the rate-determining step in cholesterol synthesis. They reduce the amount of endogenous cholesterol synthesized by the liver (Figure 2-4).

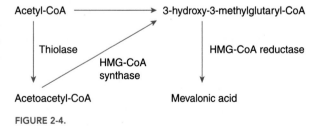

FIGURE 2-4.

■ CASE 5

A 2-day-old boy is brought to the emergency department by his mother because of frequent vomiting. The child was delivered at home to a 40-year-old mother who received no prenatal care. The mother reports that since birth the boy has been vomiting greenish material immediately after eating. He has also become lethargic and progressively less responsive. On physical examination the boy is found to have several abnormalities, including prominent epicanthal folds, upslanting palpebral fissures, and macroglossia. He also has thick skin at the nape of his neck.

What is the likely diagnosis?

The child most likely has Down syndrome, which can be associated with gastrointestinal disorders such as duodenal atresia or stenosis, annular pancreas, tracheoesophageal defects, and anal atresia. Duodenal atresia below the sphincter of Oddi causes bilious vomiting as seen in this patient.

What is the most common cytogenetic abnormality in patients with this condition?

Trisomy 21, resulting from nondisjunction of chromosome 21 during meiotic anaphase 1 or anaphase 2. The risk of nondisjunction increases with maternal age.

What other medical abnormalities are seen in children with this condition?

A single palmar crease; small, folded ears; a short neck; Brushfield spots (pale yellow spots on the iris); and a gap between the first and second toes. They also suffer from heart disease, most often cardiac cushion malformations (Figure 2-5), and may have ophthalmologic problems, gastrointestinal tract malformations, poor hearing, and mental retardation. Males with Down syndrome are almost always infertile.

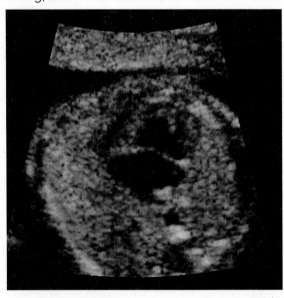

FIGURE 2-5. Ultrasound image of a fetal heart with large atrial septal defect and ventricular septal defect as indicated by the missing "cross" or crux of the heart, also known as an endocardial cushion defect. This anomaly is commonly associated with Down syndrome. (Courtesy of Wesley Lee, MD.)

What screening is available in utero for this condition?

Markers of Down syndrome in maternal blood include:

- Reduced levels of α-fetoprotein.
- Elevated levels of β-human chorionic gonadotropin (β-hCG).

Ultrasound measurements of nuchal lucency are also used. A definitive diagnosis can be made via karyotype analysis of fetal cells obtained via amniocentesis.

Later in life, what disorders is this baby at risk of developing?

Older individuals with trisomy 21 have a high risk of developing early Alzheimer disease. This may be because the amyloid-β protein implicated in Alzheimer disease is encoded on chromosome 21. They are also at increased risk of hematologic disorders, particularly acute leukemias and most commonly acute lymphoblastic leukemia.

■ CASE 6

A 5-year-old boy is brought to his pediatrician because of frequent bruising, even after minor trauma (Figure 2-6). Other than one episode of shoulder dislocation, his medical history is unremarkable. On physical examination the child has many bruises at different stages of healing. He also has hyperextensible joints, flat feet, and dental crowding.

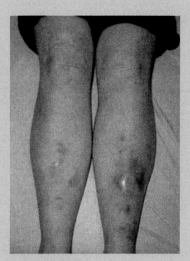

FIGURE 2-6. **Bruising on the lower extremities. Poor wound healing gives rise to "cigarette paper" scars.** (Reproduced, with permission, from Lichtman MA, et al. *Lichtman's Atlas of Hematology.* New York: McGraw-Hill, 2007: Figure XI.A.38.)

What is the most likely diagnosis?

Ehlers-Danlos syndrome is most likely. Although Marfan syndrome can cause joint hypermobility, it is unlikely to cause easy bruising. Most forms of Ehlers-Danlos syndrome are inherited as autosomal dominant mutations.

What is the etiology of the easy bruising in this child?

Mutations that affect the formation of type III collagen, which may prevent proper synthesis or posttranslational modification of collagen. The bruising is a direct result of defects in the collagen of vessel walls.

What other abnormalities may be present in individuals with this condition?

Thin, fragile skin; abnormal scar formation; aortic aneurysms; rupture of large arteries; and rupture of the bowel and uterus (pregnancy increases the risk of uterine rupture).

What are the stages of collagen synthesis?

- Protein translation on ribosomes in the rough endoplasmic reticulum.
- Hydroxylation of proline and lysine residues in the endoplasmic reticulum. This step requires vitamin C.
- Glycosylation of lysine residues to form α chains. Three α chains form a triple helix of procollagen in the Golgi apparatus.
- The procollagen is secreted by exocytosis.
- Extracellular enzymes cleave the terminal regions of the procollagen to form tropocollagen.
- Many tropocollagen units line up in a staggered arrangement and cross-link to form the final collagen fibrils.

Where are the four major types of collagen found in the body?

- Type I: Bone, skin, tendons, fascia, dentin, and the cornea.
- Type II: Cartilage, nucleus pulposus, and the vitreous body.
- Type III: Reticular collagen, found in skin, blood vessels, the uterus, granulation tissue, and fetal tissue.
- Type IV: Basement membranes.

■ CASE 7

A 6-year-old boy is followed by his pediatrician for delayed language acquisition and behavioral problems at school. He has always had a long face, large ears, and flat feet. His mother reports a normal pregnancy with adequate prenatal care and adds that she did not use drugs or alcohol during the pregnancy. Genetic analysis reveals a normal 46,XY karyotype but an abnormal-appearing X chromosome.

What is the most likely diagnosis?

This boy has fragile X syndrome. This disease occurs in individuals who have an **expansion of a CGG trinucleotide** repeat sequence on the X chromosome. This expansion results in hypermethylation of DNA in the 5′ region of the *FMR1* gene, which silences the gene by inhibiting its transcription. The FMR1 protein is an RNA-binding protein.

What is the inheritance pattern of this condition?

Fragile X syndrome is an **X-linked genetic disorder.** It is the most common inherited cause of mental retardation. The hallmark of X-linked disorders is the absence of father-to-son disease transmission. These disorders are much more common in males than in females. However, mild symptoms of fragile X syndrome appear in a significant minority of female carriers. Fragile X syndrome is not fully penetrant, and many families show a maternal transmission pattern.

What physical abnormalities are associated with this condition?

Individuals with fragile X syndrome frequently have long, narrow faces with a large jaw, large ears, and a prominent forehead. Most postpubertal males also have macroorchidism.

What are other trinucleotide repeat disorders, and why are they associated with "permutations"?

Other disorders attributable to trinucleotide repeat expansion include:

- Huntington disease (CAG expansion on chromosome 4).
- Myotonic dystrophy.
- Friedreich ataxia.

Typically, higher numbers of trinucleotide repeats result in more severe and earlier onset of the phenotypic expression of disease.

- **Permutation** occurs in patients with an intermediate number of repeats who are clinically normal but whose children are at increased risk of expressing clinical disease.
- **Anticipation** is the worsening of disease through generations because of increasing number of trinucleotide repeats.

■ CASE 8

A 5-month-old girl is brought to the pediatrician by her parents because she has been very sleepy lately and has been vomiting and sweating profusely at night. The infant's mother says that their daughter was doing fine during the first months of life but began showing these changes shortly after she began weaning from breast milk. Laboratory testing reveals a serum glucose level of 30 mg/dL, and urinalysis is positive for reducing sugar but negative for glucose.

What is the most likely diagnosis?

Fructose intolerance.

What intermediate is elevated within the liver cells in this condition?

Fructose-1-phosphate is elevated in fructose intolerance.

What enzyme is deficient in this condition?

Aldolase B is deficient in this disorder.

How does this condition cause hypoglycemia?

Aldolase B catalyzes the conversion of fructose-1-phosphate into glyceraldehyde and dihydroxyacetone phosphate (DHAP) (Figure 2-7). Its absence results in accumulation of fructose-1-phosphate in liver cells and a consequent depletion of adenosine triphosphate (ATP). A low cellular supply of ATP inhibits glycogenolysis and gluconeogenesis leading to very low serum glucose. Excess fructose is lost in the urine.

FRUCTOSE METABOLISM (LIVER)

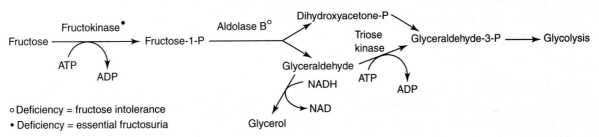

o Deficiency = fructose intolerance
• Deficiency = essential fructosuria

FIGURE 2-7. Aldolase B splitting fructose-1-phosphate into glyceraldehyde and DHAP. ADP = adenosine diphosphate; ATP = adenosine triphosphate; NAD = nicotinamide adenine dinucleotide; NADH = reduced nicotinamide adenine dinucleotide. (Reproduced, with permission, from Le T, et al. *First Aid for the USMLE Step 1: 2011*. New York: McGraw-Hill, 2011: 103.)

What is the appropriate treatment for this condition?

The condition is treated through the removal of fructose, sucrose (a disaccharide of glucose and fructose), and sorbitol from the diet.

Why did the infant exhibit no symptoms while exclusively fed breast milk?

Carbohydrates in breast milk derive largely from lactose rather than fructose.

■ CASE 9

A 12-year-old mentally retarded boy is brought into a health clinic in Peru. His parents have noted that he seems to have difficulty with his vision. Physical examination reveals bilateral dislocated lenses and a tall, thin body habitus with especially long extremities. Laboratory studies show increased levels of serum methionine and serum homocysteine.

What is the most likely diagnosis?

Homocystinuria.

What is the biochemical defect in this condition?

The most common form of inherited homocystinuria results from reduced activity of **cystathionine synthase**, an enzyme that converts homocysteine to cystathionine (Figure 2-8).

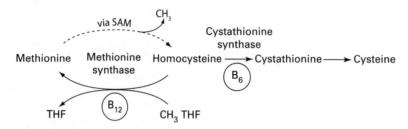

FIGURE 2-8. **Homocystinuria.** SAM = S-adenosylmethionine; THF = tetrahydrofolate. (Reproduced, with permission, from Le T, et al. *First Aid for the USMLE Step 1: 2011.* New York: McGraw-Hill, 2011: 108.)

What vitamin supplementation is appropriate in this condition?

Vitamin B$_6$ (pyridoxine) is a necessary cofactor with cystathionine synthase. Vitamin B$_6$ supplementation has been successful in many patients with this enzyme deficiency.

In addition to vitamin supplementation, what other dietary changes should be made?

The absence of cystathionine synthase means that cysteine cannot be formed from methionine. Therefore, cysteine becomes an essential amino acid. This child should be given a diet low in methionine and high in cysteine.

This boy has a marfanoid body habitus and lens subluxation, two characteristics of this condition. For which other conditions is this patient at greatly increased risk?

This child is at increased risk for **cardiovascular disease**. Elevated plasma homocysteine increases risk of coronary artery disease, stroke, and peripheral artery disease. He is also at risk for **osteoporosis**. Homocysteine inhibits collagen cross-linking and over time can cause osteoporosis.

What enzyme deficiency is most likely to be found in a patient with increased serum homocysteine but decreased serum methionine?

This could be caused by a deficiency of methionine synthase. This enzyme catalyzes the conversion of homocysteine to methionine. Like patients with cystathionine synthase deficiency, these patients often have central nervous system dysfunction and vascular disease.

■ CASE 10

A 1-year-old boy is brought to the pediatrician because his parents have recently noted a number of abnormalities. Although the child was normal at birth, he does not interact with others as his older sister did at the same age. His parents also note that he has coarse facial features. Physical examination reveals skeletal abnormalities and an umbilical hernia. Funduscopic examination shows corneal clouding. Additionally, the baby's liver and spleen are enlarged, and his joints are stiff.

What is the most likely diagnosis?

Hurler syndrome.

What is the pathophysiology of this condition?

This syndrome results from a defect in α-L-iduronidase, an enzyme essential to the degradation of dermatan sulfate and heparan sulfate. This disease is one of the **mucopolysaccharidoses**, a group of hereditary disorders characterized by defects in glycosaminoglycan (GAG) metabolism. Features that distinguish this disorder from the other lysosomal storage disorders include coarse facial features and corneal clouding. In Hurler syndrome, the GAGs are not appropriately degraded in the lysosomes and are therefore deposited in various tissues. The disease is inherited in an autosomal recessive manner.

What disease has a similar presentation but is typically milder?

Hunter syndrome is another mucopolysaccharidosis. It is due to a deficiency of iduronate sulfatase and has X-linked inheritance. Unlike Hurler syndrome, Hunter syndrome does not present with corneal clouding, but affected patients may exhibit aggressive behavior.

What are the typical findings on electron microscopy?

The lysosomal vesicles appear swollen. This is due to accumulation of partially degraded polysaccharides.

What key modification must be made in the Golgi apparatus for lysosomal enzymes, such as α-L-iduronidase, to be properly targeted to lysosomes?

Lysosomal enzymes must be covalently modified with mannose-6-phosphate (M6P) as they pass through the *cis* Golgi network to be targeted to the lysosomes. These M6P groups are then recognized by M6P receptor proteins in the *trans* Golgi network.

■ CASE 11

A 2-year-old boy with a history of mental retardation and restricted joint movement is brought to his primary care physician for a routine checkup. He is the full-term product of an uncomplicated pregnancy. A careful family history reveals that his parents are first cousins. On physical examination he is noted to have coarse facial features and clouded corneas. Blood tests revealed elevated lysosomal enzymes in the serum.

What is the significance of the consanguinity between the child's parents?

In consanguineous relationships there is an increased risk of a child's inheriting the same genetic mutation from both of his parents. There is therefore a higher incidence of autosomal recessive disorders in this population.

What is the most likely diagnosis?

This patient is suffering from **I-cell disease,** which is characterized by coarse facial features, poor tone, kyphosis, and mental retardation. These children suffer frequent upper respiratory infections, pneumonia, otitis media, and carpal tunnel syndrome. Death usually occurs in infancy or early childhood as a result of congestive heart failure or respiratory infections. I-cell disease is clinically similar to Hurler syndrome but presents with different findings at birth, including coarse facial features and restricted joint movement.

What is the fundamental molecular defect in this condition?

In I-cell disease there is a mutation in the enzyme found in the Golgi apparatus that is responsible for adding a mannose-6-phosphate group to proteins destined for lysosomes. Instead of trafficking to lysosomes, these lysosomal enzymes are secreted from the cell, and high levels are found in the blood. Because the lysosomes lack the normal hydrolytic enzymes, material accumulates in the lysosomes and is not effectively broken down.

What abnormalities would be evident by electron microscopy of cells in an affected patient?

This patient's cells would contain many vacuoles. These consist of lysosomes filled with nondegradable material.

What proteins direct movement of vesicles between the endoplasmic reticulum (ER) and Golgi apparatus?

The Golgi apparatus is responsible for modifying many different proteins and directing their trafficking. COP I proteins mediate retrograde movement of vesicles from the Golgi apparatus to the ER, whereas COP II proteins mediate anterograde transport from the ER to the Golgi apparatus.

■ CASE 12

A 35-year-old man visits a fertility specialist with his 27-year-old wife. They have been trying to conceive for more than 13 months but have been unsuccessful. The husband has no previous children but the wife has two children from a prior marriage. Their past medical history is unremarkable except for repeated sinus infections and a chronic cough in the husband. Physical examination reveals a point of maximum impulse located at the right fifth intercostal margin.

What is the most likely diagnosis?

The fact that the wife has had prior children suggests that the cause of infertility lies in the husband. Given the history, Kartagener syndrome is most likely. This is a genetic disorder with an autosomal recessive inheritance pattern.

What is the cause of their infertility?

Abnormality in *dynein*, which is an adenosine triphosphatase that acts as a molecular motor and is responsible for retrograde transport of material along microtubules. In addition, it is required for movement of cilia and flagella. If this enzyme is not functional, it results in immotile sperm.

What is the cause of the husband's recurrent sinus infections?

The cilia of the respiratory epithelium require functional dynein for motility. Without it, they are unable to transport bacteria and particles out of the respiratory tract. The retained particles and bacteria can lead to infections as well as a chronic cough with sputum production.

What abnormality might be observed on x-ray of the chest?

Situs inversus, which on the chest x-ray, the heart is found predominantly on the right side of the thorax. It may also show bronchiectasis, with signs of dilated bronchioles.

What condition is caused by a mutation in microtubule polymerization?

Chédiak-Higashi syndrome is an autosomal recessive disorder caused by a defect in microtubule polymerization resulting in impaired migration of immune cells, such as neutrophils, and impaired lysosome fusion, which results in large granules visible within the cytoplasm (Figure 2-9). These both contribute to immune deficiency. Patients present with recurrent bacterial infections with staphylococci and streptococci.

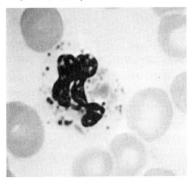

FIGURE 2-9. A neutrophil with large granules. (Reproduced, with permission, from Lichtman MA, et al. *Williams Hematology*, 7th ed. New York: McGraw-Hill, 2006: Fig. 66-5.)

There are a number of antimicrobial drugs that inhibit microtubule function. What are some examples?

Mebendazole and related drugs inhibit microtubule activity in helminths. Griseofulvin is an antifungal that acts on microtubules. A number of chemotherapeutic agents also interfere with microtubule function, such as vincristine, vinblastine, and taxols such as paclitaxel.

■ CASE 13

A 2-year-old boy is brought to the pediatrician by his mother, who is visibly upset. The mother reports that her son has recently been biting his fingers and scratching his face incessantly. She says he was normal for the first months of his life but has become increasingly irritable since about 3 months of age. The mother also mentions that her son often has "orange-colored sand" in his diapers. Laboratory studies reveal a serum uric acid level of 55 mg/dL. Urinalysis reveals crystalluria and microscopic hematuria.

What is the most likely diagnosis?

Lesch-Nyhan syndrome.

What is the biochemical defect in this condition?

Lesch-Nyhan syndrome is characterized by a deficiency in hypoxanthine-guanine phosphoribosyltransferase (HGPRT).

What is the function of the deficient enzyme?

HGPRT plays a key role in the purine salvage pathway (Figure 2-10), recycling hypoxanthine and guanine to the purine nucleotide pool. In the absence of this enzyme, purine bases are degraded into uric acid, thus causing hyperuricemia. Uric acid crystals in the urine give rise to the crystalluria.

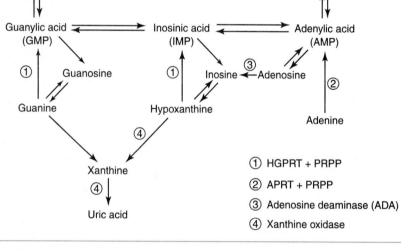

① HGPRT + PRPP
② APRT + PRPP
③ Adenosine deaminase (ADA)
④ Xanthine oxidase

FIGURE 2-10. **Purine salvage pathway.** APRT = adenine hosphoribosyltransferase; HGPRT = hypoxanthine-guanine phosphoribosyltransferase; PRPP = phosphoribosylpyrophosphate. (Reproduced, with permission, from Le T, et al. *First Aid for the USMLE Step 1: 2011.* New York: McGraw-Hill, 2011: 69.)

What is the appropriate treatment for this condition?

Allopurinol is a drug that inhibits xanthine oxidase, thus preventing the formation of uric acid from the more soluble hypoxanthine and xanthine. Hypoxanthine and xanthine can more easily be excreted in the urine. Doses should be titrated to normalize serum uric acid levels. To prevent self-injury, affected children often need lifelong benzodiazepine or barbiturate sedation, restraints, and behavioral therapy.

What associated conditions are likely if this condition is not treated?

Kidney stones, renal failure, gouty arthritis, and subcutaneous tophus deposits will result if the disorder is left untreated.

CASE 14

A 19-year-old college student comes to the university health clinic complaining of muscle aches. She recently began an exercise program to lose the 6–8 kg (13–17 lb) that she gained over the past year. After her first day of weightlifting, however, she became extremely sore. Several hours later, her urine was the color of "cherry soda pop." Physical examination is unremarkable. Laboratory tests reveal a serum creatine kinase level of 93970 IU/L. Urinalysis is negative for blood and positive for myoglobin.

What is the most likely diagnosis?

McArdle disease (type V glycogen storage disease). Other glycogen storage diseases include Von Gierke disease, which causes severe fasting hypoglycaemia; Pompe disease, which is characterized by cardiomegaly and early death; and Cori disease, which is less severe than Von Gierke and has normal lactate levels.

What is the biochemical defect in this condition?

McArdle disease is caused by a deficiency of muscle glycogen phosphorylase. Although glycogen formation is not affected, glycogen cannot be broken back down to glucose (glycogenolysis) because the α-1,4-glycosidic bonds cannot be broken in the muscle to release glucose-1-phosphate.

What are the most likely liver and muscle biopsy findings?

A liver biopsy is normal, as the defective enzyme is present only in muscle. Muscle biopsy shows accumulation of glycogen.

After the patient completes an exercise tolerance test, her lactic acid levels do not increase normally. Why?

Lactic acid is a product of anaerobic glucose metabolism. Failure of lactic acid levels to elevate after exercise is an indication of a defect in the metabolism of glycogen or glucose to lactate. This response can be seen in other disorders of glycogenolysis or glycolysis as well.

What accounts for the color of her urine?

Her muscles begin to break down during exercise because of the lack of glucose. This causes myoglobinuria as well as elevated creatine kinase. Her urine will be positive for blood on urine dipstick but will be negative for RBCs.

What is the most appropriate treatment for this condition?

Oral ingestion of sucrose before exercise has been demonstrated to improve exercise tolerance and reduce the risk of myoglobinuria.

CASE 15

A 2-year-old boy is brought to a health clinic in Mexico because of poor development as well as vomiting, irritability, and a skin rash. The boy's mother also notes that his urine has a strange "mousy" odor. Physical examination reveals the child has an eczema-like rash, is hyperreflexive, and has increased muscle tone. He has a surprisingly fair-skinned complexion compared to the rest of his family. Laboratory studies reveal a serum phenylalanine level of 28 mg/dL.

What is the most likely diagnosis?
Phenylketonuria (PKU).

What is the pathophysiology of this condition?
PKU is caused by a defect in the metabolism of **phenylalanine** (Figure 2-11). Normally, this essential amino acid is converted to tyrosine by phenylalanine hydroxylase. However, when phenylalanine hydroxylase activity is reduced or absent, phenylalanine builds up. This leads to excess phenyl ketones in the blood, resulting in the symptoms seen in this patient. PKU is inherited in an autosomal recessive fashion.

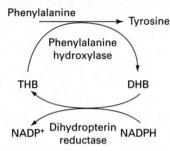

FIGURE 2-11. **Metabolism of phenylalanine.** DHB = dihydrobiopterin; NADP$^+$ = oxidized nicotinamide adenine dinucleotide phosphate; NADPH = reduced nicotinamide adenine dinucleotide phosphate; THB = tetrahydrobiopterin. (Reproduced, with permission, from Le T, et al. *First Aid for the USMLE Step 1: 2008*. New York: McGraw-Hill, 2008: 101.)

What additional physical characteristics are common at presentation?
Affected children are normal at birth but fail to reach developmental milestones. Other physical findings include failure to thrive, mental retardation, microcephaly, large cheek and upper jaw bones, and widely spaced teeth with poorly developed enamel.

What is the cofactor for the defective enzyme in this disease that, when deficient, can also lead to increased levels of phenylalanine in the blood?
A deficiency in tetrahydrobiopterin can also lead to increased blood levels of phenylalanine.

What is the appropriate treatment for this condition?
PKU is treated with decreased dietary phenylalanine (which is contained in many foods, including artificial sweeteners). In patients with PKU, tyrosine cannot be derived from phenylalanine, so it becomes an essential amino acid. Therefore, patient should also receive dietary tyrosine supplementation. Currently, screening is mandatory and performed 6 days to 2 weeks after birth using high-performance liquid chromatography.

CASE 16

A 6-month-old girl is brought to the pediatrician because she has been feeding poorly and has been lethargic for the past several months. The baby has also started breathing more rapidly than normal and recently had a seizure. Laboratory studies reveal a serum pH of 7.20, an anion gap of 19 mEq/L, elevated levels of pyruvate and alanine, and decreased levels of citrate.

What is the most likely diagnosis?
Pyruvate dehydrogenase deficiency.

What is the pathophysiology of this condition?
Glycolysis is the pathway that converts one molecule of glucose into two molecules of pyruvate. Pyruvate dehydrogenase then converts pyruvate to acetyl-CoA, which can enter the tricarboxylic acid (TCA) cycle (Figure 2-12). Without this enzyme, the cells derive much less adenosine triphosphate (ATP) from each molecule of glucose and rely more heavily on glycolysis alone. As pyruvate accumulates, some of it is converted to lactate to regenerate oxidized nicotinamide adenine dinucleotide (NAD+). The elevated lactate level is responsible for the acidemia and anion gap observed in this baby.

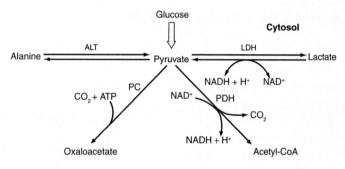

FIGURE 2-12. **Pyruvate metabolism.** ALT = alanine transaminase; ATP = adenosine triphosphate; LDH = lactate dehydrogenase; NAD+ = oxidized nicotinamide adenine dinucleotide; NADH = reduced nicotinamide adenine dinucleotide; PC = pyruvate carboxylase; PDH = pyruvate dehydrogenase. (Reproduced, with permission, from Le T, et al. *First Aid for the USMLE Step 1: 2011.* New York: McGraw-Hill, 2011: 99.)

Why are alanine levels high and citrate levels low in this condition?
Alanine levels are high because much of the excess pyruvate is converted to alanine in a reversible reaction by alanine aminotransferase. Citrate levels are low because there is little acetyl-CoA to combine with oxaloacetate to form citrate.

What is the appropriate treatment for this condition?
Treatment involves increased intake of ketogenic nutrients (foods with high fat content). The breakdown of fatty acids involves reduction of flavin adenine dinucleotide (FAD) and NAD and produces one molecule of acetyl-CoA for every two carbon atoms in the fatty acid chain. The $FADH_2$ (1-5-dihydro-FAD) and NADH (reduced NADH oxidase) can be used by the electron transport chain to produce ATP, whereas the acetyl-CoA can enter the TCA cycle. Oral citrate is also helpful for replenishing the substrates of the citric acid cycle.

Which are the only purely ketogenic amino acids?
Leucine and **lysine** are the only purely ketogenic amino acids.

■ CASE 17

A 5-month-old girl of Ashkenazi Jewish descent is brought to her pediatrician because of concerns about developmental regression. Although the baby girl was developing normally for the first 4 months of her life, she can no longer roll over by herself. In addition, she often smiled at 3 months of age but no longer does so. Funduscopic examination reveals a cherry-red spot in the macula. The remainder of her physical examination is normal.

What is the most likely diagnosis?

Tay-Sachs disease.

What is the biochemical defect in this condition?

This disease, one of the sphingolipidoses, is caused by a deficiency of **hexosaminidase A.** This enzyme is present within the lysosomes of central nervous system cells and helps degrade a lipid called GM2 ganglioside. GM2 ganglioside accumulation within the neurons leads to progressive neurodegeneration. Children become blind and deaf before paralysis ultimately sets in. Children with Tay-Sachs disease usually die by 3 years of age.

How is the gene responsible for this condition inherited?

Tay-Sachs disease is inherited in an autosomal recessive fashion. Fabry disease is the only one of the sphingolipidoses that is inherited differently; it is X-linked.

What other conditions present with similar physical examination findings?

Niemann-Pick disease, which is caused by a deficiency of sphingomyelinase, also presents with a cherry-red spot in the macula in approximately 50% of cases. These patients often present with anemia, fever, and neurologic deterioration. The prognosis of Niemann-Pick disease is poor as well; most patients die by 3 years of age. Unlike Niemann-Pick, Tay-Sachs does not involve hepatosplenomegaly and demonstrates onion-like lysosomes on microscopy. Foam cells are characteristic of Niemann-Pick.

Which of the other sphingolipidoses also has a higher prevalence among Ashkenazi Jews?

Although Tay-Sachs is considered to have a higher prevalence among Ashkenazi Jews, screening programs have significantly decreased the prevalence of Tay-Sachs in this group. **Gaucher disease,** which is caused by a deficiency of β-glucocerebrosidase, also has a much higher incidence in this population.

■ CASE 18

A 36-year-old homeless man presents to a community health clinic complaining of increasing shortness of breath. On questioning, the man admits to an extensive history of alcoholism. A review of systems reveals he has also experienced tingling and burning in his legs for the past several weeks. Physical examination reveals that he is tachycardic (heart rate of 122/min), has rales bilaterally, and has bilateral pitting edema. He also has decreased sensation in his feet and is hyporeflexive in his lower extremities. An x-ray of the chest shows an enlarged cardiac silhouette and bilateral pulmonary congestion.

What is the most likely diagnosis?

Vitamin B_1 (thiamine) deficiency. Although the patient's alcoholism presents a clear etiology, arsenic poisoning blocks thiamine utilization and can result in a clinical picture resembling thiamine deficiency; it should also be considered.

What clinical manifestations are commonly present in this condition?

This patient has the symptoms of both wet and dry beriberi. Patients with **wet beriberi** present with high-output congestive heart failure and dilated cardiomyopathy. Patients with **dry beriberi** present with peripheral neuropathy consisting of muscular atrophy and diminished sensation and reflexes. Dry beriberi presents similarly to vitamin B_{12} deficiency; however, vitamin B_{12} deficiency is usually due to a malabsorptive process, does not cause congestive heart failure, and will cause a macrocytic anemia.

The deficient factor in this condition is a cofactor for which enzymes?

Thiamine is part of thiamine pyrophosphate (TPP). TPP acts as a cofactor for transketolase (an enzyme in the hexose monophosphate shunt) (Figure 2-14A), pyruvate decarboxylase (a component of the pyruvate dehydrogenase complex), and α-ketoglutarate decarboxylase (a component of the α-ketoglutarate dehydrogenase complex) (Figure 2-14B).

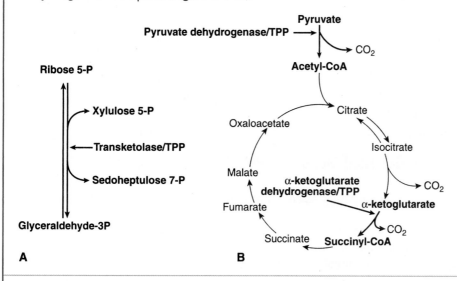

FIGURE 2-14. (A) Thiamine in the hexose monophosphate shunt. (B) Thiamine in the tricarboxylic acid cycle. TPP = thiamine pyrophosphate.

What other pathologies are commonly seen with this vitamin deficiency?

Wernicke encephalopathy is the central nervous system manifestation of thiamine deficiency. This disease classically consists of nystagmus, ophthalmoplegia, and cerebellar ataxia. When the additional symptoms of confusion/psychosis and confabulation are seen, the disease is known as **Wernicke-Korsakoff syndrome**. It is standard practice to give thiamine before glucose to any patient with suspected thiamine deficiency to prevent Wernicke-Korsakoff.

What are the most likely MRI findings?

Although degenerative changes are often seen in the cerebellum, brain stem, and diencephalon, atrophy of the mammillary bodies is most commonly noted.

■ CASE 19

A 6-month-old girl is brought to her pediatrician after having a seizure. She has a 5-month history of restlessness, vomiting, and sweating that most commonly occur between meals and subside after feeding. On physical examination, the baby is determined to be small for her age with a protuberant abdomen, liver below the costal margin, and xanthomas on the buttocks. Ultrasound shows hepatomegaly and bilaterally enlarged kidneys. Relevant laboratory values are as follows:

Serum glucose: 20 mg/dL   Lactic acid: 9 mg/dL
Anion gap: 35 mEq/L

What is the most likely diagnosis?
Von Gierke disease (type I glycogen storage disease).

What is the biochemical defect in this condition?
This is a glycogen storage disease resulting from glucose-6-phosphatase deficiency. In this disease, although the liver is able to create and break down glycogen, it is unable to release glucose into the blood, because glucose-6-phosphatase (which catalyzes the final step of this process) is deficient (Figure 2-15). The result is poor glucose control and marked fasting hypoglycemia.

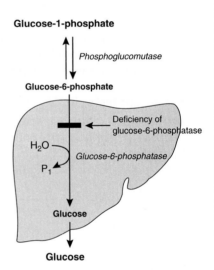

FIGURE 2-15. Glucose-6-phosphatase deficiency.

What are the most likely liver biopsy findings?
Glycogen lipid droplets and significant steatosis are most likely to be found on microscopy.

What complications are commonly associated with this condition?
- Gout can develop as a result of hyperuricemia.
- Hyperlipidemia—especially hypertriglyceridemia—is also common and can lead to xanthoma formation and pancreatitis.
- Platelet dysfunction is common and presents as easy bruising and epistaxis.
- Over time, patients may develop liver adenomas that occasionally undergo malignant transformation.
- Nephropathy often develops from the accumulation of glycogen in the kidney.

What is the appropriate treatment for this condition?
Treatment consists of frequent meals to prevent hypoglycemia. Some patients make cornstarch a central part of their diet because it is absorbed slowly and provides a steady glucose supply. Allopurinol is often used for gout. Liver transplantation is curative.

Microbiology and Immunology

CASE 1

A 19-year-old university student has been pulling all-nighters for his upcoming exams. While trying to study, he often finds himself falling asleep with his contact lenses still in. As finals week draws to a close, he is scratching his eyes often because they feel dry and painful, as if there are foreign bodies in them. He also notices that his eyes are red and that he tears up frequently.

What is the most likely diagnosis?

Keratitis caused by the free-living ameba *Acanthamoeba* is the most likely diagnosis. Conditions to consider in the differential diagnosis include herpes simplex virus (HSV), herpes zoster virus, and bacterial or fungal infection. However, HSV keratitis would present with photophobia, decreased visual acuity, and dendritic ulcer formation, which are not seen in this patient. Likewise, a bacterial or fungal source would present with accompanying systemic symptoms, and orbital cellulitis would create an ophthalmologic emergency.

What are the risk factors for developing this condition?

The number one risk factor for *Acanthamoeba* infection is **extended wearing of contact lenses.** Inadequate disinfection of the lenses with homemade saline solution and wearing lenses while swimming or showering can also predispose contact lens wearers to this infection. *Acanthamoeba* organisms can live in soil, air, and water and are resistant to chlorine.

What are other symptoms and complications of this condition?

Unlike bacterial keratitis, keratitis from *Acanthamoeba* takes days or weeks to cause symptoms. The initial symptoms are usually redness and a feeling of a foreign body in the eye. Blurring of vision may also be present. Over time, this progresses to pain, lid edema, and conjunctival injection. If untreated, increased intraocular pressure, cataracts, and even loss of vision can develop.

How is this condition diagnosed?

The diagnosis is made by **slit-lamp examination** of the eye, which shows thickened epithelium and rough corneal nerves. A characteristic ring on the cornea may also appear approximately 6 weeks after initial infection. Corneal scraping or biopsy reveals irregular polygonal cysts.

What is the appropriate treatment for this condition?

Initial treatment consists of topical antimicrobials such as miconazole and neomycin for several months. If the infection has been left untreated (ie, at the corneal ring stage), surgery, such as corneal debridement, is usually required.

What populations are at risk for this condition?

Populations include chronic disease patients, such as those with lymphoproliferative disorders, patients on chronic steroids, patients receiving chemotherapy, and patients with AIDS. In these populations, the infection is usually not of the eye but rather of the central nervous system. These patients present with changes in mental status, headache, and stiff neck. They can also develop cranial nerve palsies, ataxia, and hemiparesis (termed *granulomatous amebic encephalitis*). Treatment is urgent in such cases.

◼ CASE 2

A pathologist is sent a poorly labeled fluid sample for Gram staining. The test reveals a gram-positive rod that forms long, branching filaments that resemble fungi.

What are the possible bacterial microorganisms found in this sample?

Actinomyces and *Nocardia* both fit this description. However, although they resemble fungi on Gram stain, they are both bacteria, not fungi. They appear as characteristic gram-positive rods with long, branching filaments.

How are these two microorganisms differentiated?

Actinomyces israelii is a non-acid-fast filamentous, anaerobic organism (Figure 3-1) and has characteristic "sulfur granules." *Nocardia*, on the other hand, is weakly acid fast and an aerobic organism.

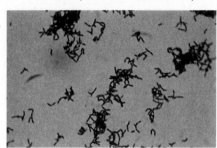

FIGURE 3-1. **Actinomyces.** (Reproduced, with permission, from Willey J, Sherwood L, Woolverton C. *Prescott's Principles of Microbiology*. New York: McGraw-Hill, 2008: Figure 28-1.)

What are the other obligate aerobic and anaerobic organisms?

The aerobic organisms are *Nocardia*, *Pseudomonas*, *Mycobacteria*, and *Bacillus* species (mnemonic: "Nagging Pests Must Breathe").

The anaerobic organisms are *Clostridium*, *Bacteroides*, and *Actinomyces* species (mnemonic: "Can't Breathe Air").

After paging the intern, the pathologist learns the sample was drained from an oral abscess. Now which of these two microorganisms is more likely?

Actinomyces is more likely because it is part of the **normal oral flora** and can cause abscesses in the mouth or gastrointestinal tract after trauma. *Nocardia* is an opportunistic infection and most often results in pulmonary symptoms due to **lung abscesses** or, rarely, central nervous system symptoms due to brain abscesses.

If this microorganism were found in a sputum sample that stained weakly acid fast, what could be inferred about the patient's immune status?

Nocardia is most often found in **immunocompromised** patients. The clinical presentation and acid-fast sputum sample resembles that of tuberculosis in this high-risk group and is commonly misdiagnosed as such in immunocompromised patients.

What is the appropriate treatment for each of these microorganisms?

Nocardia is treated with trimethoprim-sulfamethoxazole. *Actinomyces* is treated with penicillin G.

■ CASE 3

A local craftsman who makes garments from the hides of goats visits his physician because over the past few days he has developed several black lesions on his hands and arms (Figure 3-2). The lesions are not painful, but he is alarmed by their appearance. He is afebrile and his physical examination is unremarkable.

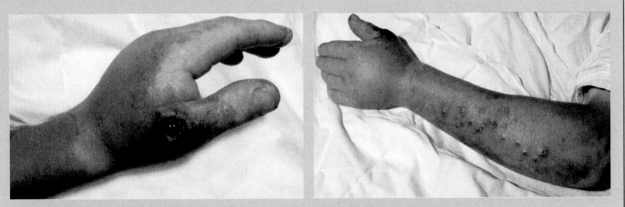

FIGURE 3-2. (Reproduced, with permission, from Wolff K, et al. *Fitzpatrick's Color Atlas & Synopsis of Clinical Dermatology*, 5th ed. New York: McGraw-Hill, 2005: 631.)

What is the most likely diagnosis?

Cutaneous anthrax, caused by *Bacillus anthracis*. The skin lesions are painless and dark or charred ulcerations known as black eschar. Cutaneous anthrax is classically transmitted by contact with the hide of a goat at the site of a minor open wound.

How will the causative microorganism appear on Gram staining?

B anthracis is a **gram-positive spore-forming rod.** The spores are resistant to many chemical disinfectants, heat, ultraviolet light, and drying and are therefore a feared agent of biological warfare.

What is the other spore-forming microorganism?

Clostridium species are the other gram-positive spore-forming bacteria. *Bacillus* and *Clostridium* species can be differentiated by their ability to neutralize oxygen free radicals. *Bacillus* species (like the other aerobic bacteria) have catalase and superoxide dismutase—enzymes that can neutralize oxygen free radicals and therefore survive in aerobic environments. *Clostridium* species do not have these enzymes and are therefore obligate anaerobic microorganisms.

What is the other primary manifestation of this infection?

B anthracis also causes pulmonary anthrax, or woolsorters' disease. In this condition, inhaled anthrax spores reach the alveoli, where they are taken up by macrophages and carried to mediastinal lymph nodes. This can result in mediastinal hemorrhage and a bloody pleural effusion. X-ray of the chest reveals a **widened mediastinum.**

▮ CASE 4

A 49-year-old woman from Alabama presents with diffuse, crampy abdominal pain that has persisted for the previous 4 days. She has had no bowel movements since the pain started and has noticed a weight loss of about 4.5 kg (10 lb) over the past month. She had a screening colonoscopy 3 months before presentation, which was negative. CT of the abdomen reveals an inflamed gallbladder and an irregular mass in the second portion of the duodenum. Stool sample reveals rough-surfaced eggs. Complete blood count and liver function test results are as follows:

White blood cell (WBC) count: 14,000/mm³
  (20% eosinophils)
Hemoglobin: 10.2 g/dL
Hematocrit: 31%
Platelet count: 250,000/mm³
Albumin: 3.2 g/dL

Aspartate transaminase (AST): 29 IU/L
Alanine transaminase (ALT): 27 IU/L
Alkaline phosphatase: 210 IU/L
Bilirubin, total: 4.0 mg/dL
Bilirubin, direct: 3.7 mg/dL

What is the most likely diagnosis?

Ascariasis, caused by *Ascaris lumbricoides,* a nematode (roundworm) found in the southern United States and tropical climates. Ascariasis is the most common helminthic infection worldwide. Eosinophilia is a classic finding in helminth infection and is due to the increased need for eosinophilic release of major basic protein.

What tests can be used to confirm the diagnosis?

Analysis of a stool sample shows eggs with a knobby, rough surface (Figure 3-3).

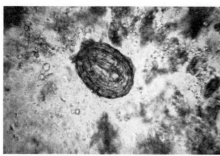

FIGURE 3-3. Ascariasis egg on stool ova and parasite test. (Courtesy of the Centers for Disease Control and Prevention. Public Health Image Library.)

What are the appropriate treatments for this condition?

As with many nematode infections, mebendazole or albendazole is the drug of choice. The bendazoles work by disrupting helminthic microtubule synthesis, which weakens cell structure.

CASE 5

A 54-year-old man with a history of tobacco use and chronic obstructive pulmonary disease (COPD) presents to the emergency department because of severe shortness of breath. The patient had a COPD exacerbation 3 weeks before the current event and began taking oral corticosteroids at that time. His symptoms resolved and he had returned to his usual state of health until 1.5 weeks later, when he again experienced cough and shortness of breath. When he developed hemoptysis 1 week ago, he was started on empiric antibiotics and underwent bronchoalveolar lavage, which revealed the presence of 45-degree branching septate hyphae (Figure 3-4).

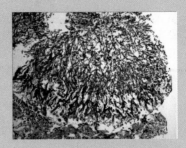

FIGURE 3-4. (Reproduced, with permission, from USMLERx.com.)

What is the most likely diagnosis?

The hemoptysis and pulmonary symptoms, along with the 45-degree septate hyphae found on lavage, indicate *Aspergillus* infection. *Aspergillus* is an opportunistic infection, secondary to the patient's recent immunosuppression from corticosteroid use.

Candida should also be considered but would appear microscopically as pseudohyphae and budding yeasts.

Mucormycosis presents with sinusitis, black nasal discharge, and can progress to hemoptysis, but lavage findings would indicate 90-degree branching nonseptate hyphae. This infection is most common in patients with type 1 diabetes mellitus.

What is x-ray of the chest likely to show?

Aspergillus can appear as a "fungus ball" or a circular mobile lung mass within preexisting cavitary lesions in the lungs. This form of *Aspergillus* infection is called an **aspergilloma**.

The patient is treated with amphotericin B. What are the drug's mechanism of action and side effects?

Amphotericin B works by binding to ergosterol, a key component of fungal membranes, thereby disrupting the integrity of the cell membrane. Its side effects can be serious and include fever, chills, kidney damage, hypotension, and arrhythmias. This grave side effect profile has given this powerful drug the nickname "Amphoterrible," and its use reserved for serious fungal infections.

The patient's symptoms improve and he is discharged a few days later. However, he returns to the hospital in 3 months with worsened respiratory function, chest pain, and decreased urine output. Could these symptoms be sequelae of the condition that caused his admission?

Yes; the patient could be suffering from **invasive aspergillosis**, which is the result of hematogenous spread of his infection to his kidneys, pericardium, and other organs, causing these diffuse symptoms. However, amphotericin B toxicity can also cause nephrotoxicity, dyspnea, and cardiac arrhythmias and therefore should be ruled out.

What patient population is at risk for invasive aspergillosis?

Neutropenic patients (because of hematologic malignancy, chemotherapy, immunosuppressive therapy, solid organ transplant, or HIV infection) are particularly susceptible to invasive aspergillosis.

If, instead of COPD, this patient had a history of severe asthma, to what type of fungal infection would he be most susceptible?

Allergic bronchopulmonary aspergillosis is an IgE-mediated hypersensitivity reaction to *Aspergillus* spores. The hyperactive inflammatory response in the airways of asthmatics predisposes them to bronchospasm and pneumonitis in response to an otherwise benign inoculation of *Aspergillus* spores.

■ CASE 6

A 41-year-old man presents to the emergency department complaining of the sudden onset of weakness, nausea, vomiting, and blurred vision. On physical examination, he has fixed, dilated pupils and a decreased gag reflex. When asked, he admits that he often eats food that he has canned himself. The patient is admitted to the hospital for further monitoring.

What is the most likely diagnosis?

Botulism, resulting from ingestion of the botulinum toxin made by the gram-positive, spore-forming bacteria *Clostridium botulinum.*

What is the pathophysiology of this toxicity?

Acetylcholine is normally released by motor neurons into the neuromuscular junction, where it binds to muscarinic receptors on the motor endplate of the muscle fiber. This binding depolarizes the membrane and subsequently contracts the muscle. Botulinum toxin binds **presynaptically** and prevents the release of acetylcholine into the **neuromuscular junction.** The result is a flaccid paralysis, or inability to contract. The binding is irreversible and it takes approximately 6 months for new synapses to form.

What is the typical course in adult patients with this condition?

Ingestion of the botulinum toxin in food usually causes symptoms within 12–36 hours. The first symptoms are gastrointestinal distress (eg, cramps and nausea), due to enteric nervous system dysfunction, followed by neurologic symptoms. The first nerves affected are the cranial nerves, causing blurred vision, decreased eye movements, and a decreased gag reflex. The paralysis is symmetric and **descending.** Autonomic nerves can also be affected, resulting in ileus, urinary retention, and orthostatic hypotension. Respiratory muscles can also be affected, necessitating ventilator support.

What is the differential diagnosis for this presentation?

The major differential includes Guillain-Barré syndrome, myasthenia gravis, and Lambert-Eaton syndrome. Unlike botulism, the paralysis seen in **Guillain-Barré syndrome** is due to a postinfectious demyelination of alpha motor neurons and is ascending. The most common infection leading to Guillain-Barré syndrome is *Campylobacter jejuni.* **Myasthenia gravis** is an autoimmune condition caused by antibodies created against the muscarinic acetylcholine receptor. Patients with this condition have muscle weakness only after prolonged muscle use, classically at the end of the day. **Lambert-Eaton syndrome** is a paraneoplastic anti–calcium channel antibody syndrome that causes muscle weakness that improves with prolonged muscle use.

How can this toxicity be acquired?

In adults, it is acquired most commonly from ingestion of **preformed toxin** in contaminated canned foods (usually home canned). In infants, ingestion of **bacterial spores** found in honey can result in toxicity referred to as "floppy baby syndrome."

CASE 7

A patient with diabetes presents to her physician with a white, flaky, adherent substance on the skin under her breasts. Another patient, a woman who has just completed a course of oral antibiotics, presents with itching and copious vaginal discharge that resembles "cottage cheese." A third patient, with AIDS, presents with white exudate on his oral mucosa and soft palate. The physician diagnoses the same causative microorganism for all three cases.

What is the most likely diagnosis?

The fungus *Candida albicans* can result in systemic or superficial fungal infection (candidiasis). Skinfold infection, vaginitis (yeast infection), and oral thrush are common manifestations of local candidiasis and present as a white, flaky, cheesy exudate on the affected surface.

Where is the microorganism that causes this condition normally found?

C albicans is part of the normal flora of mucous membranes of the gastrointestinal tract, respiratory tract, and women's genital tract. Overgrowth, due to an imbalance in normal flora from women taking **antibiotic** therapy or patients who are **immunocompromised,** causes candidiasis.

What laboratory tests can help confirm the diagnosis?

A potassium hydroxide preparation (**KOH mount**) is used for skin or tissue scrapings. **Pseudohyphae** and **budding yeast** (Figure 3-5) are observed in the tissues. Pseudohyphae are seen in culture at 20°C (68°F), and germ tube formation is seen at 37°C (98.6°F). For (rare) systemic disease (eg, invasive candidiasis found primarily in neutropenic patients), blood cultures are positive for the fungus.

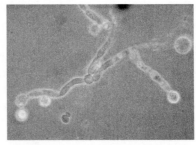

FIGURE 3-5. KOH mount of *Candida albicans.* (Reproduced, with permission, from Wolff K, et al. *Fitzpatrick's Color Atlas & Synopsis of Clinical Dermatology,* 5th ed. New York: McGraw-Hill, 2005: 717.)

What populations other than immunocompromised patients are at risk for serious forms of this condition?

Intravenous drug users are at higher risk for candidal endocarditis.

What are the appropriate treatments for this condition?

Fluconazole or nystatin is used for superficial infections, and amphotericin B or fluconazole can be used for systemic infections.

CASE 8

A 49-year-old woman who recently immigrated to the United States from Nicaragua presents to the clinic with difficulty swallowing, constipation, and abdominal pain. She says her last bowel movement was more than a week ago. Physical examination reveals tachycardia and a distended abdomen. An electrocardiogram (ECG) shows Mobitz type I heart block.

What is the most likely diagnosis?

Chagas disease, or American trypanosomiasis, caused by the protozoan *Trypanosoma cruzi.*

What is the vector of the responsible protozoan?

The vector is the reduviid bug, also known as the "kissing bug" because the bite is painless.

What is the classic sign associated with the acute form of this condition?

The Romaña sign is painless, unilateral periorbital edema and conjunctivitis that results from acute Chagas disease. This sign is specific but not sensitive for acute *T cruzi* infection (Figure 3-6).

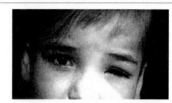

FIGURE 3-6. **Romaña sign.** (Reproduced, with permission, from Goldsmith R, Heyneman D. *Tropical Medicine and Parasitology.* Originally published by Appleton & Lange. Copyright © 1989 by The McGraw-Hill Companies, Inc.)

Where in the world is this condition commonly found?

Chagas disease is commonly found in the southern United States, Mexico, and Central and South America (ie, only in the Western hemisphere).

What is the pathophysiology of this condition?

This woman is experiencing chronic Chagas disease, which is most often characterized by heart block, ventricular tachycardia, and dilated cardiomyopathy. Dilatation of the esophagus and colon (megaesophagus and megacolon) can cause difficulty swallowing and constipation. The acute phase of the disease can be characterized by a hard red area called a **chagoma** at the parasite's site of entry into the host, accompanied by fever and meningoencephalitis. In endemic areas, the acute phase is seen more frequently in children.

What is the appropriate treatment for this condition?

Nifurtimox and benznidazole are used to treat acute cases. However, there is no effective treatment for chronic Chagas disease. For chronic heart disease, supportive measures for congestive heart failure, antiarrhythmics to prevent recurrent ventricular tachycardia, and pacemaker implantation for heart block are used. For gastrointestinal disease, dilation of the esophageal sphincter, changes in diet, the use of laxatives and/or enemas, and in some cases eventual resection of the megacolon are used.

What other disease is caused by the protozoan species that causes this condition?

The protozoa *Trypanosoma gambiense* and *Trypanosoma rhodesiense* cause African sleeping sickness. This illness is characterized by lymphadenopathy, recurrent fevers due to antigenic variation, somnolence, and possibly coma. It is transmitted by the **tsetse fly,** whose bite is painful.

■ CASE 9

A 24-year-old American man is traveling in rural India during the monsoon season. Over the course of a few hours, he develops severe watery diarrhea. In the next 30 hours, he has approximately one episode per hour of liquid stools that appear clear with small white flecks of mucus. He also has occasional episodes of vomiting. He quickly becomes lethargic and generally ill with crampy abdominal pain but is afebrile. He attempts to rehydrate himself during the illness, and the symptoms resolve within approximately 48 hours.

What is the most likely diagnosis?

This patient has cholera, a potentially fatal dehydrating illness caused by *Vibrio cholerae.* This microorganism is a gram-negative, curved, motile, polar flagellated rod (Figure 3-7) that resembles "shooting stars" on Gram stain. Symptomatic cholera usually manifests in epidemics, and it is endemic to developing regions in Africa, Asia, South and Latin America, and recently the Middle East.

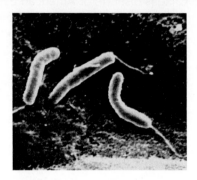

FIGURE 3-7. *Vibrio cholerae* under scanning electron micrograph. Note the curved shape and single polar flagella. (Reproduced, with permission, from Ryan KJ, Ray CG. *Sherris Medical Microbiology*, 5th ed. New York: McGraw-Hill, 2010: Figure 32-1.)

What is the primary differential diagnosis?

Watery diarrhea induced during travel within a foreign country makes the noninvasive enterotoxigenic *Escherichia coli* (ETEC) infection the primary differential diagnosis ("traveler's diarrhea"). However, ETEC diarrhea is not associated with white mucous flecks and generally is not as voluminous as the diarrhea induced by cholera.

How does the microorganism involved in this condition exert its effect on the gastrointestinal tract?

V cholerae is ingested through fecally contaminated water. It secretes an exotoxin (cholera toxin) that binds to the surface of intestinal epithelium. This toxin ADP-ribosylates adenylyl cyclase, thus increasing levels of cyclic adenosine monophosphate (cAMP) within the intestinal mucosa. This causes increased chloride secretion and decreased sodium absorption, leading to a massive secretory loss of fluids and electrolytes.

What are the clinical manifestations of this condition?

The hallmark of cholera is **rice-water stools,** so described because the small white flecks of mucus resemble grains of rice. The onset of this diarrhea typically occurs 1–3 days after infection. Vomiting and abdominal cramping is common, but fever is rare because *V cholerae* itself is noninvasive and thus remains in the gastrointestinal tract. Many infections are asymptomatic, but severe cholera can lead to extreme dehydration that can cause death within hours due to the excretion of electrolytes leading to renal failure, arrhythmias from hypokalemia, and metabolic acidosis from bicarbonate loss.

What is the appropriate treatment for this condition?

Oral rehydration solution (ORS), which has reduced mortality rates from 50% to < 1%. A typical preparation of ORS contains glucose, potassium chloride, sodium chloride, and sodium bicarbonate. Glucose facilitates sodium absorption from the gut, which allows for the concurrent absorption of water. Antibiotics are of limited use in stopping the diarrhea, although early use of doxycycline can reduce the volume of diarrhea and decrease the duration of bacteria excretion by 1 day.

CASE 10

A 3-year-old boy is brought to his pediatrician with a fever, tachypnea, and a cough productive of rusty sputum. He has a history of recurrent lung and skin infections. He has had several fungal infections of his skin, as well as an abscess that formed where he scraped his arm. An x-ray of the chest shows a normal thymic shadow but some hilar lymphadenopathy. Further questioning of the parents reveals a maternal male cousin who died at 5 years of age from severe pneumonia and a maternal uncle who has had two surgeries for intracranial fungal infections.

What is the most likely diagnosis?

The most likely diagnosis is **chronic granulomatous disease** (CGD), an X-linked inherited immunodeficiency syndrome. This patient is predisposed to bacterial and fungal infections. The normal thymic shadow suggests normal T-cell maturation, which effectively rules out a diagnosis of severe combined immunodeficiency or DiGeorge syndrome. The strong family history of male involvement on the maternal side indicates an X-linked hereditary condition and suggests CGD as the likely diagnosis in this patient.

Infections with which organisms could be particularly severe and problematic in this patient?

Patients with CGD are at risk for serious infections with catalase-positive bacteria, including *Staphylococcus aureus*, *Aspergillus* species, and *Burkholderia cepacia*.

Why are patients with this condition especially susceptible to catalase-positive organisms?

Reduced nicotinamide adenine dinucleotide phosphate (NADPH) oxidase, which is required for production of reactive oxygen species, is deficient in patients with CGD. The radicals are used by neutrophils during the oxidative burst to kill engulfed organisms. Many bacterial species make free radicals as by-products of their metabolism. These free radicals contribute to the toxic environment in the neutrophil lysosomes. However, catalase-positive bacteria such as *S aureus* can neutralize these free radicals, leaving the patient unprotected against these organisms. The primary method of host immunity is containment of the offending organism, leading to numerous granulomatous formations (Figure 3-8).

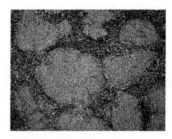

FIGURE 3-8. **Multiple noncaseating granulomas in a lymph node of a patient with sarcoidosis, similar to that seen in a patient with CGD.** (Reproduced, with permission, from USMLERx.com.)

What laboratory test can confirm this diagnosis?

The nitroblue tetrazolium test can detect the presence of a respiratory burst in neutrophils. In normal individuals the test is positive, but in patients with CGD the test is negative because the superoxide free radical is not produced.

What medical treatments are available for this condition?

Infections must be treated aggressively with appropriate antimicrobials. Trimethoprim-sulfamethoxazole can be used as long-term prophylaxis. In addition, interferon-α, an immunomodulator, is used in patients with CGD.

What therapy or procedure provides a definitive cure for this patient?

Bone marrow transplantation provides a source of functional neutrophils with the ability to create oxygen free radicals to effectively kill organisms engulfed by phagocytosis.

CASE 11

An 85-year-old man is hospitalized for community-acquired pneumonia. He is treated with penicillin, and over the next week he feels that he is slowly recovering. On hospital day 10, he develops a low-grade fever, watery diarrhea, and lower abdominal pain.

What is the most likely diagnosis?

Antibiotic-associated colitis or pseudomembranous colitis caused by *Clostridium difficile* superinfection (or overgrowth). *C difficile* is a gram-positive, spore-forming anaerobe. It should be noted that most antibiotic-associated diarrhea (without fever) is osmotic, resulting from decreased carbohydrate digestion secondary to a loss of gut flora. However, *C difficile* infection will present with fever and leukocytosis, and can be a very serious complication of prolonged antibiotic use.

What are the manifestations of this condition?

Approximately 20% of hospitalized patients are asymptomatically colonized with *Clostridium difficile* and then become carriers. Patients with symptoms upon colonization usually present with a low-grade fever, watery diarrhea, lower abdominal pain, leukocytosis, and a recent history (within 10 weeks) of antibiotic use. In severe cases, inflammation of the peritoneum can result from microperforation in the diseased colon. These patients present with signs of peritonitis such as rebound tenderness and involuntary guarding. On colonoscopy, they likely have **pseudomembranes** on the colon, which are raised yellow-white plaques created by the *C difficile* toxins (Figure 3-9). Risks include ileus and toxic megacolon, which can grossly perforate and cause death. Emergent colectomy is indicated and can be a lifesaving procedure if performed in a timely manner.

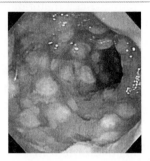

FIGURE 3-9. **Yellowish pseudomembranes in colon representing pseudomembranous colitis caused by *Clostridium difficile* infection.** (Reproduced, with permission, from Fauci AS, et al. *Harrison's Principles of Internal Medicine*, 17th ed. New York: McGraw-Hill, 2008: 1837.)

What population of patients is susceptible to this condition?

Infection is most often seen in elderly hospitalized patients. *C difficile* produces resistant spores, which are commonly found on hospital objects and on the hands of health care workers. Common alcohol-based hand sanitizers are ineffective at eliminating *C difficile* spores. *C difficile* colonizes the gastrointestinal (GI) tract (usually the colon) after the normal gut flora is killed or altered by antibiotics. The antibiotics most commonly associated with this disease are the penicillins, cephalosporins, and clindamycin. Once it has colonized the GI tract, *C difficile* releases toxins (toxins A and B) that permeate and destroy intestinal epithelial cells, respectively. A new, more virulent strain of this bacterium that produces a binary toxin is associated with the use of fluoroquinolones.

How is this condition diagnosed and treated?

Definitive diagnosis can be made with a cytotoxicity assay, an enzyme-linked immunosorbent assay for *C difficile* toxin A, or polymerase chain reaction. First-line treatment is with oral metronidazole or vancomycin. Fecal transplantation is an emerging therapy that aims to replenish the missing gut flora in patients with *C difficile* overgrowth by introducing normal fecal bacteria from a healthy patient. Pilot studies reveal a high success rate of this procedure, but further testing is needed before it becomes standard of care.

CASE 12

A 5-year-old girl is brought to the clinic with a 3-month history of worsening vision and behavioral difficulty in school. She immigrated to the United States from Guatemala with her mother and a younger sibling 2 years previously. Her mother received no prenatal care and, through a translator, reports that the patient was delivered without complication at home. As an infant, the girl had a "wartlike" perioral maculopapular rash and three or four recurrent right-sided ear infections. Physical examination reveals that the girl is in the 30th percentile for weight and the 35th percentile for height. Additional observations include fundi that are notable for nummular keratitis, prominent notching of her upper two incisors and molars, and outward bowing of the tibia bilaterally.

What is the most likely diagnosis?

Congenital syphilis. This infection is one of the so-called **ToRCHeS** infections (**T**oxoplasmosis, **o**ther infections, **R**ubella, **C**ytomegalovirus, **H**erpes simplex virus, **S**yphilis), the most common causes of congenital infection.

What is the causative microorganism in this condition?

Treponema pallidum.

What symptoms are commonly found in patients with this condition?

Congenital syphilis is a cause of hydrops fetalis, or stillbirth due to fluid accumulation in the fetus. If the newborn survives, it can develop various abnormalities, including the classic facial anomalies (tooth abnormalities known as Hutchinson incisors and mulberry molars, saddle nose, frontal bossing, and short maxilla), as well as recurrent ear infections and interstitial keratitis, leading to vision problems.

In the newborn, what tests can help confirm the diagnosis?

Serum rapid plasma reagin (RPR) test: Umbilical cord blood may show false-positive results because of maternal titers but remains the best screening tool for detecting syphilis infection.

Serum analysis and lumbar puncture can be performed for **Venereal Disease Research Laboratory (VDRL) testing.** VDRL testing detects anticardiolipin antibodies that are produced by patients with syphilis. The serum VDRL is used for screening purposes. VDRL testing from cerebrospinal fluid (CSF) samples is used to detect central nervous system involvement of the disease, known as neurosyphilis. Other CSF findings such as pleocytosis (increased number of cells) and elevated protein levels also suggest infection. The presence of anticardiolipin antibodies is not specific to syphilis and can return false-positive results in patients with Epstein-Barr virus, systemic lupus erythematosus, rheumatoid arthritis, and other autoimmune or inflammatory conditions.

What are the appropriate treatments for this condition?

Benzathine penicillin G for 10–14 days is the first-line treatment for syphilis.

CASE 13

A pathologist is performing an autopsy on a 56-year-old university professor who suffered a rapid demise from an undiagnosed neurologic disease. Approximately 1 year previously, the patient presented to a psychiatrist with symptoms of psychosis. Shortly thereafter, his symptoms advanced to include unsteadiness and involuntary movements, and the patient ultimately became immobile and unable to speak. A sample of brain tissue is shown in Figure 3-10.

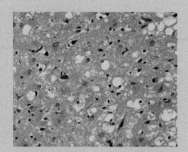

FIGURE 3-10. (Courtesy of the Centers for Disease Control and Prevention. Public Health Image Library, content provider Teresa Hammett.)

What is the most likely diagnosis?

Creutzfeldt-Jakob disease (CJD) is a prion disease characterized by rapidly progressive dementia with ataxia, myoclonus, and death within 1 year.

What are the classic brain histology findings in this condition?

On histology, prion disease presents with dramatic neuronal loss with numerous vacuoles in the gray matter resembling a porous sponge. This is therefore known as spongiform encephalopathy.

How does the causative agent in this condition differ from other pathogens?

Prions do not contain RNA or DNA; they are composed only of abnormally folded proteins.

How is this condition transmitted?

Disease can be transmitted by central nervous system (CNS) tissue containing prions (transmission has been seen secondary to corneal transplants, ingestion, and implantable electrodes or other intracranial surgery with contaminated instruments as prions are not destroyed by autoclaving). Prion disease can also be inherited.

What other condition is associated with this type of pathogen?

Prions cause two degenerative CNS diseases in humans: CJD and **kuru**, a slowly progressive, fatal disease found among tribes in Papua, New Guinea, who practice cannibalism.

How does the structure of normal prions differ from that of pathologic prions?

Normal prions have α-helix conformations, whereas pathologic prions are composed of an abnormal isoform of β-pleated sheets. The new structure renders them undegradable, and buildup leads to neuronal toxicity. Further, the abnormal prions cause normal prions to change conformation into β-pleated sheets, leading to the severe contagiousness of the disease.

CASE 14

A 32-year-old man with AIDS presents to the emergency department with complaints of worsening headache, fever, and a stiff neck. Lumbar puncture is performed, and analysis reveals an elevated opening pressure, increased protein level, and decreased glucose level. Special staining of the spinal fluid reveals budding yeast.

What is the most likely diagnosis?

Cryptococcal meningitis is the most common fungal cause of meningitis and is prevalent among patients with AIDS.

What laboratory tests can help confirm the diagnosis?

Serology is most commonly used; latex agglutination detects polysaccharide capsular antigen. The microorganism can also be cultured on **Sabouraud agar. India ink** stains the heavy polysaccharide capsule and reveals budding yeast (Figure 3-11).

FIGURE 3-11. *Cryptococcus neoformans.*

What microorganism causes this disease?

Cryptococcus neoformans is heavily encapsulated yeast. It is found only as a yeast; it is not a dimorphic microorganism.

CD4+ cell counts are typically at or below what level when infection with this microorganism occurs?

C neoformans usually infects severely lymphopenic patients with CD4+ cell counts < 50 cells/mm^3.

How does this microorganism cause illness?

C neoformans is found in pigeon droppings and in soil. When inhaled, the yeast causes a local infection in the lung; this infection can be asymptomatic or can result in pneumonia. Hematogenous spread to the central nervous system (CNS) can result in meningitis and brain abscesses. As in other common causes of meningitis, the capsule is thought to be an important virulence factor for gaining access into the CNS.

What is the appropriate treatment for this condition?

Patients who are not immunocompromised can be treated sufficiently with amphotericin B and flucytosine for the meningitis. Patients with AIDS require long-term suppression with fluconazole after induction with amphotericin B and flucytosine. In these patients long-term suppression may be stopped if the patient responds to highly active antiretroviral therapy (HAART) and has repeated measurements demonstrating high CD4+ counts.

HIV/AIDS patients with CD4+ cell counts < 50 cells/mm^3 are at risk for what other infections?

AIDS patients with a CD4+ cell count < 50 cells/mm^3 are at risk for cytomegalovirus retinitis, esophagitis, and *Mycobacterium avium-intracellulare*, which produces disseminated gastrointestinal and pulmonary disease. Prophylaxis includes ganciclovir and azithromycin, respectively.

What cerebrospinal fluid findings are expected in this condition?

Like viral meningitis, fungal meningitis has an elevated WBC count with a lymphocytic predominance. However, all other laboratory results mimic those of bacterial meningitis: increased opening pressure, increased protein, and decreased glucose in cerebrospinal fluid (Table 3-1).

TABLE 3-1	Cerebrospinal Findings in Meningitis			
	PRESSURE	CELL TYPE	PROTEIN	GLUCOSE
Bacterial	Increased	Increased PMNs	Increased	Decreased
Fungal/tuberculosis	Increased	Increased lymphocytes	Increased	Decreased
Viral	Normal/Increased	Increased lymphocytes	Normal	Normal

PMN, polymorphonuclear neutrophil; TB, tuberculosis.
(Reproduced, with permission, from Le T, et al. *First Aid for the USMLE Step 1: 2011.* New York: McGraw-Hill, 2011: 177.)

▮ CASE 15

A 42-year-old woman who works in a pork processing plant presents to her physician with new-onset seizures and bilateral lower extremity weakness. CT of the head (Figure 3-12) reveals several calcified regions and cystic masses but no solid mass lesion or evidence of bleeding. A complete blood count reveals mild anemia and a WBC count of 78,000/mm³ with 12% eosinophils.

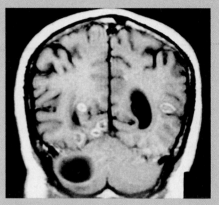

FIGURE 3-12. (Reproduced, with permission, from Rooper AH, Samuels MA. *Adams & Victor's Principles of Neurology,* 9th ed. New York: McGraw-Hill, 2009: Figure 32-8.)

What is the most likely diagnosis?

Cysticercosis, caused by *Taenia solium* (pork tapeworm), is a cestode (tapeworm) infection. When the tapeworm invades the brain, it forms small nonpurulent abscesses that can later calcify. The disease then becomes known as neurocysticercosis and is responsible for the majority of adult-onset seizures in developing nations.

How does the organism involved in this condition cause illness?

Ingestion of undercooked pork introduces larvae from pig muscle into the human gastrointestinal (GI) system. These larvae mature in the small intestine. Eggs from the adult worms are released into the feces. Ingestion of these eggs via the fecal-oral route allows eggs to enter the GI tract, where they develop into larvae. The larvae then penetrate the intestinal wall and migrate into the blood and tissues. Because humans are not a natural host for this stage of the organism, the larvae encyst into various organs.

What signs and symptoms are associated with this condition?

Infection can be asymptomatic or can cause malnutrition and abdominal discomfort. Cysticercosis can be found anywhere in the body, including the brain and eye, leading to seizures, focal neurological symptoms, and blindness.

What tests can help confirm the diagnosis?

Intestinal infection is revealed by eggs in stool. Calcified cysticerci can be observed on CT of the head when cysticercosis occurs in the brain. X-ray may reveal calcified cysticerci in other parts of the body, such as muscle.

What are the appropriate treatments for this condition?

Praziquantel is used for cysticercosis, and albendazole is used for neurocysticercosis. In addition, steroids and anticonvulsants may be given for decreasing complications of neurocysticercosis. Asymptomatic patients are rarely treated.

What are the other cestodes?

Diphyllobothrium latum is a cestode transmitted by ingestion from freshwater fish that causes vitamin B$_{12}$–deficient macrocytic anemia. *Echinococcus granulosus* eggs are ingested from dog feces and can cause liver cysts.

■ CASE 16

A 12-year-old girl presents to clinic with a sore throat and fever. She says she feels very tired. Physical examination reveals notable cervical lymphadenopathy, but the spleen is not palpable. A heterophile agglutinin test is negative. On histology, the image shown in Figure 3-13 is seen.

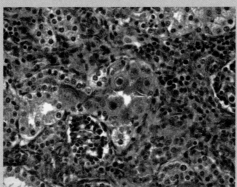

FIGURE 3-13. (Reproduced, with permission, from USMLERx.com.)

What is the most likely diagnosis?

Infectious mononucleosis syndrome resulting from cytomegalovirus (CMV) infection. CMV is a double-stranded linear virus in the family *Herpesviridae*. Infected cells have intranuclear inclusions, and on histology have an **"owl's-eye"** appearance, as seen in the center of Figure 3-13.

What is the presentation of this condition?

In the majority of people, CMV infection is asymptomatic. In those with symptoms, it usually presents with a mononucleosis-like syndrome, which includes pharyngitis, cervical lymphadenopathy, fever, lethargy, and, less often, splenomegaly. Unlike the mononucleosis syndrome seen with Epstein-Barr virus, the **heterophile agglutinin test** (monospot test) is negative. CMV can be transmitted by direct contact, blood transfusions, organ transplantation, breast milk, sexual contact, and vertically (ie, mother to fetus). It is one of the **TORCHeS** infections (**T**oxoplasmosis, **o**ther infections, **R**ubella, **C**ytomegalovirus, **H**erpes simplex virus, **S**yphilis).

What populations are at risk for complications of this condition?

The populations most at risk are those with decreased cellular immunity, such as patients with AIDS and organ transplants (especially bone marrow and lung transplants). The main complication in the transplantation population is CMV pneumonia. The main complication in the AIDS population is CMV retinitis, which usually presents when the CD4+ cell count is < 50 cells/mm^3. In both populations, prophylactic ganciclovir can be given.

How does this condition present in patients infected congenitally?

In patients congenitally infected with CMV, the complications include petechiae, jaundice, microcephaly, microsomia, retinitis, neurologic abnormalities, and deafness. At-risk fetuses are those whose mothers have a primary infection, which is seen with high IgM levels (the IgG levels could be low or high). Mothers with low IgM levels and high IgG levels likely have a secondary infection and are more likely to be able to prevent transmission from mother to fetus.

What is the appropriate treatment for this condition?

Although most patients do not need treatment, the treatment is ganciclovir, a nucleoside analog. This drug requires activation by viral kinase, which phosphorylates the drug and allows it to inhibit CMV DNA polymerase. Acyclovir is not effective against CMV.

What are the most common side effects of the treatment for this condition?

Ganciclovir is more toxic than acyclovir. Side effects include leukopenia, neutropenia, thrombocytopenia, and renal toxicity.

CASE 17

A woman who has recently returned from a city in Southeast Asia presents to her physician with sudden-onset fever, severe muscle pain in her back and extremities, and recent joint pain in her knees. Examination reveals an erythematous rash that covers her face and body and generalized lymphadenopathy.

What is the most likely diagnosis?

This woman is likely experiencing **dengue fever,** also known as "breakbone fever" because of the severe joint and muscle pain associated with it.

What is the vector for this condition?

The vector is the *Aedes aegypti* mosquito. These mosquitoes are diurnal and live near cities. They are most commonly found in pools of stagnant water. This distinguishes them from malaria-carrying *Anopheles* mosquitoes, which are nocturnal and are less populous near urban areas. Once a rare disease in the United States, dengue fever began to reappear in the 1970s, when bans on pesticides such as DDT allowed these mosquitoes to thrive. The same vector can also carry yellow fever and chikungunya.

Which microorganism causes this condition?

Dengue fever is a disease caused by a positive, single-stranded RNA virus of the *Flaviviridae* family. This family also includes St. Louis encephalitis virus, Japanese encephalitis virus, hepatitis C virus, and West Nile virus.

How does this condition differ from yellow fever?

Yellow fever virus is also a member of the *Flaviviridae* family and has a similar endemic region and transmission as dengue fever virus. However, yellow fever presents with high fever, black vomit, and jaundice and is not associated with severe joint and muscle pain.

After recovering from this condition, will the patient be immune to it in the future?

The dengue fever virus has four serotypes. The patient will develop lasting immunity to the serotype of the virus with which she was infected but not to the remaining three serotypes. This means that she could contract dengue fever four times in all.

Infection with a different serotype of this virus poses what potential complications?

The most serious complications of dengue fever are dengue hemorrhagic fever (DHF) and dengue shock syndrome (DSS), both of which can be fatal. These conditions are characterized by bleeding (often from the gastrointestinal tract or from mucosa); petechiae, ecchymoses, or purpura; thrombocytopenia; fluid leakage (manifested as pleural effusions, ascites, or hemoconcentration); and shock. Such complications most frequently occur in patients who have already been infected with another serotype of the virus. One theory underlying this phenomenon, termed **antibody-dependent enhancement,** proposes that antibodies from previous infections actually allow for increased viral replication upon reinfection with a different serotype. This has also hindered the development of a vaccine, since the vaccine must provide adequate protection against all four serotypes or it could put the patient at risk for DHF/DSS.

■ CASE 18

A 7-year-old girl who recently immigrated to the United States from Africa is brought to her primary care physician because of a sore throat and fever of 38.3°C (101°F). Physical examination reveals a grayish membrane covering her pharynx (Figure 3-14) as well as cervical lymphadenopathy.

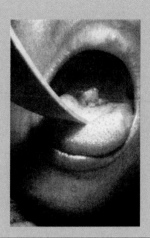

FIGURE 3-14. (Reproduced, with permission, from Connor DH, Chandler FW, Schwartz DQA, Manz HJ, Lack EE (eds). *Pathology of Infectious Diseases*, vol. 1. Stamford, CT: Appleton & Lange, 1997.)

What is the most likely diagnosis?

The child most likely has diphtheria caused by the toxin-producing, gram-positive *Corynebacterium diphtheriae*. The pathognomonic findings are the gray pharyngeal pseudomembranes on physical exam.

What should not be done when gray pseudomembranes are seen during physical examination?

Pseudomembranous lesions should never be scraped. Scraping the lesion can release the toxin, increasing the chance of serious cardiac sequelae.

How does the microorganism involved in this condition cause this presentation?

Exotoxin A is an enzyme that blocks protein synthesis by inactivating elongation factor EF-2 by ribosylating adenosine phosphate. This results in decreased mRNA translation and protein synthesis. (*Pseudomonas* toxin has a similar mechanism.)

What growth media are used to identify the microorganism involved in this condition?

Potassium tellurite agar and Loeffler coagulated blood serum media are used to isolate this microorganism. *C diphtheriae* is a gram-positive rod. In culture, it often appears in clumps described as **"Chinese characters."**

Which vaccine would have prevented this child's condition?

The inactivated form, or toxoid, is a component of the **D**iphtheria, **T**etanus, and **a**cellular **P**ertussis (DTaP) vaccine. Children in the United States are required to have the DTaP vaccine by the age of 15–18 months, with a booster shot given between 4 and 6 years of age. Recent immigrants, especially children, frequently do not have up-to-date vaccinations.

What is the appropriate treatment for this condition?

Antitoxin can inactivate circulating toxin that has not yet reached its target tissue. Penicillin or erythromycin can be given to prevent further bacterial growth and exotoxin release, thus making the patient noncontagious. The patient should receive cardiac monitoring with ECG and telemetry to monitor for myocarditis. The patient likewise needs treatment for heart failure or arrhythmia, monitoring of neurologic function for motor deficits, and supportive care to ensure a secure airway and to avoid aspiration pneumonia.

■ CASE 19

A 32-year-old man presents to his physician with extreme swelling of his legs (Figure 3-15) and scrotum. The skin associated with the swollen areas is thick and scaly. The patient admits to an episode of fever associated with enlarged inguinal lymph nodes some time ago, but he did not think much of it. His travel history is significant for spending 9 months in the tropics approximately 2 years before this presentation.

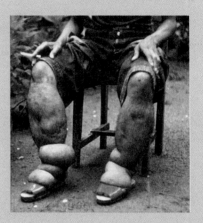

FIGURE 3-15. (Courtesy of Centers for Disease Control and Prevention. Public Health Image Library.)

What is the most likely diagnosis?

Elephantiasis is caused by the nematode (roundworm) *Wuchereria bancrofti*.

How does the organism involved in this condition cause illness?

The organism is transmitted by the bite of a female mosquito. Larvae are released into the bloodstream and travel to the lymphatics of the lower extremities and genitals, where they mature. Approximately 1 year later, adult worms, which reside in lymph nodes, trigger an inflammatory response.

What signs and symptoms are associated with this condition?

Inflammation resulting from the presence of adult worms causes **fever** and **swelling of lymph nodes.** Repeated infections cause repeated bouts of inflammation, resulting in **fibrosis** around the dead adult worms in the lymph nodes. This fibrosis can **obstruct lymphatic drainage** and lead to edema and scaly skin.

What test can help confirm the diagnosis?

Blood smears reveal larvae (**microfilariae**). Because larvae usually emerge at night, drawing blood in the evening is preferred.

What is the appropriate treatment for this condition?

Diethylcarbamazine is effective in killing the larvae but is not as effective against the adult worms. Efficacy of targeted therapy against adult worms is still unclear as there may be an increased risk of scarring with worsening lymphedema caused by host inflammatory response to dying adult worms.

■ CASE 20

A previously healthy 24-year-old man visits his physician complaining of significant weight loss, flatulence, and foul-smelling stools. He reports feeling fatigued since his return from Peru 3 months previously and has suffered abdominal cramping and intermittent loose, nonbloody stools since then. The patient's stool ova and parasite studies demonstrated characteristic trophozoites on two occasions (Figure 3-16). He was prescribed a course of drug therapy and warned that consumption of alcohol during treatment could lead to nausea and vomiting.

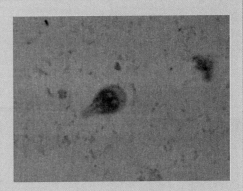

FIGURE 3-16. (Reproduced, with permission, from Le T, et al. *First Aid for the USMLE Step 1: 2011*. New York: McGraw-Hill, 2011: Color Image 5.)

What is the most likely diagnosis?

Giardiasis due to *Giardia lamblia* infection. *Giardia* appears as both a flagellated, motile, denucleated trophozoite and as a round cyst. Flatulence, foul-smelling stools, and chronic watery diarrhea in a patient with a recent travel history or exposure to well water is characteristic of *Giardia* infection. The ova and parasite test that reveals "smiley face" trophozoites are diagnostic.

What is the differential diagnosis for this patient's condition?

Entamoeba histolytica can cause a similar spectrum of symptoms but would present with bloody diarrhea instead of watery diarrhea. Infections with enterotoxigenic *Escherichia coli*, *Vibrio cholerae*, and *Campylobacter jejuni* can also cause watery diarrhea, but the onset in these cases is generally acute and will resolve within a few days.

What is the appropriate treatment for this condition?

Metronidazole is the agent used to treat giardiasis. Concurrent alcohol use with metronidazole produces a "disulfiram-like effect" (disulfiram is prescribed to discourage alcohol consumption in situations of alcohol addiction). Metronidazole interferes with the action of aldehyde dehydrogenase in ethanol metabolism, which increases serum acetaldehyde levels and thus leads to nausea, vomiting, flushing, thirst, palpitations, vertigo, and chest pain.

What is the mechanism of action of the medication used to treat this condition?

Metronidazole is effective specifically against anaerobic microorganisms. It diffuses across the cell membrane of microorganisms and is reduced in the mitochondria of obligate anaerobes to cytotoxic intermediates. These intermediates cause DNA strand breakage and generate free radicals that consequently damage the cell. Furthermore, the reduction of metronidazole creates a concentration gradient that leads to further uptake of the drug.

What are other uses of this medication?

Metronidazole is used to treat *Clostridium difficile* (anaerobe) infection in pseudomembranous colitis, amebic dysentery, bacterial vaginitis, and *Trichomonas* vaginitis and as a component of triple therapy for *Helicobacter pylori* eradication. Broadly, it is effective against most anaerobic bacteria and various protozoa.

■ CASE 21

A 23-year-old sexually active woman presents to her physician because of a painful left knee and pain with urination. Physical examination reveals a swollen, tender, erythematous left knee with decreased range of motion. Examination of her skin reveals small papules with an erythematous base on her arms. Pelvic examination is notable for purulent endocervical discharge (Figure 3-17).

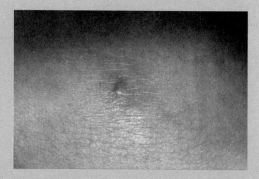

FIGURE 3-17. (Reproduced, with permission, from Tintinalli JE, et al. *Tintinalli's Emergency Medicine: A Comprehensive Study Guide*, 6th ed. New York: McGraw-Hill, 2004: 1518.)

What is the likely causative organism of this condition?

Neisseria gonorrhoeae through sexual contact with an infected partner. The vaginal infection can cause discharge and dysuria. If the bacteria disseminate, skin lesions, tenosynovitis, or septic arthritis can develop. Septic arthritis is a serious condition that must be treated aggressively to prevent permanent damage to the joint.

How are septic arthritis, reactive arthritis, rheumatoid arthritis, and osteoarthritis differentiated?

Synovial fluid WBC count is the best way to differentiate between the various types of arthritis. Osteoarthritis is the most benign and is considered a noninflammatory arthritis. The synovial fluid WBC count in osteoarthritis is < 2000 cells/mm^3.

Reactive arthritis (most commonly associated with *Chlamydia* infection leading to the classic triad of uveitis, urethritis, and arthritis) and rheumatoid arthritis are both types of inflammatory arthritis. The synovial fluid WBC count in these conditions is 2000–75,000 cells/mm^3.

Septic arthritis, which this patient has, presents with a synovial fluid WBC count of > 100,000 cells/mm^3, and Gram stain/culture of the fluid yields the causative organism.

In this patient, what is Gram stain of a cervical swab likely to show?

Gram-negative kidney-shaped cocci in pairs. However, the endocervical Gram stain is insensitive and nonspecific and is best diagnosed by nucleic acid testing.

What antibiotic is recommended for treatment of this condition?

Ceftriaxone is a first-line treatment for gonococcal infections, particularly if disseminated. Patients with gonorrhea have a high risk of coinfection with *Chlamydia trachomatis*. Therefore, patients are also empirically treated for *Chlamydia* with doxycycline or azithromycin.

If not treated early, what is a serious potential gynecologic complication of this condition?

If the infection persists, it can develop into pelvic inflammatory disease. The bacteria can ascend to the uterus, fallopian tubes, and ovaries, which can cause endometritis, salpingitis, oophoritis, and tubo-ovarian abscesses. The infection and subsequent scarring can reduce the patient's fertility, as oocytes are unable to travel through the scarred uterine tubes. In addition, untreated infection increases the risk of ectopic tubular pregnancy. In advanced stages, fibrotic adhesions between the fallopian tubes, uterus, and liver can occur in a condition is known as Fitz-Hugh–Curtis syndrome.

■ CASE 22

A 22-year-old woman presents to the emergency department in labor. This is her first pregnancy, and she has received no prenatal care. In the emergency department she has a normal spontaneous vaginal delivery of a boy. The baby appears normal at birth, but 12 hours later he begins to show signs of lethargy. He becomes tachypneic, his blood pressure drops, and his hands and feet begin to feel cold.

What infectious agents are most frequently responsible for neonatal sepsis?

Group B streptococci (GBS), *Escherichia coli,* and *Listeria monocytogenes* are common causes of sepsis, pneumonia, and meningitis in newborns. GBS often colonizes the vaginal flora of women and can be transmitted vertically during vaginal delivery. This patient's lack of prenatal care, primiparous vaginal delivery, and onset soon after birth make GBS sepsis a likely diagnosis.

What is the next step in identifying the causative agent?

In **Gram staining** of a blood sample, GBS appear as gram-positive cocci, *L monocytogenes* appears as motile gram-positive rods, and *E coli* appears as gram-negative rods.

How did the infant become infected?

These bacteria can spread through the placenta or be acquired from the birth canal during delivery. The mother may be infected or colonized but asymptomatic. However, pregnant and postpartum women are also at risk for GBS urinary tract infection or chorioamnionitis.

What prenatal testing is routinely performed to reduce the infant's risk of this infection in the birth canal?

If the patient receives good prenatal care, cultures of the mother's vagina and rectum are performed between 35 and 37 weeks of gestation to determine whether she is colonized with GBS.

What treatment is initiated if prenatal testing is positive?

Treatment of GBS in infected mothers or newborns involves the use of antepartum antibiotics such as penicillin. In mothers who are colonized vaginally or rectally, but who are not actively infected, intrapartum penicillin is recommended.

If the baby develops meningitis from this organism, what cerebrospinal fluid findings are expected?

In bacterial meningitis, the cerebrospinal fluid may show bacteria on Gram stain. In addition, the WBC count is elevated, primarily with neutrophils; the protein level is elevated; and the glucose level is reduced.

▪ CASE 23

A 3-year-old boy is brought to the pediatrician by his mother. The mother states that 2 days ago the child started refusing solid foods, preferring his bottle and applesauce. Today, the mother noticed a rash on her son's extremities and tongue (Figure 3-18), and found that he was also running a low-grade fever, which prompted her to bring him to the doctor.

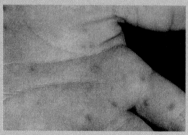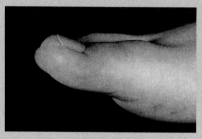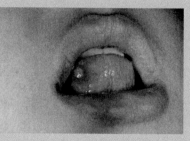

FIGURE 3-18. (Reproduced, with permission, from Shah BR, Lucchesi M. *Atlas of Pediatric Emergency Medicine.* New York: McGraw-Hill, 2006: Figure 3-65.)

What is the most likely diagnosis?

This is a case of hand-foot-mouth disease, caused by **coxsackie A virus.** This syndrome presents with a tender rash on the palms, soles, and often the buttocks and painful vesicles on the oral mucosa. This patient's avoidance of solid food strongly suggests involvement of the oral mucosa.

What other microorganisms are included in this family that caused this condition?

The *Picornaviridae* are a family of **single-stranded positive-sense RNA viruses.** The members of this family cause a wide array of illness, possibly because of the high virulence of positive-sense single-stranded RNA, which can be directly translated into protein products by host ribosomes. Members of the *Picornaviridae* family include:

- Poliovirus
- Echovirus
- Hepatitis A virus
- Coxsackie viruses
- Rhinovirus

What other conditions can this microorganism cause?

Herpangina, which presents with sore throat, red vesicles on the back of the throat, pain with swallowing, and fever. Herpangina is a mild, self-limited disease that presents in children and usually results in complete recovery. Less commonly, coxsackie A virus can cause petechial and purpuric rashes, which may also have a hemorrhagic component.

What illnesses may be caused by the group B coxsackie viruses?

The coxsackie B virus may cause aseptic meningitis, myocarditis, pericarditis, dilated cardiomyopathy, orchitis, and epidemic pleurodynia (fever, headache, spasms of the chest wall muscles, and pleuritic pain). Nephritic syndrome may also occur after a coxsackie B virus infection.

What other infections commonly presents with a rash of the palms and soles?

Other than Coxsackie **A** virus, **R**ocky mountain spotted fever caused by *Rickettsia rickettsii* and secondary **S**yphilis commonly present with a rash on the palms and soles (mnemonic: **CARS**).

■ CASE 24

An 18-year-old woman presents to clinic with a fever and headache. She also complains of vaginal itching and dysuria. When asked, she says that she recently became sexually active. Physical examination reveals tender inguinal lymphadenopathy and red, pustular, painful vesicles on her labia majora (Figure 3-19).

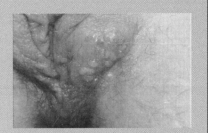

FIGURE 3-19. (Reproduced, with permission, from Klausner JD, Hook EW III. *Current Diagnosis & Treatment of Sexually Transmitted Diseases.* New York: McGraw-Hill, 2007: 86.)

What is the most likely diagnosis?

Herpes simplex virus type 2 (HSV-2). The pathognomonic findings for herpes infections are painful vesicles. Both HSV-1 and HSV-2 can cause genital herpes, but more than 80% of genital lesions are due to HSV-2.

What are the characteristics of this pathogen?

HSV-2 is a member of the Herpesviridae family, which are double-stranded DNA viruses and include: HSV-1, varicella-zoster virus (VZV), Epstein-Barr virus (EBV), cytomegalovirus, human herpesvirus-6, and human herpesvirus-8. They can be recognized by multinucleated giant cells on Tzanck smear and by eosinophilic intranuclear inclusions.

What is the differential diagnosis of painful genital lesions?

Chancroid caused by *Haemophilus ducreyi* infection. Lymphogranuloma venereum caused by *Chlamydia trachomatis* and granuloma inguinale caused by *Klebsiella granulomatis* also cause painful genital lesion.

What is the typical course of this infection?

HSV-2 is transmitted by direct contact of the virus with mucosal surfaces or open skin surfaces. It can also be transmitted from mother to newborn during delivery. Approximately 80% of infected patients are asymptomatic. The primary infection often presents with constitutional symptoms such as fever, headache, malaise, and myalgia. Later, genital vesicles may appear that can rupture and leave behind painful ulcers. Other genital symptoms include itching and tender inguinal lymphadenopathy. Like other viruses in the family, HSV-2 becomes latent and can be reactivated. Triggers for reactivation include fever, trauma, emotional stress, sunlight, and menstruation. Upon reactivation, there is often a viral prodrome that involves tenderness, pain, and burning at the future site of vesicle eruption. The lesions last 4–15 days before crusting over and reepithelializing.

Where do herpesvirus species remain latent?

In the peripheral nervous system ganglia. HSV-1 tends to remain latent in the trigeminal ganglion, reactivating and causing oral herpes or "cold sores." HSV-2 and VZV tend to remain latent in the dorsal root ganglia of the sensory afferents. This gives rise to the pathognomonic dermatomal distribution of reactivated zoster infections.

What is the treatment for this condition?

The treatment for HSV-2 is acyclovir, a nucleoside analog that acts by inhibiting viral DNA polymerase when it is phosphorylated by viral thymidine kinase. However, because efficacy requires viral thymidine kinase activity, any herpesvirus lacking a functional thymidine kinase will be resistant.

■ CASE 25

A 9-year-old girl is brought to a public clinic by her mother. The family immigrated to the United States from Guatemala 3 years previously. Her mother reports the girl seems very small for her age and has been continually lethargic for quite some time. Physical examination reveals a small girl with a thin, scaphoid abdomen. Relevant laboratory findings are as follows:

Hematocrit: 36%
Mean corpuscular volume: 73 fL
WBC count: 11,000/mm³
Differential: 35% segmented cells, 1% bands, 33% lymphocytes, 21% eosinophils

What is the most likely diagnosis?

Hookworm, or nematode, infection. The findings of eosinophilia and microcytic anemia with recent immigration from an endemic area are highly suggestive of this condition.

What is the next step in confirming the diagnosis?

Stool ova and parasite tests can confirm the presence of characteristic small, round eggs and occasional worms approximately 1 cm in size. Stool ova and parasite tests can also be used to delineate the species of helminth.

What are the species of hookworms?

Ancylostoma duodenale, Necator americanus, and *Ancylostoma braziliense* are the most common hookworms. Of the three, *A duodenale* and *N americanus* cause the classic gastrointestinal symptoms and microcytic anemia seen in this patient. *A braziliense,* however, can manifest as a condition known as cutaneous larva migrans, in which the larva migrate to the subcutaneous tissue and create pruritic, serpiginous tracts underneath the skin.

What other helminth is known to cause anemia?

Diphyllobothrium latum, a tapeworm, causes vitamin B_{12} deficiency leading to a macrocytic anemia.

How does this infection cause disease in humans?

Percutaneous infection occurs generally through the soles of the feet and is acquired commonly from sandboxes. The larvae pass into the lungs, and 8–21 days later they cross the pulmonary vasculature and enter the airways. They ascend to the pharynx and are swallowed. By the time they reach the small intestine, the larvae have become adult worms. The adults "hook" onto the mucosa and feed on the host's blood with the help of an orally secreted factor X inhibitor. This results in the microcytic anemia. The females produce eggs that are passed through the stool and deposited in the soil.

What are the appropriate treatments for this condition?

Since hookworm is a helminthic infection, mebendazole and albendazole are the first-line agents. These agents disrupt helminthic microtubule synthesis, leading to structural weakening and death of helminthic cells. Pyrantel pamoate can be used as a second-line agent.

■ CASE 26

A 46-year-old woman visits her physician complaining of "feeling poorly," with fever, chills, muscle aches, dry cough, and sore throat. She has had these symptoms for several days with no significant improvement. She works as a secretary and says these symptoms have been "going around the office." Physical examination reveals small, tender cervical lymphadenopathy, swollen nasal mucosa, and an erythematous pharynx.

What is the most likely diagnosis?

Infection with influenza virus.

What are the defining structural features of this class of microorganisms?

Orthomyxoviruses are helical, enveloped, negative, single-stranded RNA viruses. Their primary virulence factors are hemagglutinin and neuraminidase. Hemagglutinin aids in the viral entry into host cells whereas neuraminidase aids in progeny release from infected host cells. The isotypes of these two proteins determine the virulence of each particular strain of virus and are the targets of the influenza vaccine.

The patient has had a similar infection in the past. Why is her immune system not protecting her from this illness?

The isotype of hemagglutinin and neuraminidase is constantly changing because of a phenomenon known as **antigenic drift.** This is the result of random small mutations that cause changes in the antigenic structure of the virus. These mutations result in antigen structures that are only partially recognized by the host immune system.

What characteristic of this microorganism's genome makes deadly epidemics possible?

Influenza A virus infects diverse species including birds, horses, and swine; by contrast, influenza B and influenza C infect only humans. With its segmented genome, influenza A can swap segments of RNA between animal and human strains (a process known as reassortment), leading to new human strains with novel surface antigens not recognized by the immune system. This type of change is termed **antigenic shift** and was responsible for the "swine flu" or hemagglutinin isotype 1 and neuraminidase isotype 1 (H1N1) influenza A virus outbreak in 2009.

What pharmacologic agents can be used as prophylaxis against this infection?

Amantadine and rimantadine block viral penetration by inhibiting the M2 protein responsible for uncoating and can be used to treat influenza A infection. However, these drugs are rarely used anymore because of the high levels of resistance that have developed against them. Instead, zanamivir and oseltamivir (neuraminidase inhibitors) are used to treat both influenza A and influenza B infections. These agents are most effective if started within 48 hours of symptom onset. The influenza vaccine should be given in October or November, before the start of flu season. It takes approximately 2 weeks for the body to make antibodies to the viruses. The vaccine generally has four strains; the Centers for Disease Control and Prevention determine which among them is likely to be the most infectious each season. The new "swine flu" H1N1 strain was included in the 2010 influenza vaccine.

■ CASE 27

A 25-year-old man is brought to the emergency department by ambulance after a motor vehicle collision. He is lucid but has severe bleeding from his leg. His wife is with him and reports that the patient is generally healthy, although he had several bouts of "lung and ear infections" as a child. He also has a history of milk allergy and periodically suffers from diarrhea. In the emergency department he is given 1 unit of type-matched RBCs. Soon afterward he develops a red, itchy rash over most of his body (Figure 3-20) and begins to have difficulty breathing. His blood pressure drops despite continuous fluid infusion.

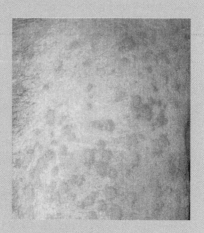

FIGURE 3-20. (Reproduced, with permission, from Kasper DL, et al. *Harrison's Principles of Internal Medicine*, 16th ed. New York: McGraw-Hill, 2005: 287.)

What is the likely cause of this patient's repeated infections and allergic reaction to the blood transfusion?

This patient is having an anaphylactic reaction. IgA is a common component in blood products. This patient likely has hereditary IgA deficiency, and therefore has developed IgG antibodies against IgA. He is particularly susceptible to gastrointestinal infections, especially giardiasis, for which secretory IgA plays an important protective role. IgA deficiency can occur as an isolated syndrome or may involve concurrent IgG deficiency, which increases the risk of sinopulmonary infections.

What is the next step in management of this condition?

Because of the patient's severe anaphylactic reaction to the transfused blood products, it is imperative to discontinue transfusion and administer epinephrine injection. Epinephrine counteracts the bronchospasm and vasodilation that is causing his respiratory difficulty and decreasing blood pressure.

What is the cause of the patient's milk allergy?

In the absence of intestinal IgA, large proteins are more likely to enter the bloodstream whole. An IgG antibody reaction to these proteins can then cause an allergic reaction. (This is different from lactose intolerance, which is not a true allergy and involves a deficiency of lactase.) For the same reasons, patients with IgA deficiency are at increased risk of developing antibodies against wheat proteins and thus celiac disease.

What are the stages in B-cell development that lead up to IgA secretion?

Pluripotent stem cells first differentiate into lymphoid stem cells, then to pro-B cells, then to pre-B cells. Pre-B cells contain the IgM (mu) heavy chains intracellularly but no surface IgM. The next step is formation of immature or naive B cells that express surface IgM. After stimulation by antigen, the immature cells can mature into IgM-secreting cells or, with CD4+ T-cell stimulation (CD40 ligand—CD40 receptor activation), can class switch to express IgG, IgA, or IgE antibodies. After class switching, the cells can undergo affinity maturation to select for antibodies with higher binding affinities for the antigen and subsequently form plasma cells that secrete the specialized antibodies.

■ CASE 28

A 43-year-old man with HIV infection presents to the HIV clinic with multiple purple-red plaques and papules distributed across his skin (Figure 3-21). The patient says he feels fine and denies fever, chills, malaise, or headache. A complete blood count reveals his CD4+ cell count is 180 cells/mm³.

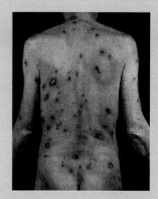

FIGURE 3-21. (Reproduced, with permission, from Wolff K, Goldsmith LA, Katz SI, Gilchrest BA, Paller AS, Leffell DJ. *Fitzpatrick's Dermatology in General Medicine*, 7th ed. New York: McGraw-Hill, 2008: Figure 128-3.)

What is the most likely diagnosis?

This is Kaposi sarcoma, an angiogenic neoplasm prevalent in HIV-positive patients. Kaposi sarcoma is caused by **human herpesvirus-8** (HHV-8), a member of the Herpesviridae family. Members of this family are DNA viruses with a double-stranded, linear genome in an enveloped, icosahedral capsid.

What important alternative diagnosis must be ruled out?

An important alternative diagnosis for such skin lesions in HIV patients is bacillary angiomatosis (BA), which typically presents with systemic symptoms such as fever, chills, and malaise. However, because BA is caused by *Bartonella henselae* it is nonneoplastic and can readily be treated with antibiotics.

How does the microorganism cause the characteristic discolored skin lesions?

HHV-8 has a tropism for endothelium cells and is thought to induce vascular endothelial growth factor, which causes irregular vascular channels to develop in the skin. RBCs extravasate into these spaces, causing the characteristic purple-red skin lesions as seen in Figure 3-21.

What other diseases are associated with this microorganism?

Kaposi sarcoma is not limited to the skin; the gastrointestinal tract, oral mucosa, lungs, lymph nodes, and other visceral organs may be infected. HHV-8 also infects B lymphocytes and has been linked to **body-cavity B-cell lymphoma** (a non-Hodgkin lymphoma subtype) and to **Castleman disease** (a lymphoproliferative disorder that may progress to lymphoma).

What other patient population is at increased risk for developing this infection?

Transplantation patients, who, like patients with HIV, are chronically immunosuppressed, have a higher incidence of infection than the general public.

What are the appropriate treatments for this condition?

Daunorubicin or doxorubicin is the treatment of choice. Both cause DNA breaks by two mechanisms: (1) intercalating into the DNA double helix, and (2) creating oxygen free radicals that damage DNA. A major adverse effect of their use, however, is cardiotoxicity. In HIV-positive patients, the first goal is to boost immunity by starting highly active antiretroviral therapy, which often leads to improvement of the disease.

What other preventive health measures should be taken in this patient since his CD4+ cell count is < 200 cells/mm³?

The patient should be started on trimethoprim-sulfamethoxazole therapy for *Pneumocystis jiroveci* pneumonia and toxoplasmosis prophylaxis.

■ CASE 29

A 17-year-old boy who recently immigrated to the United States from India presents to the emergency department with complaints of spiking fevers, weight loss, and lethargy. On examination he is cachectic with a gray skin tone, and he is found to have pronounced splenomegaly and mild hepatomegaly. Laboratory tests reveal pancytopenia. Microscopic examination of a bone marrow aspirate reveals parasites in the histiocytes.

What is the most likely diagnosis?

This patient is suffering from kala azar, or visceral leishmaniasis. Visceral leishmaniasis is caused by the protozoan *Leishmania donovani* and is characterized by spiking fevers, hepatosplenomegaly, and pancytopenia.

Is the organism found in the amastigote or promastigote form in the infected human?

The form found in the **human host** is the **amastigote,** which is small and round and has a flagellum that is difficult to visualize. The prominently flagellated form of the parasite is found in the **insect vector** and is known as the **promastigote.**

What is the vector of this pathogen?

Humans are infected with *Leishmania donovani* through the bite of a sandfly. It can also be transmitted by intravenous drug use or blood transfusion.

On the blood smear, some macrophages contain basophilic inclusions. What are these inclusions?

These inclusions are called Donovan bodies and consist of the amastigote form of the parasite.

What is the appropriate treatment for this condition?

Treatment is sodium stibogluconate or pentamidine.

What diseases are caused by other blood-borne flagellates?

Trypanosomes are another flagellated parasite that can be found in the blood. *Trypanosoma cruzi* is transmitted by the reduviid bug and is found in South America and causes Chagas disease. *T gambiense* and *T rhodesiense* are transmitted by the tsetse fly and are the cause of African sleeping sickness.

◼ CASE 30

A 64-year-old man with a past history of smoking and well-controlled diabetes mellitus presents to the emergency department with a 3-day history of low-grade fevers, mild diarrhea, and nonproductive cough. He works as a maintenance worker in a local apartment complex. Workup includes a Gram stain of sputum, which shows prominent polymorphonuclear leukocytes but no microorganisms. X-ray of the chest reveals diffuse, patchy bilateral infiltrates (Figure 3-22). Relevant laboratory findings are as follows:

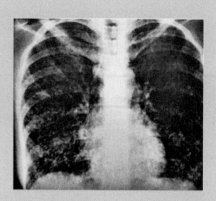

FIGURE 3-22. (Reproduced, with permission, from Le T, et al. *First Aid for the USMLE Step 1: 2008.* New York: McGraw-Hill, 2008: Image 126A.)

Hemoglobin: 14 g/mL
Sodium: 128 mEq/L
Hematocrit: 40%
Chloride: 100 mEq/L
Platelets: 200,000/mm³
Potassium: 4.2 mEq/L
WBC count: 15,000/mm³
Bicarbonate: 17 mEq/L

Blood urea nitrogen:
    16 mg/dL
Glucose: 110 mg/dL
Creatinine: 1.2 mg/dL
Urinalysis: 2+ proteinuria;
    no glucose, ketones, or
    blood

What is the most likely diagnosis?

Legionnaire's disease, an infection caused by the gram-negative rod *Legionella pneumophila*. Any patient presenting with diarrhea and pneumonia-like symptoms has *Legionella* until proven otherwise. This patient has evidence of interstitial, or atypical, pneumonia, which makes the diagnosis even more likely.

What is the differential diagnosis for atypical pneumonia?

The common differential diagnosis for atypical pneumonia is first and foremost viral infection, followed by *Chlamydia*, *Mycoplasma*, or *Legionella* infection.

What test can help confirm the diagnosis?

Urinary *Legionella* antigen test can establish the diagnosis. *Legionella* is unique in that it is the only form of community-acquired pneumonia that can be diagnosed with a urine test.

What risk factors does the patient have for developing this condition?

The patient's history of diabetes and smoking predisposes him to *Legionella* infection. Given his occupation as a maintenance man, he likely works with air conditioning systems. As this microorganism grows in infected water sources, the patient's occupation places him at risk.

What are the appropriate treatments for this condition?

Legionella responds best to antibiotics that can achieve a high intracellular concentration, such as macrolides (eg, erythromycin, clarithromycin, and azithromycin) and tetracyclines. *Legionella* produces β-lactamase, so cephalosporins and penicillins are ineffective.

■ CASE 31

A 41-year-old woman who is a recent immigrant from Mexico presents to a local clinic complaining of "white spots" on her body. She says she first noticed the lesions about 1 month ago and thought they were from the sun, but they have gradually increased in number and have not improved despite her new job indoors. Physical examination reveals multiple, asymmetrically distributed, circular, hypopigmented lesions on the patient's arms, abdomen, and back (Figure 3-23). The lesions are sharply demarcated, with raised, erythematous borders and atrophic, scaly centers. The lesions are anesthetic, and there is no hair growth within any of the hypopigmented areas. Biopsy of the lesions demonstrates granuloma formation within the dermal nerves of the forearm.

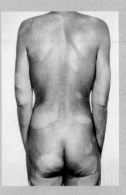

FIGURE 3-23. (Reproduced, with permission, from Wolff K, et al. *Fitzpatrick's Color Atlas & Synopsis of Clinical Dermatology*, 5th ed. New York: McGraw-Hill, 2005: 657.)

Under what conditions does the causative microorganism grow?

Both lepromatous and tuberculoid leprosy are caused by *Mycobacterium leprae,* an acid-fast bacillus that cannot be grown in vitro. *M leprae* is an obligate intracellular bacillus that, like other mycobacteria, contains mycolic acid in its cell wall. *M leprae* grows best in cooler temperatures (eg, skin, peripheral nerves, testes, upper respiratory tract).

How does this patient's condition differ from a more severe form?

This patient has tuberculoid leprosy, which is largely confined to the skin (hypopigmented macules) and peripheral nerves. Cell-mediated immunity is intact, and patients' T cells recognize *M leprae* (positive lepromin skin test). Lepromatous leprosy holds a much worse prognosis because patients have ineffective cell-mediated immunity (negative lepromin skin test). Skin lesions and nerve involvement are much more extensive than in the tuberculoid form, and there may be involvement of the testes, upper respiratory tract, and anterior chamber of the eye.

What is the appropriate treatment for this condition?

Both tuberculoid and lepromatous leprosy can be treated with a course of oral dapsone. The tuberculoid form is reliably cured by a short course of this medication. Patients with lepromatous leprosy have an exceptionally high bacterial load and may require an extended or even lifelong course of chemotherapy. Alternate therapies for leprosy include rifampin or a combination of clofazimine and dapsone.

What are the side effects of treatment?

Dapsone can cause agranulocytosis, so patients should be monitored initially with weekly or biweekly complete blood counts.

Rifampin can turn body fluids such as sweat, tears, and urine a red-orange color. Rifampin therefore can be remembered as the "Gatorade drug," referring to commercials that showed athletes with colored sweat from drinking Gatorade. This can startle patients (and rightly so) if they are not counseled before commencing therapy.

■ CASE 32

The mother of a 1-week-old girl calls her pediatrician because the infant has been fussy all morning. The infant's temperature is 39°C (102.2°F), and the mother is asked to bring the infant to the hospital for further workup and treatment. The workup includes cerebrospinal fluid (CSF) analysis, hematology studies, and cultures. Empiric antibiotic therapy is initiated. Later, upon microscopic examination of the CSF, microorganisms with tumbling end-over-end motility are visualized.

What is the most likely diagnosis?

Meningitis due to *Listeria monocytogenes* infection. This microorganism, identifiable by its classical tumbling motility, is a gram-positive rod and a common cause of meningitis in newborns and the elderly (Table 3-2).

TABLE 3-2	Age Group Preference of Most Common Infectious Agents Causing Meningitis			
ORGANISM	NEWBORN	INFANT/CHILD	TEEN/ADULT	ELDERLY
Streptococcus pneumoniae		X	X	X
Neisseria meningitidis		X	X	
Enterovirus		X	X	
Escherichia coli (gram-negative rod)	X			X
Listeria	X			X
Group B streptococcus	X			

How is the pathogen in this condition transmitted?

L monocytogenes is transmitted through ingestion of unpasteurized dairy products such as milk, cheese, and ice cream.

What microorganisms should empiric antibiotic therapy target?

Group B streptococcus, *Escherichia coli,* and *L monocytogenes* are the most common causes of sepsis and bacterial meningitis in infants younger than 1 month of age. Therefore, empiric therapy should be aminopenicillin or vancomycin for gram-positive infection and aminoglycosides, antipseudomonal penicillins, or third- or fourth-generation cephalosporins for gram-negative infection.

How does this microorganism evade the host immune response?

L monocytogenes is a facultative intracellular bacterium able to survive in the macrophages of neonates and immunosuppressed patients. In an immunocompetent host, activation of macrophages destroys phagocytosed *Listeria*.

What other population is at particular risk for developing the same infection?

Pregnant patients are at increased risk of developing a serious illness from *Listeria* known as granulomatosis infantiseptica. It can cause various complications to the mother and baby from premature rupture of membranes and intrauterine fetal demise. The elderly and immunocompromised are also at increased risk for this infection.

CASE 33

A 30-year-old woman presents to clinic with abdominal pain, a low-grade fever, and a sensation of abdominal fullness. She says the symptoms have been going on for some time and have been gradually worsening. On physical examination she appears jaundiced with notable scleral icterus. She says she is originally from South America. X-ray of the abdomen is shown in Figure 3-24.

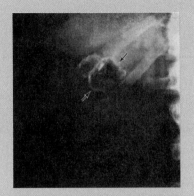

FIGURE 3-24. (Reproduced, with permission, from Tanagho EA, McAninch JW. *Smith's General Urology*, 17th ed. New York: McGraw-Hill, 2008: Fig 14-5.)

What is the most likely diagnosis?

The patient most likely has a hydatid cyst, which is a liver cyst due to *Echinococcus* infection.

How is this infection transmitted?

Echinococcus is a tapeworm that is transmitted by food or water contaminated with feces containing eggs from the tapeworm. Infection is not endemic to the United States and so is most commonly seen in immigrants or those with a travel history to endemic areas.

What is the typical presentation of this infection?

Echinococcus causes slow-growing cysts in the liver. As a result, symptoms are often gradual in onset and include abdominal pain, cough, low-grade fever, a sense of abdominal fullness, hepatomegaly, and obstructive jaundice. Leakage of cysts can cause flushing and urticaria, whereas rupture can cause anaphylaxis and death. Other organs that can be involved include the lungs and the brain. In the lungs, the presentation includes chronic cough, dyspnea, hemoptysis, and pleuritic chest pain. In the brain, presentation includes headache, dizziness, increased intracranial pressure, and hydrocephalus.

How is this condition diagnosed?

On x-ray of the abdomen, a rim of calcification around the cyst is able to distinguish hydatid cyst from amebic and pyogenic cysts. However, the diagnosis usually cannot be made with radiology alone and requires an enzyme-linked immunosorbent assay (ELISA). In addition, 25% of patients have eosinophilia.

What is the treatment for this condition?

The treatment for *Echinococcus* infection is usually surgical and involves aspiration of cyst contents followed by excision. However, during drainage, the interventional radiologist or surgeon must be careful not to rupture the cyst as this can lead to anaphylaxis. Therefore, many physicians prefer to inject formalin or ethanol into the cyst to kill the organism before aspirating. In some cases, therapy with a combination of albendazole and mebendazole is sufficient.

What other organisms are classified as cestodes?

Diphyllobothrium latum is a cestode transmitted by ingestion from freshwater fish that causes vitamin B_{12}–deficient macrocytic anemia. *D latum* is treated with praziquantel. *Taenia solium* larvae are ingested from undercooked pork and can cause calcified cysts in various organs including the brain (cysticercosis or neurocysticercosis). Cysticercosis is treated with praziquantel, whereas neurocysticercosis is treated with albendazole.

■ CASE 34

While doing a rotation in Ghana, a medical student encounters a patient who has been having nearly continuous high-grade fevers with occasional chills and sweats. Physical examination reveals a palpable spleen. A drop of the patient's blood placed in a copper sulfate solution reveals anemia. Over the next few days, while waiting for medication to arrive, the patient's level of consciousness waxes and wanes, and he is somnolent at times.

What is the most likely diagnosis?

Malaria due to *Plasmodium falciparum.* The symptoms give a clue as to the species. The patient's altered mental status is consistent with a diagnosis of *P falciparum* malaria, since this is the only strain that commonly has cerebral involvement. This patient's continuous fever and irregular chills and sweats are also characteristic of *P falciparum* malaria. Early in infection, irregular fevers are common in all types of malaria, but the fever can become periodic in well-established cases of non-*falciparum* disease. For example, *P vivax* and *P ovale* cause episodes of fever, chills, and sweats every 48 hours. With *P malariae,* these episodes occur every 72 hours. Splenomegaly is a common finding in malaria due to work hypertrophy from increased RBC breakdown.

What phase of the microorganism's life cycle results in the development of anemia?

RBC lysis occurs during the erythrocytic cycle, when the products of asexual replication inside the RBCs (the **merozoite** form) are released. The immune response to the merozoites, and resulting cytokine release, is responsible for the fever, chills, and sweats.

What are the likely peripheral blood smear (PBS) findings?

A PBS is likely to show ring-shaped trophozoites inside the RBCs (see Figure 3-25), and there may be several trophozoites per RBC. **Schizonts**, the large, multinucleated cells formed from the trophozoite by multiple cycles of nuclear division, may be visible in the erythrocytes in non-*falciparum* malaria, but are very rarely seen in *falciparum* disease. Outside the RBCs, oblong **gametocytes**, diagnostic for *P falciparum,* may also be visible.

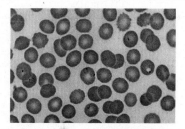

FIGURE 3-25. Malaria, *Plasmodium vivax.* Blood film shows trophozites (ring forms) in red cells. (Reproduced, with permission, from Lichtman MA, et al. *Lichtman's Atlas of Hematology.* New York: McGraw-Hill, 2007: Figure III.A.21.)

What is the treatment of choice for this condition?

Chloroquine is the drug of choice in the few areas where there is no resistance. Its major mode of action against *Plasmodium* is inhibition of the enzyme responsible for polymerizing heme. This results in the accumulation of free heme, which is toxic to the protozoan. Quinidine in combination with doxycycline or pyrimethamine/sulfadoxine is commonly used as first-line treatment for chloroquine-resistant *P falciparum.* Other effective drugs include mefloquine and atovaquone-proguanil.

What conditions provide protection again this condition?

Sickle cell trait and glucose-6-phosphate dehydrogenase (G6PD) deficiency both protect against malaria. The hypothesis is that increased fragility of the erythrocytes in these diseases does not allow for *Plasmodium* species to effectively replicate.

■ CASE 35

A 49-year-old man presents to the emergency department after a syncopal episode. He denies any chronic health problems and states that he stays fit by walking several miles through the local park every day. Physical examination shows bradycardia and a 12-lead ECG is ordered (Figure 3-26). On review of systems, the patient states that he has had low-grade fevers over the past few days and an area of induration in his left groin surrounded by an erythematous ring.

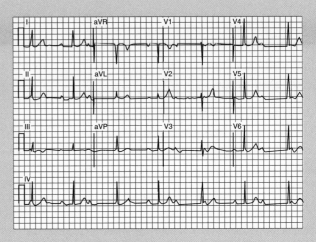

FIGURE 3-26. (Reproduced, with permission, from Fauci AS, et al. *Harrison's Principles of Internal Medicine*, 17th ed. New York: McGraw-Hill, 2008: Figure e21-6).

What is the most likely diagnosis?

Third-degree atrioventricular (AV) block secondary to Lyme disease. This condition is caused by *Borrelia burgdorferi*, a gram-negative spirochete that is poorly grown in culture and too small to be seen under regular light microscopy. Fluorescence may be used to visualize the corkscrew-shaped bacterium. However, the diagnosis is usually made clinically, supported by serology. Early local infection may present with a bull's-eye rash (**erythema chronicum migrans**) after several days. The early disseminated stage may develop as early as a few days later and presents with cardiac conduction abnormalities (Lyme carditis), cranial nerve palsies (especially cranial nerve VII), and meningitis. Up to 43% of patients with Lyme carditis develop complete heart block.

What other conditions can cause this condition?

Damage to the heart's conduction system by fibrosis, ischemia, cardiomyopathy, myocarditis, or iatrogenic damage (eg, after valve replacement) may cause complete heart block. Digitalis, calcium channel blockers, and β-blockers may produce a temporary conduction abnormality.

What is the route of infection?

Lyme disease is an arthropod-borne infection. The *Ixodes* **tick** transmits *B burgdorferi*. Mice and deer are reservoirs for the disease.

What is the prognosis for this patient?

The prognosis is good. The conduction abnormalities secondary to Lyme carditis are self-limited and short lived and often resolve within days to weeks. It is uncommon for residual conduction abnormalities to persist after the infection has been cleared.

What is the appropriate immediate treatment for this patient?

The patient's ECG demonstrates bradycardia at a rate of 40/min. The episode of syncope indicates that cerebral perfusion is inadequate at this heart rate. Consequently, transvenous pacing may be initiated, but a permanent pacemaker is not needed. Antibiotic treatment for Lyme carditis consists of intravenous ceftriaxone until the PR interval is < 300 ms, at which point oral antibiotics may be initiated. The same regimen applies to Lyme disease with neurological features. Doxycycline or amoxicillin is used for primary infection and Lyme arthritis only.

■ CASE 36

A mother brings her 14-year-old son to the pediatrician because the child has been experiencing flulike symptoms and conjunctivitis for the past 3 days. The child is pale and febrile at 39.9°C (102.7°F), and his respiratory rate is 25/min. His buccal mucosa has multiple blue-gray spots, and he has a maculopapular rash (Figure 3-27). His mother states that the rash started on his face but has spread to his torso. The physician notes that the skin lesions blanch with pressure. The mother states that her son is usually healthy and has never needed any medications or vaccinations.

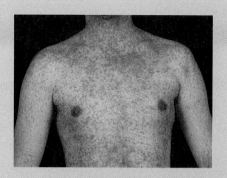

FIGURE 3-27. (Reproduced, with permission, from Wolff K, Johnson RA. *Color Atlas & Synopsis of Clinical Dermatology*, 5th ed. New York: McGraw-Hill, 2005: 788.)

What is the most likely diagnosis?

This child has **measles,** one of the most transmissible viral infections. Measles is caused by an RNA virus that is a member of the genus *Morbillivirus* and the family Paramyxoviridae. Transmission occurs by respiratory droplets and the incubation period is approximately 10 days. Two of this patient's symptoms are typical of measles: **Koplik spots** and **blanching rash** with **cephalocaudal spread.**

What should be considered in the differential diagnosis?

Flulike symptoms may also be caused by infection with rhinoviruses, parainfluenza or influenza, adenovirus, or respiratory syncytial virus. Common causes of rash include *Mycoplasma pneumoniae,* human herpesvirus-6, rubella, Rocky Mountain spotted fever, scarlet fever, or a drug reaction. However, none of these rashes have cephalocaudal spread and none feature Koplik spots.

What are potential neurologic sequelae of this condition?

Approximately 1:1000 patients with measles develop encephalitis, which is rapidly fatal in 15% of cases and leads to permanent neurological damage in 25% of patients. Infection with *Morbillivirus* can trigger acute disseminating encephalomyelitis, an autoimmune attack on the central nervous system, which is lethal in up to 20% of cases. Survivors often suffer mental retardation and epilepsy. Approximately 7–10 years after a measles infection, subacute sclerosing panencephalitis may develop; this infection, although rare, is almost always fatal.

What tests can confirm the diagnosis?

Anti-measles IgM is seen in patient serum approximately 48 hours after the onset of the rash. A mucosal biopsy may demonstrate **Warthin-Finkeldey cells** (multinucleated giant cells with inclusion bodies in the nucleus and cytoplasm).

What is the appropriate treatment for this condition?

There is no treatment for active infection; care is limited to supportive measures. Measles is a reportable disease and the patient must be placed in isolation. If other children in the family have not received the measles-mumps-rubella vaccine, it is likely that they will develop measles as this virus is *highly* transmissible.

■ CASE 37

A 19-year-old college sophomore presents to the university health center with a 7-day history of sore throat, headache, and fatigue. He has a temperature of 37.7°C (99.9°F). Physical examination reveals enlarged, tender cervical lymph nodes in both the anterior and posterior cervical chain. The spleen is found to protrude 5 cm under the costal margin with inspiration. Upon examination of his oropharynx, gray-green tonsillar exudate is noted (Figure 3-28).

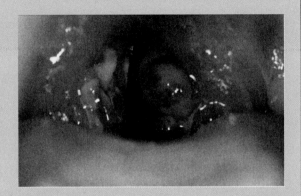

FIGURE 3-28. (Reproduced, with permission, from Knoop KJ, et al. *The Atlas of Emergency Medicine*, 3rd ed. New York: McGraw-Hill, 2010: Figure 5-37. Photo contributor: Lawrence B. Stack, MD.)

What is the most likely diagnosis?

Infectious mononucleosis is most frequently caused by Epstein-Barr virus (EBV), a member of the Herpesviridae family.

What should be considered in the differential diagnosis?

Several diseases present with symptoms similar to mononucleosis. However, streptococcal infection of the oropharynx is usually not associated with splenomegaly, and cytomegalovirus pharyngitis tends to be mild if clinically apparent at all. Low-grade fever, lymphadenopathy, and splenomegaly may also be seen in lymphoma. Lymphoproliferative disorders generally do not present with tonsillar exudate.

What are the peripheral blood smear (PBS) findings?

Infectious mononucleosis leads to lymphocytosis. The WBC count is often elevated (12,000–18,000/mm³) with more than 50% lymphocytes. Up to 10% "atypical" lymphocytes containing large amounts of cytoplasm may be seen. However, these findings may also be seen in other infections (eg, cytomegalovirus, rubella, and toxoplasmosis), in some malignancies, and as a result of drug reactions.

Which malignancies are associated with EBV infection?

Burkitt lymphoma is endemic to Africa and primarily affects children. The disease is a B-cell lymphoma and often presents with a tumor of the jaw. This tumor often has a "starry sky" appearance under light microscope. **Nasopharyngeal carcinoma** is one of the most common cancers in southern China, and evidence supports EBV as its primary causative agent.

What treatments are available for this condition?

Symptomatic treatment, usually with nonsteroidal anti-inflammatory drugs, is usually used. Although EBV might be expected to be susceptible to acyclovir since it is a herpesvirus, studies have shown that acyclovir produces reduction of oral shedding of the virus but no other significant clinical benefit. Ampicillin should be avoided, not just because it is ineffective against viruses but because it can precipitate a rash.

▌CASE 38

A 55-year-old woman presents to the emergency department with confusion and lethargy. On physical examination she is found to be tachypneic and tachycardic, and her breath smells somewhat like nail polish remover. A review of her electronic medical record reveals that she was diagnosed with type 1 diabetes mellitus at 12 years of age. She is admitted to the hospital and treated for diabetic ketoacidosis, and her symptoms begin to improve. However, 4 days after admission she develops fever, mucoid nasal discharge, and periorbital swelling (see Figure 3-29). While cultures are pending, she is treated with empiric antibiotics but fails to improve.

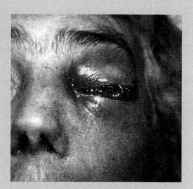

FIGURE 3-29. (Courtesy of the Centers for Disease Control and Prevention's Public Health Image Library.)

What is the most likely diagnosis?

Mucormycosis.

What is the microscopic appearance of the fungus involved in this condition?

The zygomycetes are nonseptate, branching fungi, with wide (> 90-degree) branch angles and large hyphae. By contrast, *Aspergillus* tends to have narrow, septated hyphae and branches in acute angles.

What patient populations are at increased risk for this condition?

The fungus is ubiquitous in nature and spores can be transmitted in air. Most patients are exposed to these spores several times per year, but an intact immune system is usually sufficient protection. Therefore, mucormycosis is typically seen in diabetic patients with poor glucose control or those with ketoacidosis. Neutropenic patients, burn victims, and patients treated with iron-chelating drugs are also at risk.

What is the pathogenesis of this condition?

The fungi grow along blood vessels and invade their walls. Protruding hyphae are highly thrombogenic, resulting in ischemia and necrosis of distal tissues, which, in turn, provide nutrients for continued fungal growth. Necrosis compromises the integrity of the bony walls of the sinuses and the cribriform plate, allowing fungal growth into paranasal sinuses, the bony orbit around the eye, or the brain. This rhinocephalic form of infection is rapidly progressive and carries a high mortality rate. Other forms include pulmonary, gastrointestinal, cutaneous, and disseminated infection.

What is the appropriate management for this condition?

Surgical debridement of infected and necrotic tissue is paramount. Reversal of the permissive condition (in this case ketoacidosis) should be initiated in conjunction with potent antifungal therapy with amphotericin B. However, despite optimal management, this condition still carries a high mortality rate.

■ CASE 39

A 21-year-old man from Guatemala presents to his physician with a 2-day history of painful unilateral testicular swelling. The patient complains of minimal fever and myalgia about a week earlier. Physical examination reveals swollen and painful parotid glands. No vaccination history is available, but the patient does not believe that he received any shots when he was younger.

What is the most likely diagnosis?

Orchitis secondary to mumps. In rare instances, orchitis can affect both testes and lead to sterility.

How is this condition transmitted?

The mumps virus is a member of the Paramyxoviridae family of single-stranded RNA viruses. It is not stable enough to be aerosolized but can be transmitted by droplets (eg, sneeze). The virus has a 2- to 3-week incubation period, after which the infection results in painful inflammation and edema of glandular tissues including the parotid gland, testes, and ovaries.

What other clinical syndrome can result from infection with this microorganism?

If the viral infection spreads to the meninges, **aseptic meningitis** may develop. This can be differentiated from bacterial meningitis by analysis of the cerebrospinal fluid (CSF):

Viral meningitis
CSF protein ~150 mg/dL
Normal CSF glucose
CSF lymphocytes

Bacterial meningitis
CSF protein > 300 mg/dL
Low CSF glucose
CSF neutrophils

Most viral meningitides are self-limited and require only symptomatic treatment. Other common pathogens are coxsackievirus and echovirus. Mumps meningitis is rare in the United States because of vaccination.

How is the underlying condition diagnosed?

For the most part, the diagnosis of mumps can be made clinically. Supportive laboratory values include elevated amylase due to infection in the parotid glands. In uncertain cases, viral polymerase chain reaction assay may also be used.

What is the appropriate treatment for this condition?

The treatment is supportive and directed at reducing pain. Analgesics, compression, and icing of the parotid gland can be useful. In children, aspirin should be avoided as it has been linked to Reye syndrome. Vaccination with live attenuated mumps virus as part of the measles-mumps-rubella vaccine is used to prevent disease.

■ CASE 40

An 18-year-old college freshman is brought to the university health center by his dormitory roommate. The patient complains of 2 days of fever, several episodes of vomiting and joint and muscle pain. His temperature is 38.9°C (102°F). Physical examination reveals a petechial rash on the lower extremities, photophobia; both Kernig and Brudzinski signs are positive.

What is the most likely diagnosis?

This patient likely has *Neisseria meningitidis* meningitis, a gram-negative, kidney-shaped diplococci infection.

What test can confirm the diagnosis?

Culture of meningococcus from cerebrospinal fluid (CSF) or blood. Lumbar puncture shows an elevated WBC count (with mainly polymorphonuclear cells), decreased glucose levels, and normal to high protein levels. Bacteria are visible on Gram stain. This pathogen can also be cultured on Thayer-Martin media (chocolate agar with antibiotics to kill competing bacteria). *N meningitidis* is oxidase positive and ferments both maltose and glucose.

What are Kernig and Brudzinski signs?

Kernig sign is considered positive when the patient resists straightening of the knee joint while the hip is flexed. Brudzinski sign is considered positive when the patient, while supine, lifts his legs when the neck is flexed by the examiner. Neither test is very sensitive, but a positive result is suggestive of meningeal irritation either by blood or inflammation.

What are the most important virulence factors and toxins of this microorganism?

N meningitidis has thin protrusions called pili that help it attach to nasopharyngeal epithelial cells. Once attached to the nasopharynx, the pathogen secretes IgA protease to neutralize the predominant antibody idiotype found on mucous membranes. *N meningitidis* also features a capsule that protects it from other host defenses such as complement and phagocytosis. As with all gram-negative bacteria, *N meningitidis* has lipopolysaccharide, a potent endotoxin, in its cell wall.

What is the appropriate treatment for this condition?

Intravenous penicillin G or ceftriaxone must be administered immediately. Bacterial meningitis can be fatal within hours, so empiric antimicrobial treatment must be started before culture results or other confirmatory tests become available. Rifampin is recommended as prophylactic treatment for contacts of the patient, especially if they are immunocompromised or have not been vaccinated.

■ CASE 41

A 35-year-old man presents to a medical mission near the Benue River in Nigeria complaining of itchy skin. Physical examination shows depigmentation several nodules on his thorax, hips, legs, and elbows; and thickening of the skin (Figure 3-30). Visual testing reveals decreased visual acuity in his right eye.

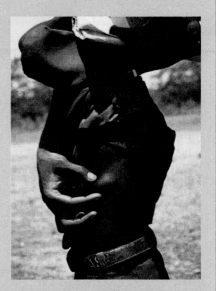

FIGURE 3-30. (Reproduced, with permission, from Brooks GF, et al. *Jawetz, Melnick, & Adelberg's Medical Microbiology*, 25th ed. New York: McGraw-Hill, 2010: Figure 46-21.)

What is the most likely diagnosis?

Onchocerciasis (river blindness) is caused by *Onchocerca volvulus*, a nematode (roundworm) found near rivers. Onchocerciasis is the leading cause of blindness in the developing world. Of the 18 million people infected worldwide, 99% of cases are in Zaire and Nigeria.

How is this condition transmitted?

The bite of a female black fly transmits larvae (microfilariae) into the host's skin. Humans are the only known definitive host of this parasite.

What is the pathogenesis of the causative organism?

The larvae become adults within 6–12 months, and subsequent fibrosis around the adult worms results in subcutaneous nodules, which protect the parasite from the host's immune system. The parasites mate in the tissue, releasing microfilariae that can migrate to the eye where they cause keratitis and subsequent sclerosis.

What tests can help confirm the diagnosis?

A skin biopsy may show larvae under the microscope, whereas nodules contain the adult filariae. The microfilariae in the eye may be visible on slit-lamp examination. Serologic tests such as enzyme-linked immunosorbent assay, polymerase chain reaction assay, and direct antigen testing are also available but require a laboratory, which is often not available to physicians treating the primary patient population.

What are the appropriate treatments for this condition?

Ivermectin is effective against the larvae (microfilariae). It must be given every 6–12 months until the patient is asymptomatic. The subcutaneous nodules containing adult worms can be surgically removed.

■ CASE 42

A 30-year-old man presents to the emergency department complaining of chills, myalgia, and extreme throbbing pain in his right shin. He fractured his tibia 3 weeks ago and required external fixation. His temperature is 40°C (104°F), blood pressure is 130/80 mm Hg, and heart rate is 80/min. Physical examination reveals that his right leg is red, tender, warm, and swollen over the anterior tibia just inferior to the knee. X-ray of the extremity demonstrates periosteal elevation and changes consistent with soft tissue swelling adjacent to the tibia. The patient is admitted, and blood and bone biopsy cultures are pending.

What is the most likely diagnosis?

Osteomyelitis. *Staphylococcus aureus* is responsible for approximately 90% of pyogenic osteomyelitis cases. *S aureus* expresses receptors for the bone matrix, thus allowing it to adhere to bone and produce a focus of infection. Many affected adults have a history of compound fracture or surgery.

What patient populations are susceptible to this condition?

Osteomyelitis can be a sequela of trauma, as is the case in this patient, but is also often found in intravenous drug abusers (direct injection of bacteria) and patients with diabetes who have poorly controlled blood glucose. Bacteremic patients (typically children) may develop osteomyelitis as a consequence of hematogenous spread.

How does a subperiosteal abscess lead to accelerated bone necrosis?

A subperiosteal abscess separates the bone from its blood supply in the periosteum, leading to ischemic injury and necrosis.

A history of sickle cell disease would increase this patient's risk of infection from which pathogen?

Patients with sickle cell disease have an increased risk of developing *Salmonella* osteomyelitis because of the reduced immune clearance of this pathogen.

What are the typical imaging findings?

Periosteal elevation is often found on plain film radiography. This finding, however, can lag up to 2 weeks behind the onset of the infection. MRI is sensitive but not specific as it cannot distinguish osteomyelitis from other causes of marrow edema, such as normal postsurgical changes. Negative MRI findings essentially exclude osteomyelitis.

■ CASE 43

A 4-year-old boy is brought to the pediatrician because of perianal itching, which is worse at night. He attends preschool during the day, where he shares toys and play areas with other children. The patient's mother recalls her son playing with another child who had been "scratching his backside" and wonders if there is a connection.

What is the most likely diagnosis?

Pinworm infection caused by *Enterobius vermicularis,* a nematode (roundworm).

What is the life cycle of this organism?

After **fecal-oral transmission,** the eggs hatch in the small intestine. Adults mature in the ileum and large intestine and mate in the colon. Females exit the rectum at night to lay eggs in the perianal area. This irritates the perianal area, inducing the host to scratch. Scratching transfers eggs onto hands, greatly increasing the likelihood of transmission to another host.

What sequelae may this infection have?

Intense scratching may compromise the integrity of the perianal skin, predisposing the patient to dermatitis or folliculitis due to dermal invasion of fecal bacteria.

What test can help confirm the diagnosis?

Adhesive tape test: The physician places adhesive tape over the perianal area and then removes and examines the tape. The presence of eggs under light microscopy indicates pinworm infection.

What are the appropriate treatments for this condition?

Mebendazole or albendazole is first-line therapy. Pyrantel pamoate can also be helpful. Individual cases are easily treated, but institutional outbreaks (eg, in preschool) are more difficult to treat because undertreated patients quickly reinfect others who had already been cured.

■ CASE 44

A 52-year-old woman with AIDS presents to her physician with difficulty breathing. She has experienced slowly worsening dry cough and dyspnea for approximately the past week. Her most recent CD4+ cell count is 175 cells/mm^3. In the office, her oxygen saturation is 92%. The patient says that she is not currently taking any medications because she is "tired of taking pills." An x-ray of the chest is taken (Figure 3-31).

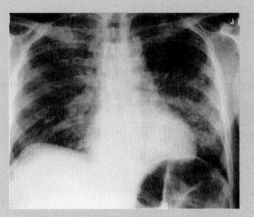

FIGURE 3-31. (Reproduced, with permission, from Fauci AS, et al. *Harrison's Principles of Internal Medicine*, 17th ed. New York: McGraw-Hill, 2008: Figure 200-1A.)

What is the most likely diagnosis?

Pneumocystis jiroveci (formerly *carinii*) **pneumonia** causes interstitial pneumonia in certain patient populations. Once thought to be a protozoan, *P jiroveci* is now recognized as a fungus (yeast).

What patients are most at risk for developing a clinical infection with this microorganism?

Most individuals are exposed to *P jiroveci* during childhood but develop no symptoms. However, immunocompromised patients (including patients with AIDS who have low CD4+ cell counts) and malnourished infants may develop severe clinical disease. *Pneumocystis* pneumonia in steroid-treated immunocompromised patients is most often seen as steroids are being withdrawn.

What are the likely x-ray findings?

"Ground-glass" bilateral infiltrates are commonly seen on x-ray of the chest (see Figure 3-31). In these patients, **hypoxia** is often **out of proportion** to the radiographic findings.

What tests can help confirm the diagnosis?

Sputum samples, bronchoalveolar lavage, or lung biopsy treated with **silver stain** demonstrate cysts and dark oval bodies contained within the cyst (**sporozoites**).

What is the appropriate treatment for this condition?

Treatment is primarily with trimethoprim-sulfamethoxazole. In immunocompromised patients, trimethoprim-sulfamethoxazole or dapsone may be used as prophylaxis when CD4+ cell counts fall below 200 cells/mm^3. In patients with severe hypoxia, steroids should be given as adjunctive therapy to prevent worsening respiratory status due to the inflammatory response induced by treatment.

■ CASE 45

A 20-year-old woman returns from a day hike in a densely wooded area and develops a rash that evening. The next day she presents to her physician. The patient has never developed a rash like this before and has hiked in this wooded area several times. Physical examination reveals that the rash (Figure 3-32) is mostly on the legs, arms, and hands—areas the patient says "were not covered by clothing." She is afebrile.

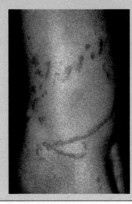

FIGURE 3-32. (Reproduced, with permission, from Wolff K, Johnson RA. *Fitzpatrick's Color Atlas and Synopsis of Clinical Dermatology*, 6th ed. New York: McGraw-Hill, 2009: Figure 2-8.)

What is the most likely diagnosis?

Phytodermatitis secondary to poison ivy. This rash is characterized by vesicles < 5 mm in diameter. However, vesicles often coalesce in severe rashes.

Which type of hypersensitivity reaction is occurring in this patient?

Type IV hypersensitivity reactions (delayed or cell-mediated) include contact hypersensitivity from poison ivy, transplant rejection, hypersensitivity pneumonitis, granulomatous hypersensitivity reactions, and the tuberculosis skin test (Table 3-3). Type IV reactions are also important in the control of mycobacterial and fungal infections.

TABLE 3-3	The Four Types of Hypersensitivity Reactions		
	MECHANISM	PATHOGENESIS	EXAMPLE
Type I	IgE-binding antigen	Massive histamine release	Peanut allergy (anaphylaxis)
Type II	IgG-binding cell surface protein	Tissue damage by immune system	Myasthenia gravis, Hashimoto thyroiditis
Type III	Specific antigen:antibody ratio	Precipitation of immune complexes in vessel walls activates complement	Poststreptococcal glomerulonephritis
Type IV	T cell mediated	Local release of inflammatory cytokines	Poison-ivy rash, tuberculin test

Was this the patient's first exposure to poison ivy?

A key feature of type IV hypersensitivity is that the patient must be sensitized to the antigen before development of hypersensitivity on subsequent exposure. The tuberculin skin test relies on the principle of prior sensitization to assess for previous exposure to tuberculosis.

CASE 46

A 27-year-old man presents to a medical mission in Tanzania with a complaint of paralysis of his lower extremities. He says he had a mild fever about 2 weeks previously, which resolved. Several days ago, the fever recurred and this time was followed by nuchal rigidity and then paralysis of both legs. Physical examination demonstrates 0/5 strength and hyporeflexia of the lower extremities. Sensation to pain, temperature, position, and light touch seems to be unaffected.

What is the most likely diagnosis?

Poliovirus, a **picornavirus,** can cause subclinical gastrointestinal infection, aseptic meningitis, or poliomyelitis. **Poliomyelitis** results in the classic flaccid paralysis (fasciculations, areflexia, and muscle wasting) secondary to destruction of the lower motor neurons in the anterior horn cells of the spinal cord. Similar symptoms may be seen in cauda equina syndrome, botulism, and Guillain-Barré syndrome.

What is the morphology of the microorganism responsible for this condition?

Poliovirus is a **single-stranded, positive-sense RNA virus** with an icosahedral coat. Like other viruses that infect the gastrointestinal tract, it lacks an envelope.

How is this condition transmitted?

Poliovirus is spread by the fecal-oral route. The virus can attach to and infect host cells in the pharynx and ileum. It can then disseminate hematogenously to lymphoid tissue during a primary "minor" viremia, which is typically asymptomatic. In a minority of patients, there is a secondary or "major" viremia that likely allows the virus to spread to the central nervous system (CNS). During the second viremia, patients experience mild symptoms and low-grade fever. Subsequent CNS disease typically occurs 11–17 days after exposure.

What treatments are available to prevent this condition?

Two vaccines are available to prevent this condition. The **Salk vaccine** consists of formalin-killed virus and elicits an IgG response. This is the form used in the United States. The **Sabin vaccine** is a live attenuated virus. Its major disadvantage is that it may revert to its natural form on rare occasions, leading to illness. However, its major advantage is that the recipient sheds attenuated viruses, thereby vaccinating household contacts secondarily. The attempt to eradicate polio failed because of the fear among some populations that the vaccine had been designed by colonial powers to sterilize the African people. Since then, poliomyelitis has resurged in several African countries.

■ CASE 47

An 18-year-old man with cystic fibrosis (CF) and a history of multiple respiratory infections is brought to the emergency department after recent onset of dyspnea, chills, and cough productive of purulent sputum. His mother reports he has been lethargic and recorded his temperature at 39°C (102.2°F). Physical examination reveals a poorly responsive man in moderate respiratory distress. Laboratory studies are notable for a WBC of 17,000/mm³, with a left shift on the differential. Sputum culture yields gram-negative, non-lactose-fermenting bacilli.

What is the most likely diagnosis?

Pseudomonas aeruginosa infection. *P aeruginosa* is a **gram-negative, aerobic, oxidase-positive, rod-shaped** bacterium with a single flagellum. As an opportunistic pathogen, it causes infection in patients with impaired defence mechanisms, especially immunocompromised individuals and burn victims. It commonly lives in water or wet environments and can be particularly problematic for patients on ventilators. It is a major cause of respiratory failure in patients with CF.

What other infections does this microorganism cause?

Community-acquired infections include otitis externa ("swimmer's ear"), endocarditis (seen in intravenous drug users), osteomyelitis, and pneumonia. **Nosocomial infections** may present as bacteremia, leading to sepsis in burn victims and neonates. Ventilator-associated pneumonia and infections secondary to Foley catheter placement may also be due to *P aeruginosa*.

What is the pathology of chronic respiratory infection with this microorganism in patients with CF?

Pseudomonas can colonize the lungs of patients with CF. These patients cannot effectively clear the pathogen as the thickened mucous is not easily expectorated. The patient's immune response causes a chronic inflammatory state that eventually results in progressive loss of pulmonary function.

What virulence factors contribute to acute infection with this microorganism?

Pseudomonas has a host of virulence factors that contribute to pathology in acute infection. These include pili and a flagellum for host invasion; lipopolysaccharide (endotoxin); exotoxins A, S, and U; elastase; and various cytotoxins.

What are the appropriate treatments for this condition?

Pseudomonas is frequently resistant to multiple-drug regimens, so therapy guided by antimicrobial susceptibility testing is essential. In addition to its intrinsic resistance to many antibiotics, it is able to acquire resistance rapidly during treatment. Potentially useful antibiotics include ceftazidime, cefepime, ciprofloxacin, aztreonam, imipenem, piperacillin-tazobactam, and the aminoglycosides. These drugs are usually employed in combinations of two drugs of different classes. Topical (eg, inhaled) as well as systemic antibiotic therapy are utilized in CF patients. Colistin is a drug of last resort for severe cases of multidrug-resistant *Pseudomonas* infection.

CASE 48

A 10-year-old boy is camping with his family in the Adirondack Mountains when he is bitten on the leg by a raccoon. The animal was not provoked by the boy but attacked him unexpectedly. His family brings the boy to the nearest emergency department.

What condition is this boy at risk of contracting?

Rabies. If left untreated, rabies results in a nearly 100% mortality rate. Rabies causes only a few deaths per year in the United States but is significantly more dangerous in countries with unvaccinated domestic animals. For example, rabies-infected dog bites cause tens of thousands of deaths each year in India.

What is the morphology of the pathogen that causes this condition?

Rabies is caused by a rhabdovirus, a single-stranded RNA virus enveloped by a bullet-shaped capsid, covered by glycoprotein "spikes." The spikes bind to acetylcholine receptors, a property that may contribute to virulence.

What is the pathogenesis of this condition?

Animals transfer the virus to humans through bites that inoculate the host. The virus remains local for a period of days to months, then binds to acetylcholine receptors on neurons and travels to the central nervous system (CNS), utilizing axonal retrograde transport mechanisms. In the CNS, the virus infects neurons, including Ammon horn cells of the hippocampus. Rabies carries a significant person-to-person transmission risk through bites or mucous membrane exposure.

What signs and symptoms are associated with this condition?

Spasms of the pharyngeal muscles cause dysphagia, which leads to painful swallowing and accidental aspiration. This often leads to hydrophobia, a fear of water. Excess autonomic stimulation can cause hypersalivation. The buildup of saliva accounts for the apparent "foaming at the mouth." As rabies multiplies in the CNS, nonfocal neurological symptoms result, including confusion, agitation, hallucinations, and sensitivity to bright light (photophobia). Focal neurological deficits include cranial nerve palsies. Encephalitis can give rise to seizures, and inflammatory edema eventually leads to coma, then death.

How is the condition diagnosed and treated?

Identifying cytoplasmic inclusions called **Negri bodies** in tissues obtained from brain biopsy, polymerase chain reaction for viral RNA, and serology are diagnostic. In the event of a bite by an infected animal, the **human diploid cell vaccine** (a live attenuated virus) is administered. Additionally, **human rabies immune globulin (IgG)** is used to confer passive immunity to the patient. Both treatments are effective only in the lag period between the bite and onset of symptoms. Once symptoms appear, there is no effective treatment.

■ CASE 49

A 30-year-old man who recently joined a gym complains of itching between his toes. Physical examination reveals pustules on the fingers of both hands and white macerated tissue between the toes (Figure 3-33). The patient says the pustules have been itchy and appeared about a week after the itching between the toes began.

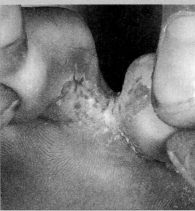

FIGURE 3-33. (Reproduced, with permission, from Wolff K, et al. *Fitzpatrick's Dermatology in General Medicine*, 7th ed. New York: McGraw-Hill, 2008: Figure 188-14.)

What is the most likely diagnosis?

Ringworm (tinea pedis) infection. Although caused by the same group of fungi, each dermatophytosis is named after the region of the body that it infects: tinea cruris (perineum and creases of inner thigh; "jock itch"), tinea pedis ("athlete's foot"), tinea capitis (scalp), tinea unguium (nails), and tinea corporis (body).

What three microorganisms are often responsible for this presentation?

Microsporum, *Trichophyton*, and *Epidermophyton* are three filamentous fungi that cause **dermatophytosis**.

How is the microorganism transmitted?

After contact with an infected host, the keratinized epithelium of warm, moist skin is colonized. The infection expands radially and is characterized by curvy (wormlike) circular borders. Thus, it is termed "ringworm," despite the fact that the causative microorganism is actually a fungus.

What tests can help confirm the diagnosis?

Branched hyphae are observed on potassium hydroxide preparation (**KOH mount**). This fungus is not dimorphic. A sample from the lesions on the patient's feet will likely demonstrate the organism.

What is the appropriate treatment for this condition?

Topical azoles (eg, fluconazole), butenafine, terbinafine, or griseofulvin is used for treatment.

■ CASE 50

A 13-year-old boy, who had been camping in the Appalachian Mountains with his family, was brought to the emergency department because of a headache, rash, and the abrupt onset of a high fever. The rash began on his palms and soles but spread up his ankles and arms (Figure 3-34). On physical examination he was found to have palpable purpura on his wrists and lower legs.

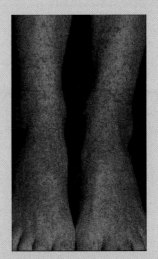

FIGURE 3-34. (Reproduced, with permission, from Wolff K, Johnson RA. *Fitzpatrick's Color Atlas and Synopsis of Clinical Dermatology*, 6th ed. New York: McGraw-Hill, 2009: Figure 26-2.)

What infections frequently cause a rash on the palms and soles?

Infections with *Rickettsia rickettsii, Treponema pallidum*, and coxsackievirus A can all cause a rash in this distribution.

What is the most likely infectious agent in this case?

This patient is most likely infected with *R rickettsii*. The clinical course is typical for Rocky Mountain spotted fever, which is characterized by fever with abrupt onset and a rash that spreads from the extremities toward the trunk. Palpable purpura is a poor prognostic sign, as it indicates active vasculitis and leakage of blood into the skin. The rash in syphilis and coxsackievirus is typically more gradual in onset. However, syphilis should never be excluded because of the patient's age, as it is occasionally seen in sexually abused children.

How is this pathogen transmitted to humans?

R rickettsii is acquired from *Dermacentor* tick bites.

What other diseases are caused by these organisms?

Endemic typhus (also known as murine typhus) is caused by *R typhi*. This illness presents with vasculitis leading to headache, fever, chills, and myalgia. Epidemic typhus is caused by *R prowazekii* and often presents with high fevers, hypotension, and delirium. It often occurs in conditions of crowding and after disasters (eg, refugee camps). Both diseases are caused by arthropod-borne agents: endemic typhus is transmitted by fleas, whereas epidemic typhus is transmitted by the human body louse.

What laboratory technique can be used to identify the cause of this patient's illness?

Diagnosis is made clinically. Direct fluorescent antibody or polymerase chain reaction testing of a skin biopsy of one of the petechial lesions will confirm the diagnosis, but not early enough to guide therapy. Rocky Mountain spotted fever antibody testing can also be used to confirm the diagnosis after recovery.

What is the appropriate treatment for choice for organisms of this class?

Tetracyclines are most frequently used in rickettsial infections. The rickettsiae are obligate intracellular organisms, as they require coenzyme A and nicotinamide adenine dinucleotide from the host cell; they also lack the peptidoglycan cell wall targeted by many antibiotic classes. Tetracyclines can enter cells and act on ribosomal targets.

■ CASE 51

In the month of January, a 2-year-old girl is brought to her pediatrician by her parents because of a 3-day history of watery, nonbloody diarrhea, nausea, vomiting, and abdominal pain. Physical examination reveals the child is slightly tachycardic, with sunken eyes and poor skin turgor.

What is the most likely diagnosis?

Rotavirus infection is the most common infectious cause of diarrhea in infants and young children and a major cause of acute diarrhea in the United States during the winter. It is also the most common cause of gastroenteritis in infants globally.

What is the pathogenesis of this infection?

Rotavirus is transmitted via the fecal-oral route and infects villus cells of the proximal small intestine. The virus replicates intracellularly and eventually causes lysis in host cell. Cell destruction results in a significant decrease in intestinal surface area and consequently absorption from the intestinal lumen, thus causing watery diarrhea. Rotavirus does not cause inflammation and the stool is nonbloody.

What is the appropriate treatment for this condition?

Treatment is supportive through rehydration. Suspected rotavirus can be confirmed by enzyme-linked immunosorbent assay of a stool specimen. In practice, this is generally reserved for epidemiological investigations. Stool ova and parasite examinations and bacterial cultures are sometimes obtained to exclude more serious causes of diarrhea that might require antibiotic treatment.

In what age group is this condition usually seen?

Infection is not commonly seen before 6 months of age, as children have passive immunity from IgA from the mother's breast milk. By 3 years of age, most children worldwide have developed lifelong immunity from prior infection. Therefore, it is most common between these two ages.

■ CASE 52

A 21-year-old college student presents to the clinic with fever, hives, headache, weight loss, and cough. On review of systems, she reports doing field research in Egypt over the summer. She recalls an intense itching sensation while collecting samples in a river. Physical examination reveals lymphadenopathy and hepatosplenomegaly.

What is the most likely diagnosis?

The patient likely acquired **schistosomiasis**, caused by a type of **trematode (fluke)**, from contact with contaminated water. The three main flukes are *Schistosoma japonicum* (in East Asia), *S mansoni* (in South America and Africa), and *S haematobium* (in Africa).

What other species are intermediate hosts of this pathogen?

Snails are the intermediate host for all trematodes. Reservoirs include primates (*S mansoni* and *S haematobium*) and domesticated animals (*S japonicum*).

In which human organs are the organisms found?

S japonicum and *S mansoni* reside in the intestines, where organisms mate in the mesenteric veins and release eggs into the feces as well as the portal circulation. *S haematobium* resides in the bladder, where organisms mate in the vesicular (bladder) veins and release eggs into the urine.

How is this condition diagnosed?

Examination of the urine (*S haematobium*) and stool (all three species) reveals eggs.

What are the chronic manifestations of this condition?

After the initial **"swimmer's itch,"** which is a dermatitis that occurs as the organism initially penetrates the skin; there is a lag period of 4–8 weeks. **Katayama fever** occurs as the adult organisms lay eggs. The eggs trigger a granulomatous immune response, fibrosis, and inflammation. For example, eggs that pass into the portal system become foci for granulomatous inflammation of the liver, eventually leading to fibrosis. Complications include portal hypertension (*S japonicum* and *S mansoni*), pulmonary artery hypertension, chronic abdominal pain, and central nervous system injury. *S haematobium* can increase the risk for developing squamous cell **bladder cancer.**

What is the appropriate treatment for this condition?

Praziquantel is the treatment of choice.

CASE 53

A 9-year-old boy is brought to the emergency department with a 5-day history of abdominal pain and diarrhea. He is admitted to the hospital for intravenous fluid replacement and further workup. One day before admission he noticed that his stool appeared bloody. His stool is found to be positive for Shiga-like toxin. After 4 days his abdominal pain begins to subside but he notices that his urine is grossly bloody. Peripheral blood smear (PBS) (Figure 3-35A) and biopsy of his kidney (Figure 3-35B) are obtained.

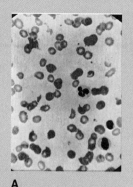
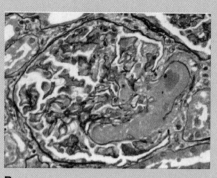

A   B

FIGURE 3-35. **(A) Peripheral blood smear showing fragmented RBCs. (B) Biopsy of the kidney showing fibrin thrombi within the glomerular vessels typical of patients with this condition.** (Image A reproduced, with permission, from Lichtman MA, et al. Williams Hematology, 7th ed. New York: McGraw-Hill, 2006: Figure 35-2. Image B reproduced, with permission, from Fauci AS, et al. Harrison's Principles of Internal Medicine, 17th ed. New York: McGraw-Hill, 2008: Figure 9-21.)

What is the most likely causative organism?

Enterohemorrhagic *Escherichia coli* (EHEC) serotype O157:H7. Infection with this organism most commonly occurs through consumption of undercooked meat or contaminated vegetables.

What is the mechanism of action of Shiga toxin and Shiga-like toxin?

These toxins are similar. One is produced by *Shigella* and the other by *E coli* O157:H7. They bind to host ribosomes and cleave a particular glycosidic bond, which inhibits ribosome function. The reduction in cellular translation triggers events that lead to apoptosis.

What is the cause of the blood in the patient's urine?

The patient has developed hemolytic-uremic syndrome. This is a complication of infection with *Shigella* and EHEC in which the toxin damages the renal vascular endothelium, compromising vascular integrity. Several schistocytes are apparent on the PBS and the kidney biopsy shows a fibrin thrombus (Figure 3-35B).

What is the classic triad of findings associated with this condition?

In hemolytic-uremic syndrome the triad of findings is renal damage, hemolytic anemia, and thrombocytopenia.

What other conditions could feature a similar PBS?

The PBS shows schistocytes (Figure 3-35A). When RBCs are forced past a partial microvascular obstruction, they become damaged and assume the characteristic schistocyte shape. Other conditions in which schistocytosis may be seen are thrombotic thrombocytopenic purpura (TTP) and disseminated intravascular coagulation (DIC). In TTP, an autoantibody destroys ADAMST13, an enzyme responsible for cleaving large multimers of von Willebrand factor (vWF), which is more prone to cause coagulation of blood. By contrast, DIC is caused by an overabundance of tissue factor in the blood, triggering the coagulation cascade. Increased levels of tissue factor may be seen in severe trauma, cancers, or sepsis. DIC has a mortality rate of up to 55%.

What serum markers should be measured to follow the progression or recovery of this patient?

The platelet count is a useful marker for this syndrome. In addition, the blood urea nitrogen and creatinine levels should be measured to follow renal recovery. The hemoglobin and hematocrit should be followed to assess the need for transfusion.

■ CASE 54

A 59-year-old woman presents to her physician with prominent scattered erythematous papules (Figure 3-36) on the right side of her forehead. She says she has had a "burning" pain and general hypersensitivity in that area for the past 2 days. On review of systems, she denies headaches, mental status changes, or recent infections. Neurological examination indicates that her pain is localized to the right supraorbital area and the right aspect of the dorsum of her nose.

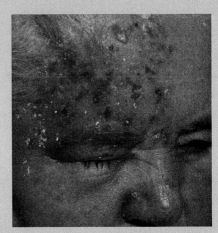

FIGURE 3-36. (Reproduced, with permission, from Wolff K, Johnson RA. *Fitzpatrick's Color Atlas and Synopsis of Clinical Dermatology*, 6th ed. New York: McGraw-Hill, 2009: Figure 27-46.)

Which nerve relays the painful sensation in this patient?

Sensory information from the face is relayed by the trigeminal nerve to the ventral posterolateral nucleus of the thalamus. Specifically, the area described by the patient is the left V1 dermatome.

What infectious agent may be responsible for this woman's pain?

This woman is suffering from herpes zoster, or "shingles," a late complication of prior infection with varicella zoster virus, one of the herpesviruses.

What are the characteristic distribution patterns of this condition?

The virus remains latent in the ganglia of sensory nerves after the primary infection. When reactivation occurs, virions are transported to the dermatome innervated by this sensory nerve using axonal transport mechanisms. Therefore, the characteristic shingles rash is always confined to a dermatome and does not cross the midline.

What are the likely findings on histologic examination of these vesicles?

A **Tzanck smear** may demonstrate multinucleate giant cells, which are typical for infection with varicella and herpes simplex viruses. This test is rarely used for diagnosis, having been superseded by more specific molecular tests such as polymerase chain reaction.

What are the appropriate treatments for this condition?

Acyclovir is activated by viral thymidine kinase to inhibit viral DNA polymerase. Valacyclovir and famciclovir have a similar mechanism and longer half-lives. These drugs target herpesviruses and may provide relief, speed recovery, and prevent postherpetic neuralgia. The drug doses for varicella are substantially higher than for herpes simplex virus. Primary infection with varicella and zoster can be prevented by vaccination. A zoster vaccine is available for the elderly population; however, its use remains controversial.

What are the advantages of a live attenuated vaccine?

Three general types of vaccinations are available: live attenuated, killed, or passive. Passive vaccination is the transfer of antibodies and is limited by antibody half-life in the bloodstream. A killed vaccine can stimulate only a humoral response as the virus cannot replicate within cells; therefore, no viral proteins can be displayed on major histocompatibility complex receptors. Live attenuated virus vaccine stimulates both arms of the immune system (humoral and cell mediated) as it leads to limited viral replication. Live attenuated vaccines should be avoided in pregnancy as only the humoral arm of the mother's immune system can protect the fetus across the placental barrier.

▪ CASE 55

A 36-year-old woman from Alabama presents with abdominal pain and diarrhea of 3 days' duration. She denies nausea, vomiting, or fever. She has no sick contacts or significant travel history. A complete blood count shows eosinophilia. A stool sample reveals larvae. On further questioning, she describes that she frequently gardens in her backyard while barefoot.

What is the most likely diagnosis?

Strongyloidiasis, caused by *Strongyloides stercoralis,* a nematode (roundworm).

What is the life cycle of this parasite?

Larvae in the soil penetrate the skin, usually the sole of the foot (fecal-cutaneous transmission). Local itching at the entry site promotes scratching, which aids larval entry into the bloodstream. Once in the blood, the larvae settle in the respiratory tree and travel up the trachea into the pharynx to be swallowed. They enter the small intestine, where the larvae mature into adults. Female adults invade the intestinal wall and lay eggs. During passage through the gastrointestinal tract, the eggs hatch into larvae. Most of these larvae pass with the stool and can continue the life cycle in the soil; some, however, directly penetrate the colonic wall or perianal skin and, uniquely, continue the life cycle within the original host. These continually migrating parasites are responsible for the eosinophilia commonly seen in chronic *Strongyloides* infections.

What other two organisms demonstrate the same route of transmission in humans?

Necator americanus (New World hookworm), and *Ancylostoma duodenale* (Old World hookworm).

What is the pathogenesis of hyperinfection syndrome?

Hyperinfection syndrome, caused by uncontrolled autoinfection, can increase parasitic burden and widely disseminated disease. This is more common in individuals with defective eosinophil function, such as patients treated with steroids or cytotoxic chemotherapeutic agents that cause granulocytopenia.

What tests can help confirm the diagnosis?

Stool sample reveals larvae (not eggs as in hookworm infection). Blood samples reveal eosinophilia. *Strongyloides* antibody testing can also be valuable in patients with unexplained eosinophilia, as larvae are not always detectable in the stool.

What are the appropriate treatments for this condition?

Ivermectin or thiabendazole.

CASE 56

A 52-year-old man from Michigan presents with worsening cough, fever, chills, and pleuritic chest pain. He was diagnosed with community-acquired pneumonia at a hospital but seeks a second opinion. He recently developed multiple ulcerated sores on his skin, which began as pimple-like lesions. X-ray of the chest reveals segmental consolidation. Biopsy of a skin lesion reveals big, broad-based, budding yeasts.

What is the most likely diagnosis?
Blastomycosis, one of the systemic mycoses.

To what areas are the systemic mycoses endemic?
Three forms of systemic mycoses are endemic to the United States. **Coccidioidomycosis** (also called desert bumps, San Joaquin Valley bumps, or valley fever) is specific to the southwestern United States. **Histoplasmosis** is endemic to the Mississippi and Ohio River Valleys and is found in bird and bat droppings. **Blastomycosis** is found east of the Mississippi River (and in Central America). **Paracoccidioidomycosis** is found in rural Latin America.

Which diagnostic tests can differentiate between the mycoses?
Systemic mycoses are caused by dimorphic fungi, which grow as molds in the cold (eg, in the soil) and as yeast at higher temperatures (eg, in tissues at 37°C [98.6°F]). The exception is coccidioidomycosis, which is a spherule in tissue. Therefore, growing cultures on Sabouraud's agar at multiple temperatures aids in the diagnosis. In addition, a tissue biopsy revealing broad-based budding yeast is diagnostic for blastomycosis. Tissue biopsy demonstrating yeast cells within macrophages is diagnostic of histoplasmosis. A biopsy showing "captain's wheel" morphology of budding yeast is diagnostic of paracoccidioidomycosis. Serologic testing for antifungal antibodies is also useful in some patients, and a histoplasma antigen test is the diagnostic test of choice for systemic (but not localized) *Histoplasma* infections.

What are the typical x-ray findings?
These diseases can mimic tuberculosis, forming **granulomas,** which appear as small calcium deposits on x-ray.

What is the appropriate treatment for this condition?
Systemic infection is treated with itraconazole or amphotericin B.

■ CASE 57

A 13-year-old girl is brought to the physician's office by her mother. Her mother says the girl had a sudden onset of fever a few days ago, with a temperature of 39.4°C (103°F), lightheadedness, nausea, vomiting, and watery diarrhea. Physical examination reveals a desquamating rash of her palms and soles. She has no sick contacts, and there is no evidence of ingestion of unsafe food. Upon questioning, the patient says she began menstruating a little more than a month ago.

What is the most likely diagnosis?

Toxic shock syndrome (TSS).

What microorganism is the most likely cause of this condition?

Staphylococcus aureus is the most common cause, although β-hemolytic group A streptococci can cause a similar presentation. The most common nidi of infection are high-absorbency tampons worn for a prolonged period of time and cutaneous wounds.

What are the distinguishing characteristics of the responsible microorganism?

S aureus is a gram-positive coccus. It is catalase-positive and coagulase-positive and may produce an enterotoxin. Figure 3-37 provides a useful laboratory algorithm for differentiating the gram-positive bacteria.

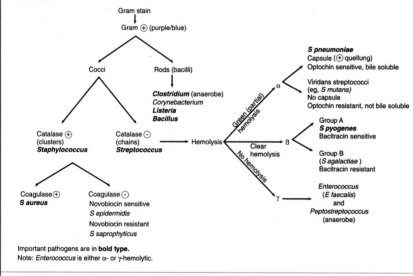

FIGURE 3-37. Algorithm for differentiating gram-positive bacteria. (Reproduced, with permission, from Le T, Bhushan V, Tolles J. *First Aid for the USMLE Step 1: 2011.* New York: McGraw-Hill, 2011: 144.)

What is the pathophysiology of this condition?

The exotoxin (TSST-1) acts as a "superantigen" and is responsible for this presentation. Superantigens activate large numbers of T cells at once by simultaneously binding directly to T-cell receptors and major histocompatibility complex (MHC) molecules, regardless of the peptide presented by MHC. Activated T cells then release large amounts of inflammatory cytokines, which are responsible for the manifestations of TSS.

What other conditions should be considered in the differential diagnosis?

The differential for desquamating disease is limited. Toxic epidermal necrolysis should be suspected; this is an exacerbation of Stevens-Johnson syndrome that may be a serious adverse reaction to certain medication. Additionally, scalded skin syndrome leads to desquamation of the skin. In this condition, an infection with *S aureus* producing exotoxin A and B causes detachment of the epidermal layer from the dermis. Lastly, pemphigus vulgaris features autoantibodies against desmosomes, leading to flaccid blister formation that may look like desquamation in severe cases.

What is the appropriate treatment for this condition?

Removal of the infected wound dressing or tampon is the first step, followed by supportive care. Antibiotics that cover both *Staphylococcus* and *Streptococcus* will kill these bacteria and stop the production of additional exotoxin. However, it is the toxin, not the bacteria, that is responsible for the symptoms. In severe cases, intravenous immunoglobulin is also given.

■ CASE 58

A 54-year-old man with HIV infection presents to the emergency department after suffering a grand mal seizure. He has no known personal or family history of seizures. He is afebrile and his vital signs are stable. Funduscopic examination reveals yellow cotton-like lesions on his retina. Findings on physical examination are otherwise unremarkable. CT scan of the head demonstrates multiple ring-enhancing lesions in the cerebral cortex. Laboratory findings reveal a CD4+ cell count of 53 cells/mm³.

What is the most likely cause of this patient's seizure?

Toxoplasma gondii infection.

How did this patient likely become infected with this microorganism?

It is likely that this man (like most individuals) has been latently infected with this protozoan for many years. However, his immunocompromised status has resulted in disease reactivation. Humans are most often infected by ingestion of cysts in undercooked meat or by fecal-oral transmission of cat feces. Cats may shed the protozoan and pregnant women are discouraged from cleaning the litter box as inhaled aerosolized particles are sufficient to cause infection.

Why is this condition dangerous in pregnancy?

Primary infection with *T gondii* in a pregnant woman can allow parasites to cross the placenta. This leads to congenital problems in the newborn, including mental retardation, microcephaly, chorioretinitis, intracerebral calcifications, and blindness. It is one of the **ToRCHeS** infections (**To**xoplasmosis, other infections, **R**ubella, **C**ytomegalovirus, **H**erpes simplex virus, **S**yphilis).

Given this patient's ring-enhancing lesions on CT scan, what other conditions should be included in the differential diagnosis?

This patient is also at an increased risk of lymphoma, cryptococcosis, and tuberculosis, all of which appear as ring-enhancing lesions on CT scan (although less likely to cause multiple lesions) and can also cause seizures.

What is the appropriate treatment for this condition?

First-line treatment is a regimen of pyrimethamine and sulfadiazine.

■ CASE 59

A 55-year-old man with end-stage renal disease is scheduled to undergo kidney transplantation. While on the operating table, the donor kidney is connected to the patient's blood supply. Within minutes of perfusion, the transplanted organ becomes extremely erythematous. After a short period of time, the kidney becomes ashen gray and urine production ceases. The surgeon immediately removes the organ.

What caused the transplanted organ to fail?

Hyperacute rejection occurs within minutes of the transplantation. Rejection is due to preformed antibodies that recognize graft antigens. The patient's serum must be tested for antibodies that bind to a biopsy of the graft tissue before transplantation. There are three types of graft rejection (Table 3-4).

TABLE 3-4	The Three Types of Graft Rejection	
TYPE	MECHANISM	TIME FRAME
Hyperacute	Preformed antibodies to graft antigens elicit an immediate immune response	Within minutes of graft perfusion
Acute	Cell-mediated attack elicited by donor MHCs on graft tissue	As soon as 1 week after transplantation but can recur any time, especially if patient is no longer immunosuppressed
Chronic	Fibrosis of graft blood vessels	Years

What would histology show in a kidney that had undergone this complication?

The kidney would show fibrinoid necrosis of the small vessels and thromboses.

What would histology show in a kidney that had undergone acute or chronic forms of this complication?

Acute rejection is primarily cell mediated, although antibodies can also cause damage to graft tissue. A biopsy reveals T-cell and macrophage infiltrates as well as blood vessel and parenchymal damage. Chronic rejection is characterized by vascular damage. Damage to graft blood vessels can be due to antibody binding, complement activation, T-cell activation, and cytokines. The result is intimal proliferation, causing narrowing of the vessel lumen and tissue ischemia. Examination of the graft shows a small, scarred kidney.

Patients who undergo bone marrow or hematopoietic cell transplantation are at risk of another potential complication, graft-versus-host disease (GVHD). What is the mechanism of GVHD?

During bone marrow transplantation, the donor's immune system is essentially introduced into the host's body. As donor-derived T cells have not become immunotolerant toward host antigens, GVHD can occur when grafted T cells bind to host antigen and become activated, damaging host tissue. The most frequent sites of injury are the skin, liver, and gastrointestinal tract. By contrast, GVHD can be exploited in the treatment of certain haematological malignancies. For example, the host's immune system is tolerant toward the malignant plasma cells in multiple myeloma. Allogenic bone marrow transplantation may cause an immune reaction against the cancerous cells.

■ CASE 60

A 45-year-old man visiting rural Brazil develops fever, headache, pain in his knees and back, and nausea and vomiting. After 3 days these symptoms resolve, and he decides not to seek medical help. However, 2 days later the symptoms return, and he develops epigastric pain and yellowing of his skin. His vomitus is now dark in color.

What is the most likely diagnosis?

Yellow fever is endemic in South America and parts of Africa. It is characterized by an initial febrile illness, during which time serum aspartate aminotransferase and alanine aminotransferase levels begin to rise, followed by a remission of symptoms. Approximately 15% of infected patients experience a return of symptoms 2–3 days later, developing further liver dysfunction (resulting in jaundice and coagulopathy), renal damage, and myocardial damage.

What type of virus is responsible for this patient's condition?

The yellow fever virus is a **flavivirus.** These viruses have **positive, single-stranded RNA** genomes and icosahedral, enveloped capsids.

What are the most likely liver biopsy findings?

The characteristic finding on liver biopsy is midzone hepatocellular death, with sparing of cells bordering the central vein and portal tracts. **Councilman bodies** are found in the affected hepatocytes. These are eosinophilic inclusions that represent condensed chromatin. Typically, there is no inflammatory response. Liver biopsies are usually not done because of their concomitant coagulopathy.

Enzyme-linked immunosorbent assay (ELISA) may be useful in confirming the diagnosis by detecting antibody to the virus. How does ELISA work?

ELISA is a technique often used for serologic testing. It involves coating the surface with the desired antigen (in this case, yellow fever viral particles) and then placing the patient's serum on the surface, followed by a secondary antibody (antihuman antibody) that is linked to an enzyme. If the patient's serum has antibody to the antigen, the secondary antibody will bind. The linked enzyme can be detected by a reaction that produces an alteration in color with a colorimetric agent (eg, horseradish peroxidise). The color change can be quantified by spectroscopy. Detection of antibody to yellow fever virus in a patient with exposure can support a clinical diagnosis of the disease.

■ CASE 61

A 34-year-old Haitian nurse complains to her physician of occasional rust-colored sputum and fever of 6 months' duration. She also notes her clothes fit more loosely than they used to. She does not have a history of smoking or asbestos exposure. Her only medication is an oral contraceptive. An x-ray of the chest is shown in Figure 3-38. A radiology report expresses concern about the structure indicated by the arrow.

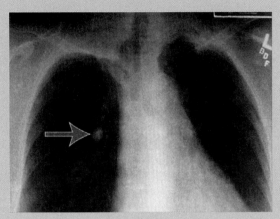

FIGURE 3-38. (Reproduced, with permission, from Tintinalli JE, et al. *Tintinalli's Emergency Medicine: A Comprehensive Guide*, 7th ed. New York: McGraw-Hill, 2011: Figure 70-1.)

What is the most likely diagnosis?

This patient's symptoms and x-ray of the chest suggest primary tuberculosis (TB). Associated findings include a positive purified protein derivative (PPD) test, positive culture, and/or positive acid-fast staining of bacteria from sputum samples. Primary TB is often seen in the lower lobes of the lung with enlargement of the associated lymph node, whereas reactivation TB tends to cause cavitation in the apices.

What type of lesion does the x-ray show?

Primary lesions are usually found in the lower lobes as Ghon foci. If there is lymph node involvement, the lesions are termed Ghon complexes (see arrow in Figure 3-38). Reactivation (secondary) TB lesions are usually seen in the apical and posterior portions of the upper lobes.

How is the microorganism that causes this condition cultured and stained?

Mycobacterium tuberculosis is cultured on **Lowenstein-Jensen agar.** It is an acid-fast bacterium and therefore stains with **Ziehl-Neelsen stain.**

What is the appropriate treatment for this condition?

The standard treatment lasts for 6 months. Rifampin, Isoniazid, Pyrazinamide, and Ethambutol (**RIPE**) are used for the initial phase of therapy (usually 2 months), followed by rifampin and isoniazid for an additional 4 months. Susceptibility testing is necessary to guide the choice of agents. More drugs may need to be used in multidrug-resistant TB. Because emergent drug resistance is often due to medication nonadherence, the United States has installed "observed therapy" programs in which TB patients take their medication in the presence of a healthcare provider. Prophylactic treatment is with isoniazid.

What are the main side effects of treatment with these agents?

Rifampin colors urine, feces, sweat, and tears a reddish-orange color. It also upregulates the cytochrome P450 isoenzyme system, increasing the metabolism of many drugs, including oral contraceptives. If the patient stays on her current dose of birth control pills and remains sexually active, she is more likely to become pregnant while taking rifampin. Isoniazid causes peripheral neuropathies; vitamin B_6 reduces this adverse event. Rifampin, isoniazid, and pyrazinamide are associated with liver toxicity. Ethambutol can cause retrobulbar optic neuritis, which impairs visual acuity and color vision; patients should receive frequent ophthalmologic examinations during the treatment period.

Pharmacology

▪ CASE 1

A 22-year-old woman is brought to the emergency department by her roommate who found the woman lethargic and covered in vomit. The roommate explains that the woman has been depressed lately and that she has a history of epilepsy that is controlled with medications. On examination, the patient is sweaty, jaundiced, and lethargic, with marked right upper quadrant tenderness. Transaminase values are markedly elevated (aspartate aminotransferase: 12,450 U/L). A serum toxicology screen is sent.

This woman most likely overdosed on what medication?

Acetaminophen accounts for more overdose deaths in the United States than any other drug. Anticonvulsant medications can increase the toxicity of acetaminophen (phenytoin and carbamazepine both induce the isoenzyme CYP2E1, which metabolizes acetaminophen into hepatotoxic metabolites).

What is the pathogenesis for this condition?

At therapeutic doses, a small quantity of acetaminophen is metabolized by hepatic cytochrome P450 into a hepatotoxic intermediate, N-acetyl-p-benzoquinone imine (NAPQI) (see Figure 4-1A). Glutathione rapidly conjugates with NAPQI to form nontoxic compounds. At toxic doses, glutathione storage is depleted and hepatic damage ensues (see Figure 4-1B).

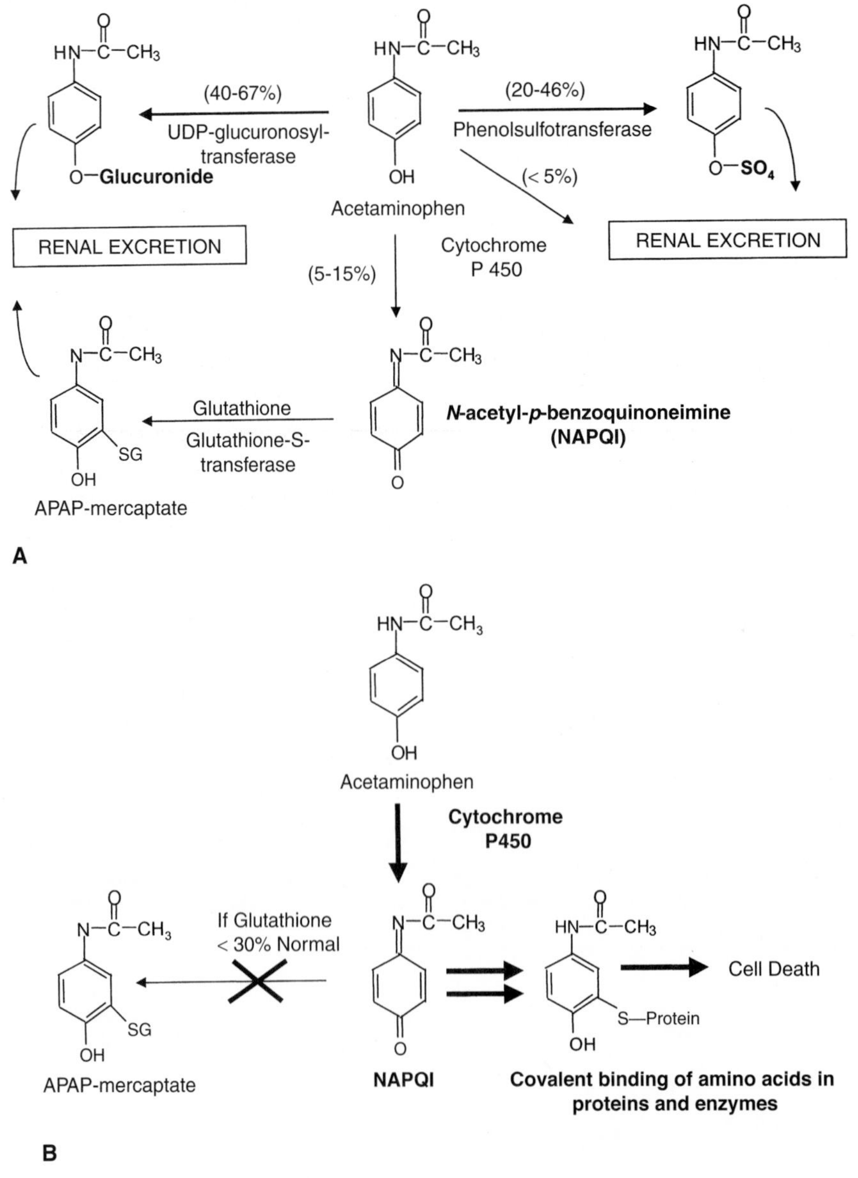

FIGURE 4-1. A and B: Acetaminophen metabolism. (Reproduced, with permission, from Tintinalli JE, et al. *Tintinalli's Emergency Medicine: A Comprehensive Study Guide,* 6th ed. New York: McGraw-Hill, 2004: 1089.)

What is the mechanism of action of the antidote?
N-acetylcysteine (NAC), the antidote, works via several pathways. NAC enhances the conjugation of NAPQI into nontoxic compound, in part by increasing glutathione.

Given the patient's presentation, approximately how long ago was the overdose?
There are four stages in an acetaminophen overdose:

- Stage 1 (< 24 hours after ingestion): Nonspecific complaints such as nausea and vomiting; sometimes asymptomatic and normal lab values.
- Stage 2 (1–3 days): Subclinical elevations in liver and/or renal function tests; resolution of stage 1 symptoms.
- Stage 3 (3–4 days): Peak of abnormal liver function tests and a return of stage 1 symptoms; clinical evidence of hepatic dysfunction; sometimes fatal. The patient in this case was most likely in this stage.
- Stage 4 (> 4 days): Recovery stage, if other stages are survived; complete by approximately day 7 if there is no underlying disease.

What histologic regions of the liver would be most affected in this case?
The centrilobular zone (zone III—the area surrounding the central hepatic venule of a lobule, furthest from the branch of the hepatic vein; see Figure 4-2) is most involved because it has the highest concentration of CYP4502E1. Histologic recovery takes approximately 3 months.

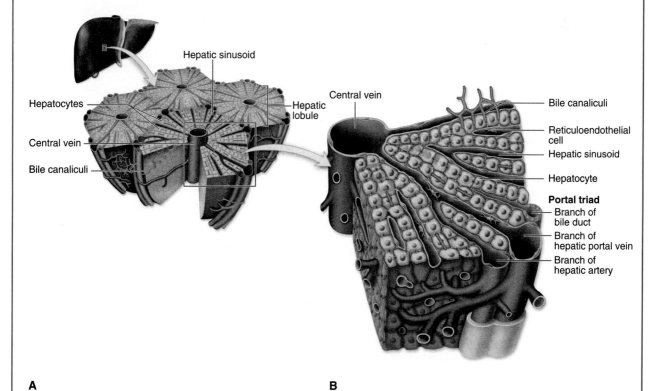

A   **B**

FIGURE 4-2. **(A) Hepatic lobules; (B) hepatocytes and sinusoids.** (Adapted, with permission, from Mescher AL. *Junqueira's Basic Histology: Text and Atlas*, 12th ed. New York: McGraw-Hill, 2010: Figure 16-11.)

▮ CASE 2

A 45-year-old woman is brought to the emergency department by the police for unusual and disruptive behavior. She is muttering to herself and does not make eye contact or answer any of the physician's questions but is otherwise cooperative. The patient's temperature is 38°C (100.4°F). A throat examination yields the findings shown in Figure 4-3. Her urine and serum drug screens are negative for acetaminophen, salicylates, and drugs of abuse. She is HIV negative. Her CBC shows:

WBC count: 2000/mm³   Basophils: 2%
Neutrophils: 1%   Hemoglobin: 12 g/dL
Monocytes: 15%   Lymphocytes: 74%
Eosinophils: 8%   Platelet count: 270,000/mm³

What is the most likely diagnosis, given the findings in Figure 4-3?

Figure 4-3 shows the characteristic whitish plaques of oral candidiasis (thrush) on the buccal mucosa. The lymphoreticular disorders in this patient suggest agranulocytosis. Nystatin "swish and swallow" is used to treat thrush.

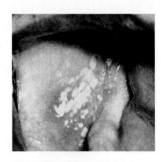

FIGURE 4-3. (Courtesy of James F. Steiner, DDS, as published in Knoop KJ, et al. *Atlas of Emergency Medicine*, 2nd ed. New York: McGraw-Hill, 2002: 177.)

Given her presentation, what medication is the patient likely to be taking?

This patient is acutely psychotic and suffering from agranulocytosis (lack of granulocytes [neutrophils, eosinophils, and basophils]). **Clozapine**, an antipsychotic, causes agranulocytosis in 1%–2% of patients and will usually do so in the initial months of treatment.

What is the appropriate management for this patient?

First, the medication causing neutropenia should be discontinued immediately, which should cause neutropenia to resolve within 1–3 weeks. Treatment may include granulocyte colony–stimulating factor, which has been shown to restore immune function in some neutropenic patients with serious infections.

What are the main differentials for white plaques in the oral cavity?

Although thrush is the most common cause, oral leukoplakia and oral hairy leukoplakia (OHL) should also be considered. Oral leukoplakia is a precancerous lesion representing hyperplasia of squamous epithelium. OHL (which is not considered to be premalignant) is seen in HIV patients and is caused by the Epstein-Barr virus. It usually occurs on the lateral part of the tongue and, unlike thrush, cannot be scraped off.

■ CASE 3

A 37-year-old homeless man is brought to the emergency department by the police. He was seen yelling and stumbling and says that he feels bugs crawling all over him. Physical examination reveals tachycardia, diaphoresis, tachypnea, tremor of the hands, and normal-sized pupils.

What is the most likely diagnosis?

The first step in reaching a diagnosis in this case is determining whether the patient's presentation is due to substance abuse/withdrawal or to a psychiatric condition such as schizophrenia. The constellation of physical symptoms here suggests a sympathomimetic toxidrome. The specific sensation of feeling bugs crawling over him, called formication, is highly suggestive of alcohol withdrawal.

What is the appropriate treatment for this condition?

Alcohol withdrawal is treated with benzodiazepines, usually chlordiazepoxide, diazepam, or lorazepam.

What are other indications of the treatment?

Benzodiazepines have many indications, including anxiety, status epilepticus, night terrors, and somnambulism. Benzodiazepines act by increasing the **frequency** of the γ-aminobutyric acid (GABA)$_A$ chloride channel opening. GABA$_A$ is a ligand-gated chloride channel; GABA$_B$ is linked via G-proteins to potassium channels.

How do benzodiazepines differ from barbiturates?

Barbiturates increase GABA$_A$ (see Figure 4-4) signaling by increasing the **duration** of chloride channel opening, which causes hyperpolarization. Barbiturates are contraindicated in porphyria and are used primarily for their sedative effects. Importantly, barbiturates have a greater risk of coma and respiratory depression than benzodiazepines. In clinical practice, benzodiazepines have largely replaced barbiturates.

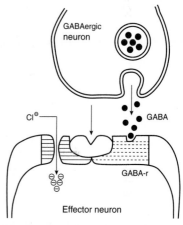

FIGURE 4-4. GABA receptors at work.

Is there an antidote for benzodiazepine overdose or for barbiturate overdose?

Benzodiazepine overdose can be reversed with flumazenil, a competitive antagonist at the GABA receptor. However, flumazenil is used only in a controlled setting due to the risk of unmasking seizures in benzodiazepine-naïve patients. **Barbiturate overdose is more dangerous** because there is no reversal agent. Therefore, symptomatic management and ventilator support are the only treatments for barbiturate overdose.

What is the time course of events that can occur in this condition?

Symptoms of alcohol withdrawal often start 4–10 hours after alcohol cessation (when the blood alcohol concentration drops < 100 mg/dL) and can include symptoms of autonomic hyperactivity (increased respiratory rate, temperature, pulse, sweating), headache, tremors, agitation, and hallucinations. Severity of symptoms usually peak at day 2–3. The most concerning event of alcohol withdrawal is delirium tremens (DT), which is defined by hallucinations, disorientation, hypertension, tachycardia, and fever in the setting of alcohol withdrawal. DT is usually seen 2–4 days after the last drink and can cause life-threatening seizures.

CASE 4

A 36-year-old man is brought to the emergency department by his wife, who explains that he has felt lightheaded, dizzy, and weak. When asked about his medical history, she states that he switched to a new medication to treat his depression. When asked about symptoms of his depression, she states that he had been overeating and oversleeping and had a strange sensation of heaviness in his arms and legs. Physical exam reveals a blood pressure of 80/45 mm Hg.

What class of drug has the patient recently started?

The signs described by the wife indicate atypical depression. Monoamine oxidase inhibitors (MAOIs) are frequently used to treat patients with atypical depression (but not those with typical depression), especially after other medications have failed.

What is the mechanism of action of this class of drugs?

MAOIs (phenelzine, tranylcypromine, selegiline) increase the availability of monoamines such as epinephrine, norepinephrine, and dopamine (MAO_A affects all of these, whereas MAO_B affects only dopamine). They do so by inhibiting MAO, which breaks down such compounds.

What caused this patient's symptoms?

Symptoms of dizziness and lightheadedness have a wide differential, but given this patient's blood pressure and MAOI use, they are likely due to hypotension. Orthostatic hypotension is a common side effect of MAOIs, although the mechanism is not completely understood.

The drugs that could be used to increase this patient's blood pressure act on what receptors?

For a hypotensive patient, activity should be increased on the α_1-receptor. The α_1-receptor is a $G(G_q)$ protein–coupled receptor that vasoconstricts the arteries. Conversely, activity on the α_2-receptor (also a G protein–coupled receptor, but G_i) leads to vasodilation. For this reason, midodrine is preferred to phenylephrine or epinephrine, as it is most selective for α_1. In practice, the most commonly used first-line medication for chronic hypotension is fludrocortisone, which acts by increasing sensitivity of blood vessels to catecholamines and increasing norepinephrine release.

What other precautions should a patient be given when starting this class of drugs?

In addition to the risk of hypotension, paradoxically, various factors can cause a hypertensive crisis in patients taking MAOIs, including coadministration of a sympathomimetic (including over-the-counter drugs such as ephedrine) and ingestion of foods rich in tyramine, such as certain cheeses. In the latter case, when MAO is inhibited, excess tyramine is taken up by adrenergic neurons, which must then release norepinephrine, leading to acute hypertension.

CASE 5

A 32-year-old woman with a history of asthma begins to have difficulty breathing. She has forgotten her inhaler and is brought to the emergency department, where she is noted to be in moderate respiratory distress. She is using her accessory muscles, and her oxygen saturation is 89%. She is becoming anxious because it is increasingly difficult for her to breathe. She is immediately given an inhalant treatment.

What type of drug was likely given?

Short-acting β_2-adrenergic receptor agonists (β_2-agonists) such as albuterol are a mainstay in treating acute asthma. β_2-agonists such as albuterol cause bronchodilation. Other β_2-agonists include terbutaline, metaproterenol, and ritodrine.

In what other locations can this subset of receptors be found?

β_2-adrenergic receptors are found:

- On the smooth muscle of blood vessels, where they induce vasodilation.
- On bronchioles, where they facilitate bronchodilation.
- In pancreatic α cells, where they stimulate glucagon release.
- In the central nervous system.
- On parietal cells of the gastric mucosa, where they stimulate acid secretion.
- In the uterine myometrium, where they cause uterine relaxation.

Stimulation of these receptors activates what second-messenger system?

All adrenergic receptors, including α- and β-adrenergic receptors (see Table 4-1), are G protein–linked receptors, and β_2-receptors are linked to the S class of G proteins.

TABLE 4-1	G Protein–Linked Second Messengers		
	G_I RECEPTOR	G_S RECEPTOR	G_Q RECEPTOR
Action	Adenyl cyclase $\rightarrow \downarrow$ cAMP $\rightarrow \downarrow$ PKA	Adenyl cyclase $\rightarrow \uparrow$ cAMP $\rightarrow \uparrow$ PKA	PLC $\rightarrow PIP_2 \rightarrow IP_3 \rightarrow \uparrow Ca^{2+}$
Types of receptors	α_2 M_2 D_2	$\beta_1, \beta_2, \beta_3$ H_2 D_1 V_2	α_1 M_1, M_3 H_1 V_1

What is the mechanism of action of this subclass of G receptors?

The G_s protein activates adenyl cyclase, which converts adenosine triphosphate to cyclic adenosine monophosphate, which in turn activates protein kinase A (PKA). In uterine myometrial cells, the activated PKA phosphorylates other proteins; this reduces intracellular calcium concentration, decreases activity of myosin light-chain kinase, and diminishes contractility of the uterine muscle cells.

What other classes of receptors are linked to this subclass of G receptors?

Other receptors linked to G_s include β_1, D_1, H_2, and V_2 receptors. Activation of any of these receptors leads to activation of G_s and adenyl cyclase.

■ CASE 6

A 30-year-old farmer is brought to the emergency department with severe diarrhea, shortness of breath, sweating, abdominal pain, and urinary incontinence. The patient appears confused and his speech is slurred. His brother said he saw the farmer drink liquid from an unlabeled bottle approximately 1 hour earlier.

What is the most likely diagnosis?

Organophosphate ingestion. Organophosphates are cholinesterase suicide inhibitors, which cause an excess of acetylcholine (ACh) in the synapse. Organophosphates are commonly found in insecticides and can be ingested, inhaled, or cutaneously absorbed. Organophosphorus nerve agents are a known deadly chemical weapon and have been used to this end in the past—most notably in the 1995 attack on the Tokyo subway system by a religious cult using sarin.

What symptoms can be expected in parasympathetic excess?

Symptoms resulting from parasympathetic excess can be summarized by the mnemonic **DUMBBELSS:** Diarrhea, Urinary incontinence, Miosis, Bronchospasm, Bradycardia, Excitation of skeletal muscle and central nervous system, Lacrimation, Sweating, and Salivation. Central nervous system effects, such as confusion or slurred speech, are common.

What are two treatments and their mechanisms of action?

Atropine and pralidoxime (2-PAM) can reverse organophosphate poisoning. Atropine works by inhibiting muscarinic receptors (it has little effect at nicotinic receptors), thereby decreasing the effect of acetylcholine. 2-PAM works by inhibiting the binding of organophosphates to acetylcholinesterase. A schematic of neuromuscular blockade is shown in Figure 4-5.

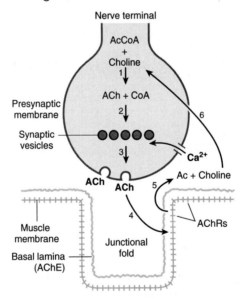

FIGURE 4-5. Representation of some of the events involved in neurotransmitter synthesis, release, and action at a prototypic synapse, the neuromuscular junction. Acetylcholine (ACh) is the transmitter at this synapse. Synthesis of ACh occurs in the presynaptic terminal from acetyl-coenzyme A (CoA) and choline (1). ACh is then incorporated into membrane-bound synaptic vessels (2). Exocytosis of ACh then occurs via the fusion of the vesicles with the presynaptic membrane, which is also mediated by an influx of Ca^{2+}, which is triggered by the action potential (3). Approximately 200 synaptic vesicles are released into the synaptic cleft in response to a single action potential. The released ACh diffuses rapidly across the synaptic cleft (4) and binds to postsynaptic ACh receptors (5), where a conformational change in the channel triggers the influx of Na^+ ions into the muscle, which depolarizes the membrane. Once the channel closes, the ACh dissociates and is hydrolyzed by acetylcholinesterase (6). (Reproduced, with permission, from Waxman SG. *Clinical Neuroanatomy*, 26th ed. New York: McGraw-Hill, 2010: Figure 3-9.)

What adverse events are associated with this treatment?

Atropine poisoning can lead to sympathomimetic adverse effects, including pupillary dilation, decreased gastrointestinal motility, increased body temperature, rapid heart rate, dry mouth, dry skin, constipation, and disorientation.

■ CASE 7

A 53-year-old woman presents to her primary care physician for a follow-up visit after having high blood pressure on her last visit. She is again found to be hypertensive and is prescribed hydralazine, a β-blocker, and furosemide. The woman takes no additional prescription or over-the-counter medications. She complains of muscle aches, joint pain, and rash. Physical exam reveals a temperature of 37.7°C (100.0°F) and a scaling erythematous rash on her face. The physician orders an autoantibody panel that yields the following results:

Antinuclear antibodies (ANA): Positive
Anti–ribonucleic protein (RNP) antibodies: Negative
Anti-Smith (Sm) antibodies: Negative
Anti-DNA antibodies: Negative
Anti-histone antibodies: Positive
Rheumatoid factor: Negative

What is the most likely diagnosis?
Rash, arthralgias, and antihistone antibodies suggest drug-induced systemic lupus erythematosus (SLE). Hydralazine is the causative drug in this case. Positive ANA is nonspecific, as there are many conditions, mostly infectious and autoimmune, that show positive ANA. However, the sensitivity of ANA for drug-induced SLE is 100%, so if ANA is negative, drug-induced SLE can be ruled out.

What other medications can cause a similar presentation?
Drugs known to induce SLE include procainamide, chlorpromazine, isoniazid, methyldopa, minocycline, penicillamine, and diltiazem.

How do spontaneous forms of this disorder differ from drug-induced forms?
Whereas hematologic abnormalities (anemias) are common in spontaneous SLE, they are unusual in drug-induced SLE. Also, rash is common in spontaneous SLE but is not frequent in drug-induced SLE.

■ CASE 8

A small biotechnology company has developed a new drug that holds promise for the treatment of osteoarthritis. Currently, it is being tested on a group of 100 patients with osteoarthritis, some of whom are receiving placebo.

In which phase of testing is this drug?

The drug is in **phase 2** of clinical testing, which entails the enrollment of a small group of patients, usually 100–300, into a trial. The trial, usually single-blinded, compares the new product to placebo as well as to an older drug that has already been proven effective.

What characterizes the phase of testing that the drug has already been through?

The first step of clinical testing, **phase 1**, involves nonblinded testing on a small group (20–30) of healthy volunteers (see Figure 4-6). The goals in this phase are to determine if the response of humans to the drug is significantly different from the response of animals (before reaching clinical trials, a drug is extensively tested on animals for toxicity, carcinogenicity, etc.) and whether the effects of the drug are a function of dose (Figure 4-7).

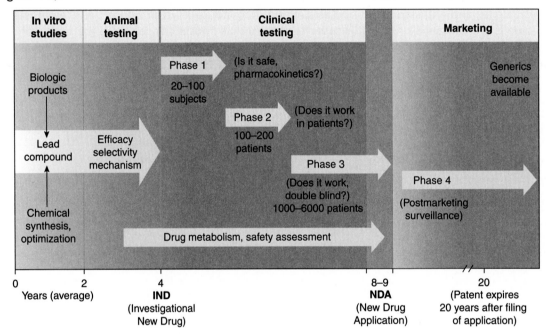

FIGURE 4-6. **Phases of the FDA review process.** (Adapted with permission from Katzung BG, Trevor AJ. *Pharmacology: Examination & Board Review,* 5th ed. Stamford, CT: Appleton & Lange, 1998: 365. Copyright © The McGraw-Hill Companies, Inc.)

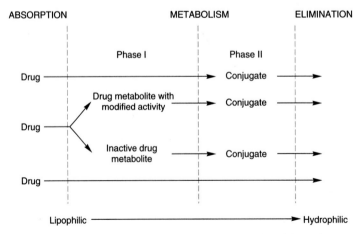

FIGURE 4-7. **Phase I and phase II reactions.** (Reproduced, with permission, from Katzung BG. *Basic & Clinical Pharmacology,* 9th ed. New York: McGraw-Hill, 2004: 52.)

What happens in the next phases of testing?

Phase 3 testing involves evaluating the drug in a trial of a large group of patients (hundreds to thousands). The trial is usually double-blinded and evaluates the overall benefit-risk relationship to provide an adequate basis for physician labeling. If phase 3 testing is successful, the company will submit a New Drug Application to the Food and Drug Administration (FDA), which will include preclinical and clinical data. The FDA will then review this material and if the drug is approved for market, phase 4 testing starts. **Phase 4 entails monitoring the drug as it is used in real conditions with large numbers of patients. This phase is important for discovering low-incidence toxicities that would not be uncovered in clinical trials.** Phase 4 is the last phase of testing and continues indefinitely.

What is a double-blinded study and why is it the most powerful type of research study?

In a **double-blinded** study, neither the subjects nor researchers know who is receiving the experimental drug and who is receiving placebo. Masking this information eliminates both observer and subject bias, which is why it is considered to be the best format for obtaining objective data.

If this drug passes all phases of testing, when will a generic form become available?

A drug patent is typically issued for 20 years, after which time generic forms become available. However, the evaluation of the application by the FDA may take several years. Up to 5 years of the review time may be added back to the patent.

■ CASE 9

A man calls the police because he hears someone moving around in the garage of his house. When the police arrive, they find an intoxicated homeless man with slurred speech collapsed by a closet full of automotive supplies. The homeless man is immediately rushed to the emergency department. Blood tests show a large anion gap acidosis and markedly elevated creatinine. Eye exam is normal.

What is the most likely diagnosis?

This could be either methanol or ethylene glycol poisoning, as both are found in antifreeze. However, the most likely diagnosis is ethylene glycol poisoning because methanol poisoning leads to ophthalmologic abnormalities such as afferent papillary defect and mydriasis. Ethylene glycol has a mildly sweet taste, which allows unintentional consumption by both children and adults, often in large quantities. Although ethylene glycol and methanol themselves are mostly nontoxic, accumulation of the metabolites (see Figure 4-8) is toxic.

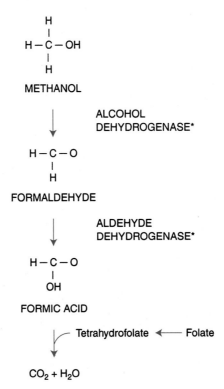

FIGURE 4-8. **Methanol metabolism.** *Blocked by ethanol and fomepizole.

Without treatment, what symptoms would likely occur?

Ethylene glycol poisoning typically follows three stages. Stage 1 is pure intoxication with dizziness and slurred speech. Stage 2 comprises metabolic acidosis, tachycardia, and hypertension due to the toxic metabolite **oxalic acid** that is formed by metabolism of ethylene glycol by alcohol dehydrogenase. Stage 3 is often kidney failure.

Why might kidney failure occur if this patient is not treated?

Alcohol dehydrogenase is an endogenous enzyme that can metabolize ethanol, methanol, and ethylene glycol to eventually produce acetate, formaldehyde, and oxalate, respectively. The calcium in the kidney can combine with the oxalate to produce calcium oxalate crystals in the kidney, which causes renal failure.

What is the treatment for toxic alcohol poisoning?

There are three possible treatments:
- **Fomepizole** (Figure 4-9) is a competitive inhibitor of alcohol dehydrogenase. It blocks metabolism of ethylene glycol (or methanol), allowing it to be excreted in a harmless premetabolic stage.
- An intravenous infusion of alcohol can be administered if fomepizole is not available.
- Hemodialysis may be needed in patients that present with ethylene glycol toxicity late enough that their kidneys are severely affected.

Of note, gastric lavage and emesis are no longer recommended methods of decontamination for any ingestion.

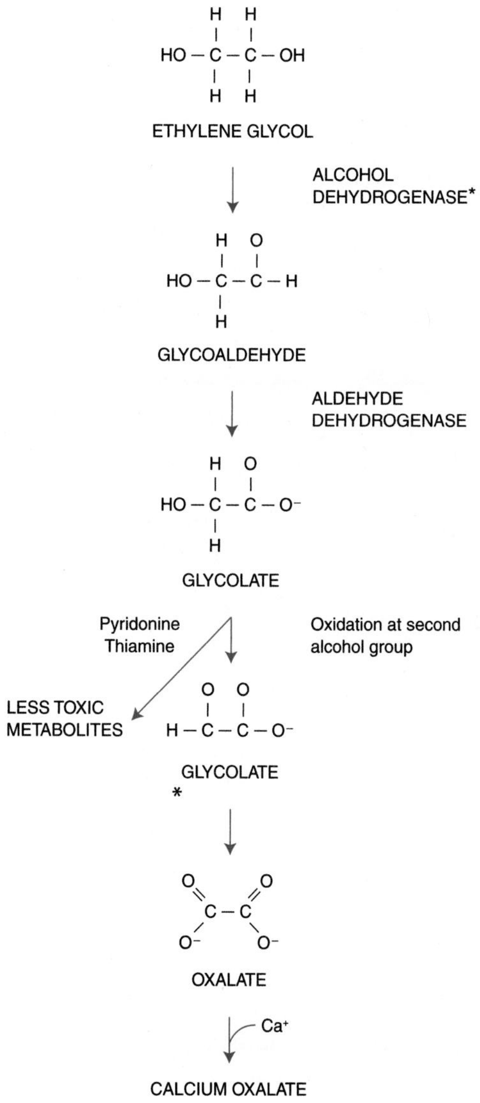

FIGURE 4-9. **Ethylene glycol metabolism.** *Blocked by ethanol and fomepizole.

▪ CASE 10

3-year-old boy is brought to the emergency department by his grandmother who states that she saw the boy playing around old paint cans in the basement. For the past several days she has noticed that his appetite has decreased and he has indicated that his tummy hurts.

What is the most likely diagnosis?

Subacute lead poisoning. In terms of presentation, abdominal colic is one of the hallmark symptoms of lead poisoning and can be followed by bloody diarrhea.

If a smear of this patient's blood were examined microscopically, what signs would help confirm the diagnosis?

Basophilic stippling of erythrocytes (see Figure 4-10) is commonly seen with lead poisoning. In addition, lead poisoning may present in the form of sideroblastic anemia. Sideroblastic anemias impair heme synthesis in developing RBCs, leading to impaired hemoglobin production and the formation of hypochromic and microcytic cells. In addition to lead poisoning, sideroblastic anemia can also be seen in alcoholism, prescription drug use (isoniazid, chloramphenicol), copper deficiency, refractory anemia, and some rare congenital diseases.

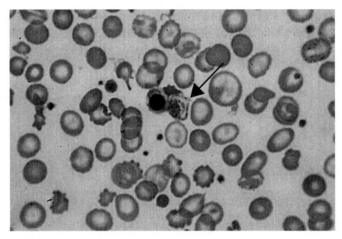

FIGURE 4-10. Stippled red cell. (Adapted, with permission, from Lichtman MA, et al. *Lichtman's Atlas of Hematology*. New York: McGraw-Hill, 2010: Figure I.C. 142.)

What neurologic complications can occur in this condition?

Lead poisoning may present with a range of neurological symptoms, including hearing loss, developmental delay, and neuropathies. Two neuropathies often seen are wrist and foot drop, reflecting radial and common peroneal neuropathies, respectively. Lead poisoning may also cause encephalopathy.

What radiographic findings might be present in chronic forms of this condition?

In chronic pediatric lead poisoning, lead deposits can form in the epiphyses of long bones.

How does treatment differ between children and adults with this condition?

In both children and adults, further prevention of lead exposure is the most important treatment. Succimer is a water-soluble analog of dimercaprol and can be used to treat children with lead poisoning as it increases the excretion of lead. For adults, the first-line treatment is ethylenediaminetetraacetic acid (EDTA) and dimercaprol.

■ CASE 11

Several new drugs are being tested for their effects on β_2-adrenergic receptors. The investigator plots an S-shaped curve of the activity of adenylate cyclase vs. drug dose in response to drug A. When the response of drug D is similarly plotted, D is found to have a lower median effective dose (ED_{50}) and a lower maximal response than A. In the presence of drug A plus drug B, the curve has the same shape but is now shifted to the right. In the presence of drug A plus drug C, the curve is not shifted, but the maximal response is lower.

Which drug, A or D, has a higher efficacy?

Efficacy refers to the maximal response a drug elicits. Thus, drug A has a higher efficacy, since it produces a higher maximal response (Figure 4-11).

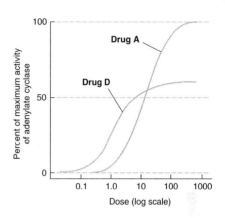

FIGURE 4-11. Dose-response curves comparing drug A and drug D.

Which drug is more potent?

Drug D is more potent (Figure 4-11). **Potency** is the amount of drug required for a specified response. Typically, potency is measured by the ED_{50}, or the dose that gives 50% of the maximal response. The *lower* the ED_{50}, the more potent the drug.

What type of antagonist is drug B?

Drug B is a competitive antagonist—that is, it binds to the same site on the receptor as does drug A (Figure 4-12A). It does not affect the maximal response the agonist can elicit, but it does increase the ED_{50}, requiring more agonist to achieve the same response, thus decreasing potency.

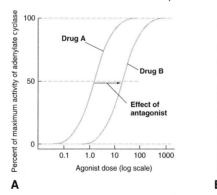
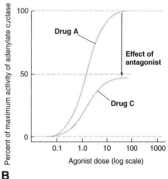

FIGURE 4-12. A and B: Dose-response curves showing drug A, drug B, and drug C.

What type of antagonist is drug C?

Drug C is a **noncompetitive antagonist** (Figure 4-12B). These drugs act by binding irreversibly to a site on the receptor distinct from the site of agonist binding. Noncompetitive antagonists do not affect the ED_{50} but do affect the maximal response (decrease efficacy) that the agonist can elicit.

How can the effect of drug B be overcome?

Since **competitive antagonists** bind at the same site as the agonist, their action can be overcome by increasing agonist dose. If enough agonist is present, the same efficacy can be reached that the agonist had in the absence of an antagonist.

■ CASE 12

The kinetics of a new pharmaceutical agent is being tested in an animal model. A dose of 50 mg of the substance is injected intravenously into a rat. The concentration of the substance in the animal's blood is measured every 30 minutes thereafter for the next 10 hours. The concentration of the drug plotted against time produces the graph shown in Figure 4-13.

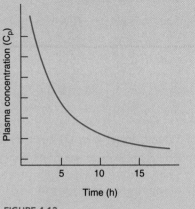

FIGURE 4-13.

Is this substance being metabolized by first-order or zero-order kinetics?

The shape of the graph shows that the drug is being eliminated by **first-order kinetics** (see Figure 4-14A), meaning that a constant **fraction** of the substance is eliminated per unit of time. As a result, the rate of elimination is proportional to the concentration of the drug. By contrast, **zero-order kinetics** (see Figure 4-14B) results in a constant **amount** of the substance being cleared per unit of time; the elimination rate is constant regardless of the **plasma concentration** (C_p), and the plot of C_p vs. time is a straight line.

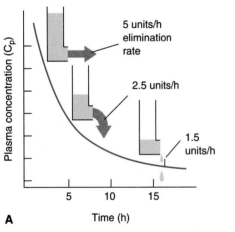
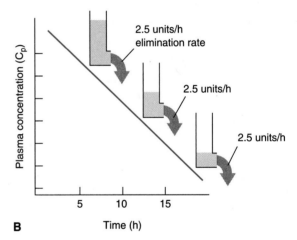

A   Time (h)   **B**   Time (h)

FIGURE 4-14. **First-order drug elimination (A) and zero-order drug elimination (B).** (Reproduced, with permission, from Katzung BG, Trevor AJ. *Pharmacology: Examination & Board Review*, 5th ed. Stamford, CT: Appleton & Lange. Copyright by McGraw-Hill, 1998: 5.)

Which drugs follow zero-order kinetics?

Nearly all medications follow first-order kinetics. Three notable exceptions are aspirin, phenytoin, and alcohol.

Why does the volume of distribution affect the half-life of a drug?

Volume of distribution (V_d) is the theoretical volume in which the total amount of drug would need to be uniformly distributed to produce the desired blood concentration of a drug. A useful equation is the following:

$$V_d = \text{Clearance} \sim t_{1/2}/0.7$$

As indicated by the equation above, $t_{1/2}$ is directly proportional to V_d. This is because the larger the V_d, the smaller the amount of drug present in the plasma compartment and therefore the smaller the amount of drug circulated through the kidneys and liver for metabolism and excretion.

What is the half-life of this substance, and how does the half-life change if a dosage of 100 mg is administered?

Half-life ($t_{1/2}$) is the time necessary to decrease the C_p of the drug by 50%. As shown in Figure 4-13, at 5 hours the C_p of the drug is half of the initial concentration, and thus $t_{1/2}$ is 5 hours. Half-life does not depend on the size of the dose being eliminated.

How would the therapeutic index of this drug be determined, and why is this important?

Therapeutic index is the ratio of a drug's toxic dose to the therapeutic dose. Safe drugs will have a high therapeutic index, indicating a large difference between the dose used to treat patients and the dose resulting in toxicity. Drugs with a low index, such as digoxin, have to be carefully monitored by checking serum levels of the drug.

$$\text{Therapeutic ratio} = \frac{LD_{50}}{ED_{50}}$$

LD_{50} = lethal dose of drug for 50% of population.

ED_{50} = effective dose of drug for 50% of population. Case 13

◼ CASE 13

A 17-year-old high school student is brought to the emergency department after feeling a tearing sensation in his knee when he was tackled playing football. After the initial consult, it is determined that the boy will need surgery to reattach a torn ligament. During anesthesia, a neuromuscular blocking drug (NMBD) is given.

In what clinical settings are NMBDs used?

The NMBDs are used for muscle paralysis during surgery or mechanical ventilation.

What are some examples of NMBD drugs?

Examples of these agents include succinylcholine, tubocurarine, and most drugs that end in "–curium" (eg, atracurium) or "–curonium" (eg, rocuronium).

For what type of receptors is this class of drug selective?

Neuromuscular agents are specific for the motor nicotinic acetylcholine receptors present at the neuromuscular junction.

What are the two types of neuromuscular blocking drugs?

There are depolarizing and nondepolarizing (of which succinylcholine is the only one commonly used) blocking agents.

What is the mechanism of action of depolarizing blocking agents?

Depolarizing agents such as succinylcholine act in two phases. Phase I consists of active depolarization of sodium channels, which can be potentiated by cholinesterase inhibitors. Phase II keeps sodium channels stuck in their depolarized state. Phase II can be **reversed** with cholinesterase inhibitors.

What is the mechanism of action of nondepolarizing blocking agents?

These drugs are mostly close relatives of tubocurarine. They act by competing with acetylcholine for nicotinic motor receptors. These drugs can be reversed using cholinesterase inhibitors.

What is an important potential risk of using succinylcholine?

The combination of inhalational anesthetics and succinylcholine may result in malignant hyperthermia (sympathetic hyperactivity, muscular rigidity, acidosis) due to the prevention of calcium release from the sarcoplasmic reticulum of skeletal muscle. This condition can be treated with dantrolene.

5

Cardiovascular

▉ CASE 1

A 75-year-old man visits his physician complaining of lower back pain. He has a history of hyperlipidemia and hypertension. On physical examination, he is obese and has moderately limited range of motion of the back. MRI shows that the abdominal aorta is dilated to 4 cm, 200% its normal size.

What is the most likely diagnosis?
Abdominal aortic aneurysm (AAA).

What are the major branches of the aorta below the diaphragm?
Blood flow to the major organs is of special concern with an AAA. The inferior phrenic arteries, celiac trunk, middle suprarenal arteries, renal arteries, superior mesenteric artery, testicular arteries, inferior mesenteric artery, lumbar arteries, and the common iliac arteries are located below the diaphragm (Figure 5-1).

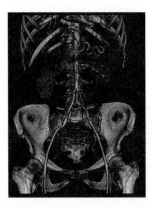

FIGURE 5-1. **3D reconstruction of CT angiogram in a healthy person.** (Reproduced, with permission, from Fuster V, et al. *Hurst's The Heart*, 11th ed. New York: McGraw-Hill, 2004: 652.)

What is the three-layer composition of muscular arteries?
- The **tunica intima** is adjacent to the lumen and includes the endothelial layer and the internal elastic lamina.
- The **tunica media** includes smooth muscle, collagen, and reticular and elastic fibers.
- The **tunica adventitia** contains blood and lymph vessels and nerves supplying the artery.

An increased risk of AAA is associated with defects in the genes coding for which proteins?
Fibrillin and **collagen.** Marfan syndrome is linked to a mutation in the fibrillin-1 gene. Ehlers-Danlos syndrome results from various defects in collagen synthesis or structure. Both syndromes are associated with an increased incidence of AAA.

Once the aortic wall is disrupted, how does coagulation proceed?
Exposure of tissue factor in the vessel wall initiates the extrinsic pathway of coagulation. Circulating factor VII comes into contact with tissue factor, activating factor X. Activated factor X helps convert prothrombin to thrombin. Thrombin then cleaves fibrinogen to fibrin, allowing fibrin deposition and cross-linking to form a clot. The functionality of the extrinsic pathway is measured by the prothrombin time and International Normalized Ratio.

What are the risk factors for this condition?
AAA occurs most frequently in males. Advanced age and smoking are the most common risk factors. Atherosclerotic lesions in the abdominal aorta are thought to increase the risk of AAA; by contrast, hypertension is thought to increase the risk of aortic dissection. Other risk factors for aneurysmal disease of the aorta include aortic infection, trauma, vasculitis, and connective tissue disorders such as cystic medial necrosis as seen in Ehlers-Danlos syndrome or Marfan syndrome.

What are the treatment options for this condition?
A small, asymptomatic AAA can be treated conservatively with frequent ultrasound surveillance and smoking cessation. Rapidly expanding aneurysms or those > 5.5 cm in diameter require surgical repair.

■ CASE 2

A 65-year-old man presents to his cardiologist for evaluation of recurrent episodes of lightheadedness, chest pain, and shortness of breath with exertion. One week earlier, he experienced an episode of syncope while walking up the stairs to his house. Doppler echocardiography demonstrates a heavily calcified aortic valve with a calculated valve area that is 40% its normal size. Echocardiogram is shown in Figure 5-2).

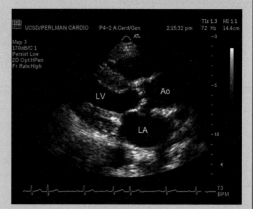

FIGURE 5-2. (Reproduced, with permission, from Fuster V, et al. *Hurst's The Heart,* 12th ed. New York: McGraw-Hill, Figure 18-59.)

What is the most likely diagnosis?

Aortic stenosis.

What factors increase the risk of this condition?

Aortic stenosis is commonly associated with older age, male gender, hypercholesterolemia, rheumatic fever, and congenital bicuspid aortic valve.

What type of murmur is caused by this condition?

The murmur of aortic stenosis is a **systolic ejection murmur** at the right upper sternal border, radiating to the neck. Signs of a severely stenosed valve include peaking of the murmur late in systole, palpable delay of the carotid upstroke, soft second heart sound, and an S_4 gallop.

How is this condition associated with congestive heart failure (CHF)?

Aortic stenosis implies narrowing of the aortic valve, causing resistance to outflow of blood. In severe stenosis (valve area < 50% of normal size), the narrowed valve causes increased pressure to build up in the left ventricle (LV), leading to concentric left ventricular hypertrophy (LVH). Although the LV initially responds to the increased pressure by thickening its walls, the increasing wall stress eventually decreases LV function, leading to CHF. LVH also compromises coronary blood flow during exertion and can lead to angina.

What complications are associated with this condition?

- **Angina:** Without intervention, 50% of patients with angina die within 5 years.
- **Syncope with effort:** 50% of patients die within 3 years.
- **Dyspnea on exertion:** 50% of patients die within 2 years.
- **Poststenotic aortic dilation:** Dilation of aortic root due to high-pressure flow through the narrow valve increases the risk of aortic dissection.

What is the appropriate treatment for this condition?

Valve replacement is recommended in patients with symptomatic, severe aortic stenosis, as 10-year survival rates after replacement are comparable with those of the normal population. Mechanical intervention, such as **balloon valvotomy,** provides only temporary symptomatic relief for patients with calcified valves and offers no survival benefit. Sodium restriction and cautious use of diuretics may be indicated in the setting of CHF. Excessive volume depletion should be avoided to prevent hypotension.

CASE 3

A 58-year-old man comes to the physician complaining of occasional chest pain that occurs with strenuous activity. He is obese and has a history of hypertension and diabetes mellitus. During the physical examination, he admits to eating most of his meals at fast food restaurants. He also reports he has little time for exercise.

What is the most likely diagnosis?

Stable angina, characterized by chest pain with exertion, is often secondary to atherosclerosis. Stable angina is chest discomfort that occurs only during activity and resolves within several minutes of ceasing the activity. Patients with stable angina have minimal or no chest pain at rest. By contrast, unstable angina is defined as chest pain that changes or worsens. Unstable angina occurs at rest or increases in frequency, severity, or duration.

What risk factors increase a person's likelihood of developing this condition?

Hypertension, diabetes mellitus, advanced age, gender, and hyperlipidemia are major risk factors for atherosclerosis. Family history and smoking are also risk factors. Obesity and lack of exercise have not been definitively linked to increased risk of atherosclerosis.

What is the pathophysiology of this condition?

Endothelial injury resulting from various factors, including hyperlipidemia, smoking, and hypertension, can lead to monocytic and lipid infiltrates into the subendothelium (fatty streaks), release of growth factors leading to smooth muscle cell proliferation into the intima (proliferative plaque), and subsequent development of foam cells and complex atheromas with calcification and ischemia of the intima (Figure 5-3).

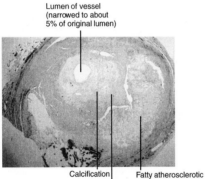

Lumen of vessel
(narrowed to about
5% of original lumen)

Calcification   Fatty atherosclerotic
                  plaque (lipid zone)
     Fibrous cap

FIGURE 5-3. Cross-section of atherosclerotic artery. (Reproduced, with permission, from Le T, et al. *First Aid for the USMLE Step 1: 2011*. New York: McGraw-Hill, 2011: 270.)

Which arteries are most commonly affected in this condition?

Atherosclerosis preferentially affects the branching points of arteries or areas of turbulent blood flow including the proximal coronary arteries, popliteal arteries, renal arteries, carotid arteries, and arteries of the circle of Willis.

What complications are commonly associated with this condition?

In addition to angina, other complications of atherosclerotic injury include aneurysms, myocardial infarction, stroke, ischemia, and ischemic bowel disease.

What are the major forms of angina?

- **Stable angina:** Chest pain with exertion; responds to nitroglycerin.
- **Unstable angina:** Chest pain at rest secondary to thrombus in a branch. May not completely respond to nitroglycerin; antithrombic agents and heparin may also be required.
- **Prinzmetal angina:** Chest pain at rest, secondary to coronary artery spasm. Treatment includes calcium channel blockers.

■ CASE 4

A 58-year-old woman comes to the physician's office complaining of feeling lightheaded for the past week. She says she can feel her heart racing in her chest. She mentions she has been staying up late for the past few weeks because of her workload. Medical history reveals well-controlled diabetes mellitus. Physical examination reveals an anxious woman with pallor and mild diaphoresis. Cardiac examination reveals an irregularly irregular beat. Vital signs are as follows:

Temperature: 36.1°C (97.0°F)
Respiratory rate: 22/min
Heart rate: 142/min
Blood pressure: 118/55 mm Hg
Glucose: 130 mg/dL

What is the likely diagnosis?

Atrial fibrillation.

What clinical and electrocardiographic abnormalities are commonly associated with this condition?

Lightheadedness, palpitations, anxiety, pallor, and diaphoresis are commonly associated with atrial fibrillation. Likewise, as in this patient, heart rate is elevated and borderline hypotension is possible. Electrocardiogram (ECG) shows an absence of P waves, irregular R-R intervals, and tachycardia, as in this patient. Irregularly irregular uncoordinated atrial contractions can lead to tachycardia and stasis of blood in the left atrium; the development of clot within the heart often ensues (Figure 5-4).

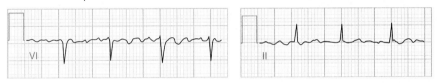

FIGURE 5-4. **ECG strip in atrial fibrillation.** (Reproduced, with permission, from Fauci AS, et al. *Harrison's Principles of Internal Medicine*, 17th ed. New York: McGraw-Hill, 2008: Figure 226-4A.)

What is the appropriate treatment for this condition?

The patient's high heart rate needs to be slowed; to this end, β-blockers, calcium channel blockers, or digoxin are indicated. Metoprolol is a $β_1$-blocker that slows conduction through the atrioventricular node, thereby slowing heart rate. Cardioversion to a normal sinus rhythm may also be considered. However, care must be taken not to promote thromboembolism, which can occur if cardioversion is performed more than 48 hours after the onset of atrial fibrillation due to stasis of blood within the atrium. A transesophageal echocardiogram can screen for a left atrial thrombus, or the patient may be given an anticoagulant like warfarin for several weeks before cardioversion is attempted.

How do heparin and warfarin work together to treat this condition?

Given intravenously, heparin activates antithrombin III. Its effectiveness is determined by partial thromboplastin time (which reflects activity of the intrinsic pathway). Given orally, warfarin impairs the synthesis of vitamin K–dependent clotting factors (II, VII, IX, and X). It is monitored by prothrombin time (extrinsic pathway).

Why does paradoxical coagulation sometimes occur after starting warfarin therapy?

Warfarin also inhibits the synthesis of protein C and protein S. Because proteins C and S inhibit factors Va and VIIIa, a deficiency in these proteins promotes coagulation.

CASE 5

A 50-year-old woman presents to her physician with a several-day history of fever, night sweats, and chills and increasing dyspnea during her regular walks. She also reports having a transient weakness in her right arm approximately 2 weeks ago, which has spontaneously resolved. She denies chest pain, arthralgia, myalgia, or rash. Medical history and family history are unremarkable. Physical examination is notable for a fever of 38°C (100.4°F), a heart rate of 90/min, and a respiratory rate of 12/min. On cardiac auscultation, a loud split S_1 and a diastolic third heart sound are heard. Rales and increased tactile fremitus are present in both lung fields.

What is the most likely diagnosis?

Cardiac myxoma of the left atrium. Most myxomas arise from the mural endocardium and measure 1–15 cm.

What conditions should be included in the differential diagnosis?

- **Endocarditis:** Constitutional symptoms are common with atrial myxomas. However, this patient's transient right-arm weakness suggests embolization. This, combined with her fevers, chills, and sweats, makes infective endocarditis a possibility.
- **Vasculitis:** A peripheral vasculitis should be considered if the patient has arthralgia, myalgia, or rash, which occur in some patients with myxomas. Polyarteritis nodosa can cause multiple arterial aneurysms.
- **Transient ischemic attack** (TIA): Although not typically associated with constitutional symptoms, transient episodes of weakness or other neurological deficits may be secondary to TIAs caused by carotid artery plaque burden. Carotid ultrasound can exclude this possibility.

The patient's rales and increased fremitus may represent atelectasis or consolidation at the lung bases.

What is the epidemiology of this condition?

Primary tumors of the heart are rare. Myxomas account for approximately 50% of benign tumors in the heart. The majority (75%) are located in the left atrium, although all chambers can be affected. The typical age of onset is 30–60 years. Familial occurrences have been reported in approximately 5% of cases via autosomal dominant transmission. These are associated with a younger age of presentation and higher rates of recurrence.

What complications may result from this condition?

Complications from left atrial myxomas can be categorized as follows:

- **Embolization** occurs in 40%–50% of cases with tumor fragments lodging in distal organs (eg, brain, heart, or extremities).
- **Infection** is rare but may lead to further complications with embolization.
- **Obstruction** of the mitral or pulmonary venous orifices may occur, resulting in pulmonary hypertension and right heart failure.

How can the results of the cardiac examination be explained?

Splitting of S_1 is accentuated as the tumor is extruded from the mitral orifice. P_2 can also be louder if the tumor obstructs the mitral orifice or pulmonary venous return. The third heart sound is produced by the tumor "plopping" within the atrium during diastole.

■ CASE 6

A 55-year-old man comes to his physician for a follow-up visit, after being hospitalized 2 weeks earlier for an inferior wall myocardial infarction (MI). The patient has a history of coronary artery disease. His ECG is shown in Figure 5-5.

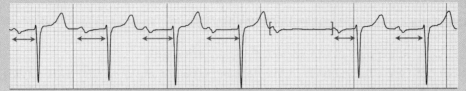

FIGURE 5-5. (Reproduced, with permission, from Knoop KJ, et al. *The Atlas of Emergency Medicine*, 3rd ed. New York: McGraw-Hill, 2010, Figure 23.15B.)

What pathology does the ECG in Figure 5-5 depict?

Second-degree atrioventricular (AV) block type I, also known as **Mobitz type I block** or **Wenckebach block**. Progressive lengthening of the PR interval from one beat to the next is seen until finally a beat is dropped (a P wave is not followed by a QRS complex).

What is the pathophysiology of this condition?

Second-degree AV block type I occurs secondary to impaired conduction at the level of the AV node, such that atrial impulses fail to reach the ventricles. Given the location of the patient's prior MI, it is possible that it may have compromised the conductive ability of his AV node. An MI involving the right coronary artery may disrupt blood supply to the sinoatrial [SA] node and atrioventricular [AV] node. By contrast, involvement of the left anterior descending coronary artery causes infarction of the His-Purkinje system.

How is this condition classified?

In **first-degree block**, the PR interval is prolonged but there are no missed beats (a QRS complex follows every P wave) (Figure 5-6A).

In **second-degree block**, there is intermittent failure of AV conduction. In a **Mobitz type I block**, the PR interval progressively lengthens until a beat is dropped (Figure 5-5). In a **Mobitz type II block**, there is a sudden loss of impulse conduction without a corresponding change in PR interval. Mobitz type II may progress to more serious arrhythmias such as complete heart block (Figure 5-6B).

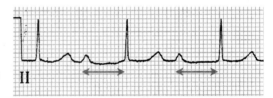

FIGURE 5-6A. **First-degree AV block.** The PR interval is fixed (double arrows) and is longer than 0.2 seconds, or five small blocks. (Reproduced, with permission, from Knoop KJ, et al. *The Atlas of Emergency Medicine*, 3rd ed. New York: McGraw-Hill, 2010, Figure 23-14B.)

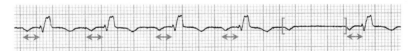

FIGURE 5-6B. **Mobitz type II second-degree heart block.** The PR interval is constant (double arrows) until the dropped beat (brackets). (Reproduced, with permission, from Knoop KJ, et al. *The Atlas of Emergency Medicine*, 3rd ed. New York: McGraw-Hill, 2010, Figure 23-16B.)

In **third-degree block** (also known as **complete heart block**), there is no conduction via the AV node; atrial impulses do not reach the ventricles, and the ventricles beat at their intrinsic pace (Figure 5-6C). On ECG, this is reflected as P waves and QRS complexes occurring independently of each other.

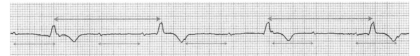

FIGURE 5-6C. **Third-degree heart block.** The P-P interval is uniform (lower double arrows) and the R-R interval is uniform (upper double arrows), but the P waves and QRS complexes are disassociated. (Reproduced, with permission, from Knoop KJ, et al. *The Atlas of Emergency Medicine*, 3rd ed. New York: McGraw-Hill, 2010, Figure 23-17B.)

What is the appropriate treatment for this condition?

Often, no treatment is necessary in asymptomatic patients with a second-degree Mobitz type I block. In symptomatic patients, atropine or isoproterenol may be used, or a pacemaker may be required.

■ CASE 7

A 2-week-old baby boy is seen in the pediatrician's office for a well-baby checkup. On physical examination, the baby's femoral pulses are weak and delayed bilaterally.

What is the most likely diagnosis?

Coarctation of the aorta occurs two to five times more often in males than in females.

In this condition, which part of the aorta is typically affected?

In the majority of cases, the lesion is in the descending aorta, distal to the origin of the left subclavian artery and in the periductal region. Disease course depends on the degree of obstruction after ductal closure, the presence of collateral circulation, and any associated cardiac anomalies. Less severe forms are characterized by an isolated aortic narrowing and the presence of adequate collateral flow. These forms progress gradually and become symptomatic between the second and third decades of life. Severe, symptomatic disease in early infancy (< 10 days of age) occurs if the coarctation is associated with additional cardiac anomalies and/or inadequate collateral flow to compensate for ductal closure. Figure 5-7 shows the anatomic features of aortic coarctation.

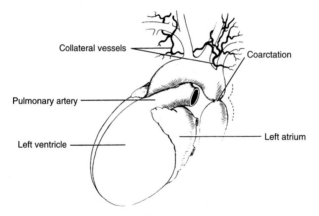

FIGURE 5-7. **Anatomic features of aortic coarctation.** (Reproduced, with permission, from Cheitlin M, et al. *Clinical Cardiology.* New York, NY: Appleton & Lange. Copyright by McGraw-Hill, 1993.)

What is the characteristic finding on physical examination?

Auscultation over the chest and/or back may reveal a midsystolic ejection murmur. A continuous murmur over the chest may also be heard in older individuals who have developed collateral circulation. Weak, delayed pulses in the lower extremities are also characteristic of coarctation.

What chromosomal abnormality is associated with this condition?

Coarctation of the aorta is associated with Turner syndrome (45,XO).

What findings on physical examination, ECG, and x-ray of the chest often develop over time in patients with this condition?

Many patients develop hypertension of the upper extremities with weak, delayed femoral pulses. If the coarctation is proximal to the point of division of the left subclavian artery, the systolic pressure in the right arm may be greater than that in both the lower extremities and the left arm.

Left ventricular hypertrophy is a common finding on ECG.

X-ray of the chest often shows an indented aorta and/or notching of the inferior surface of the ribs, usually around 7 years of age. This notching is the result of increased blood flow through the intrathoracic and intercostal vessels, which serve as collateral circulation.

CASE 8

A 2-day-old baby is observed to have purpuric skin lesions (Figure 5-8). His mother recently emigrated from a developing country. Her pregnancy is notable for a flulike illness involving a maculopapular rash of her face and body several weeks after her last menstrual period. Physical examination of the neonate reveals a low birth weight, cataracts, and a grade II/VI harsh crescendo-decrescendo systolic murmur most audible at the left upper sternal border with radiation to the axilla and back. Laboratory testing demonstrates thrombocytopenia.

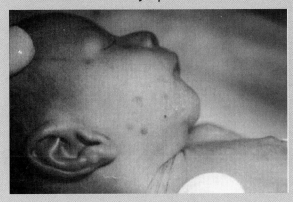

FIGURE 5-8. (Reproduced, with permission, from Lichtman MA, et al. *Lichtman's Atlas of Hematology.* New York: McGraw-Hill, 2007: Figure XI.A.56.)

What is the most likely diagnosis?

This constellation of clinical findings, including cardiac manifestations, a "blueberry muffin" rash, and the maternal history strongly suggest **congenital rubella syndrome** (CRS). Rubella virus (RV) is an RNA virus of the Togaviridae family, and it is associated with an 85% risk of congenital defects if acquired in the first 12 weeks of pregnancy. Other infections acquired in utero that can present with rash and ocular findings can be recalled with the **ToRCHeS** acronym: **T**oxoplasmosis, **o**ther infections, **R**ubella, **C**ytomegalovirus infection, **He**rpes simplex, and **S**yphilis.

What laboratory test in the neonate can help confirm this diagnosis?

Viral culture of nasal secretions or monthly serology testing for anti-rubella IgM antibody with rising titers can establish a laboratory CRS diagnosis.

What cardiac anomalies are associated with the murmur seen in this patient?

In this patient, the location of the murmur at the left upper sternal border and radiation into the lung fields strongly suggest pulmonary valve or pulmonary artery stenosis, which are common in CRS. A supravalvar or peripheral pulmonary artery stenosis is more likely in this case given the radiation and the absence of a systolic click, which would indicate an obstructed or dysplastic valve. Another common cardiac anomaly of CRS is patent ductus arteriosus. Failure of the ductus arteriosus to close produces a continuous machine-like murmur across the precordium. Prostaglandin E_2 is responsible for maintaining the patent ductus arteriosus; therefore, nonsteroidal anti-inflammatory drugs such as indomethacin are a treatment option.

What other symptoms are common in patients with this condition?

Primary rubella infection early in pregnancy results in defective organogenesis. The classic permanent abnormalities include cataracts, retinopathy, heart defects, and sensorineural deafness. Transient abnormalities include meningoencephalitis, thrombocytopenia with or without purpura, and bony radiolucencies. Since CRS is a persistent infection, more abnormalities, such as developmental difficulties and progressive panencephalitis, can occur.

What is the appropriate treatment for this condition?

Since no therapy currently exists for CRS, the focus is on prevention through vaccination. Rubella vaccine contains live, attenuated rubella virus and therefore is contraindicated in pregnant women. Rubella has been eliminated in the United States and Scandinavia but persists elsewhere because of inadequate vaccination programs.

■ CASE 9

A 56-year-old man with a history of hypertension and hyperlipidemia presents to the emergency department 2 hours after the sudden development of crushing chest pressure and pain radiating to his jaw and left arm. His ECG shows ST elevations in the precordial leads and his cardiac troponin levels are elevated. He undergoes cardiac catheterization, which reveals an occlusion in his left anterior descending (LAD) coronary artery.

Which area of the heart is affected by this obstruction?
The LAD runs along the anterior interventricular (IV) groove and supplies the anterior right and left ventricles as well as the anterior IV septum. The LAD is the most common coronary artery to become occluded.

From what vessel does the LAD originate?
The left main artery bifurcates, in most people, to the LAD and the circumflex artery (Figure 5-9).

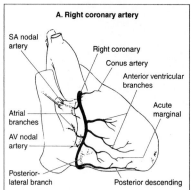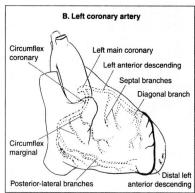

FIGURE 5-9. Arteries of the heart. (Reproduced, with permission, from Doherty GM. *Current Surgical Diagnosis & Treatment*, 12th ed. New York: McGraw-Hill, 2006: 391.)

What are the branches of the right coronary artery (RCA), and what territories do they supply?
The **RCA** first travels in the atrioventricular (AV) groove then wraps around the inferior border of the heart to the posterior IV groove. In 80% of people, the **SA nodal artery** is the first branch of the RCA. Other branches of the RCA include the right marginal, posterior descending (in 80% of people) and AV nodal arteries.

During which part of the contraction cycle do coronary arteries fill?
The coronary arteries have maximal blood flow during diastole and minimal flow during systole. This is due to their location above the cusps of the aortic valve, which obstructs flow into the coronary arteries when the valve opens during systole.

What biomarkers indicate myocardial injury?
Creatine kinase (CK) is an enzyme that is found in muscle tissue throughout the body and may become elevated from damage to muscle cells. Elevated CK levels are not specific to myocardial infarction (MI) and may be seem in rhabdomyolysis, myocarditis, and myositis.

CK-MB is an isoenzyme of CK that is expressed in higher levels in cardiac muscle and is thus more specific for myocardial necrosis.

Cardiac troponin I and T are sensitive and specific markers of damage to the heart.

What is the timing of biomarker release after myocardial injury?
CK levels rise within 4–8 hours, peak at 12–24 hours, and return to baseline by 4 days. The CK-MB isoenzyme curve peaks slightly earlier and is cleared within 48 hours.

Troponin I and T may be detected as early as 2 hours after MI but usually rise by 6 hours, peak at 12 hours, and return to baseline by 7–10 days, making the test useful to identify patients with delayed presentations of MI.

■ CASE 10

A 65-year-old woman with a 60-pack-year smoking history comes to her primary care physician with 3 months of shortness of breath and dry cough. Until recently, she was able to walk the four blocks to her local grocery store without shortness of breath; however, now she is able to walk only one block before having to stop and rest. She has been waking from sleep with difficulty breathing and feels uncomfortable lying flat in bed. Her physical examination is notable for crackles at the lung bases. There is no evidence of hepatosplenomegaly or jugular venous distention.

What is the most likely diagnosis?

Left heart failure (LHF) is evidenced by orthopnea, paroxysmal nocturnal dyspnea, dyspnea on exertion, and mild edema.

What are the common causes of this condition?

Hypertension, myocardial infarction, valvular heart disease, myocarditis, and cardiomyopathies are associated with the development of LHF.

What symptoms help differentiate right heart failure from left heart failure?

Right heart failure is characterized by compromised venous return. This can manifest as ascites, significant edema of the lower extremities, jugular venous distention, and hepatosplenomegaly secondary to liver and spleen congestion.

This patient is at risk for which other conditions?

LHF is the most common cause of right heart failure. In addition, her history of smoking increases her risk for chronic lung disease. This can lead to cor pulmonale, characterized by right ventricular hypertrophy and failure due to pulmonary congestion in patients with lung disease or pulmonary hypertension. Emphysema is commonly associated with cor pulmonale.

What are the likely findings on gross pathology?

Hemosiderin-laden macrophages in the lung are commonly seen in LHF. If LHF leads to right heart failure, patients may develop chronic passive liver venous congestion (called nutmeg liver). Congestion in the central region of the hepatic lobule causes deposition of red/brown pigment from blood cells and can lead to centrilobular necrosis.

■ CASE 11

A 75-year-old nonsmoking male, status–post recent abdominal surgery suddenly develops calf muscle pain in his left lower extremity (LLE). His hospitalization since his surgery 3 days ago has been unremarkable. The patient's medical and family histories reveal no cardiovascular disease or malignancy. On physical examination, he is afebrile and is not in acute distress. His LLE is swollen and mildly erythematous. The skin is warm to the touch and intact throughout. Homans' sign (pain on passive dorsiflexion of the foot) is negative. His right lower extremity is unremarkable. Relevant laboratory test results are as follows:

Partial thromboplastin time (PTT) 28 seconds
Prothrombin time (PT) 12 seconds
International normalized ration (INR) 0.9

What is the most likely diagnosis?

Deep venous thrombosis (DVT) is most common in the lower extremities. Hospitalized patients are at high risk for DVT and the associated complications of pulmonary embolism. Risk of DVT is higher in surgical patients than medical patients and is particularly high for patients who have had hip or knee surgery.

How is this condition diagnosed?

The level of D-dimer, a fibrin degradation product, is often elevated in DVT. Assays for D-dimer are highly sensitive and have a low false-negative rate in symptomatic patients. A negative D-dimer test therefore may exclude DVT in low-risk patients. In DVT-prevalent populations (eg, surgical patients), additional tests may be used to diagnose or confirm DVT, especially deep venous ultrasonogram with examination for the flow abnormalities (that would be present with a thrombus). Other tests include MRI and venography.

In what other conditions is D-dimer elevated?

D-dimer may be elevated in a number of inflammatory conditions including liver disease, autoimmune disease, malignancy, surgery, and in elderly patients. D-dimer therefore has a low specificity for DVT.

What are the risk factors for this condition?

Risk factors of DVT are described by the Virchow triad. **Stasis** may increase secondary to surgery, immobility, paresis, increasing age, heart failure, pregnancy, or obesity. **Vessel injury** may result from smoking, prior DVT, catheterization, or varicose veins. Numerous hereditary conditions result in **hypercoagulability**. Other hypercoagulable states include malignancy, estrogen therapy, acute medical illnesses, inflammatory bowel disease, and nephrotic syndrome.

What conditions should be included in the differential diagnosis?

Numerous conditions can mimic DVT, including the following: muscle strain or tear, lymphedema, venous valvular insufficiency, popliteal cysts, and cellulitis.

What is the anatomy of the major deep veins in the lower extremities?

The anterior tibial, posterior tibial, and peroneal veins converge at the lower popliteal fossa to form a single popliteal vein. The popliteal vein continues medially to become the superficial femoral vein. The deep femoral vein runs laterally and joins the superficial femoral and great saphenous vein in the femoral canal to form the common femoral vein. Thrombus formation in the superficial veins of the legs (thrombophlebitis) has a low risk of thromboembolization or pulmonary embolism formation and thus is not routinely treated with anticoagulation.

■ CASE 12

A 50-year-old African-American man presents to his physician complaining of worsening dyspnea on exertion, orthopnea, and paroxysmal nocturnal dyspnea. His medical history is notable for an anterior myocardial infarction (MI) 15 months ago. A holosystolic murmur is audible, particularly at the apex, along with a diastolic rumble. ECG demonstrates left ventricular hypertrophy and deep (> 1 mm), broad Q waves in V_1, V_2, and V_3. Echocardiography shows depressed ejection fraction (EF) and thinning of the left ventricular walls.

What is the most likely diagnosis?

Dilated cardiomyopathy (DCM) is defined as a left ventricular (LV) EF < 40% and a ventricular chamber with increased diastolic and systolic volumes. In this patient, it is likely of ischemic etiology. DCM is a major cause of congestive heart failure in young people. Males and African Americans are at an increased risk for DCM.

What are causes of this condition?

There are many causes of DCM, but they can be broadly categorized as primary or secondary. **Primary** causes of DCM include idiopathic or genetic factors. **Secondary** causes of DCM include ischemia, hypertension, valvular disease, drugs (alcohol, cocaine, doxorubicin), infectious disease (Chagas disease, coxsackievirus), vitamin B deficiency, and postpartum state.

What typical signs and symptoms are associated with this condition?

DCM results in depressed systolic pump function and the typical symptoms of myocardial failure, as seen in this patient. Enlargement of the ventricle dilates the annulus and displaces the papillary muscles. This can result in the holosystolic murmur of mitral regurgitation. The subsequent increase in early diastolic atrium-to-ventricle flow results in the diastolic rumble. Prior MIs are characterized by deep, broad Q waves. The presence of Q waves in the precordial leads suggests an old anterior MI.

What is the pathogenesis of this condition?

After an MI, it is hypothesized that the reduced peripheral (particularly renal) perfusion leads to fluid retention in an attempt to increase cardiac output. This ultimately results in cardiac remodeling. Figure 5-10 shows the relationship between renin-angiotensin and autonomic nervous system activation and cardiac myocyte cell death.

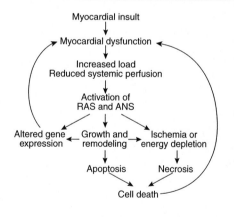

FIGURE 5-10. **The renin-angiotensin system and autonomic nervous system in the progression to myocardial failure.** (Reproduced, with permission, from Fuster V et al. *Hurst's The Heart*, 11th ed. New York: McGraw-Hill, 2004: 1892.)

What is cardiac remodeling?

Following MI, necrotic muscle cells are replaced by proliferating fibroblasts and collagen deposition. The development of scar tissue in the myocardium thins the ventricle walls, reshapes the ventricle, and ultimately adversely affects cardiac function.

What is the appropriate treatment for this condition?

Angiotensin-converting enzyme inhibitors and β-blockers are appropriate in symptomatic patients, because they slow the remodelling process and reduce myocardial workload, respectively. In so doing, they improve cardiac output and reduce mortality. Diuretics may be used in volume-overloaded patients. In some cases, anticoagulation may be required, as there is a predilection for thrombi to form in a dilated cardiac chamber. Digitalis may also improve the EF, but survival benefit is uncertain. Aldosterone antagonists have been shown to provide a mortality benefit in patients with severe heart failure symptoms.

CASE 13

A 30-year-old man is evaluated in the emergency department for a 24-hour history of chest pain, difficulty breathing, and chills. He denies any history of medical problems. On physical examination, he appears ill. His temperature is 40°C (104°F), his blood pressure is 90/50 mm Hg, and his heart rate is 110/min. Cardiac examination reveals a 3/6 diastolic murmur, but the patient denies any history of a murmur. ECG results are normal. Gram stain of a peripheral blood smear shows gram-positive cocci in clusters.

What is the most likely diagnosis?

Acute endocarditis caused by *Staphylococcus aureus*. The man's new heart murmur suggests a possible valvular lesion as the source of infection. In this case, a Gram stain that demonstrates gram-positive organisms in clusters suggests staphylococci.

Which valvular structure is most commonly affected in this condition?

In the general population, endocarditis most frequently involves the mitral valve. Common organisms include staphylococcal and streptococcal species. In intravenous (IV) drug users, however, the tricuspid valve is most commonly involved. In these cases, venous blood contaminated by nonsterile venipuncture crosses the tricuspid valve first.

What other microorganisms are associated with this condition?

Acute endocarditis develops in previously normal valves; *S aureus*, *Neisseria gonorrhoeae*, and *Streptococcus pneumoniae* are common culprits. **Subacute endocarditis** is diagnosed in previously abnormal or damaged valves and is often secondary to previous rheumatic fever. Viridans streptococci, *Staphylococcus epidermidis*, enterococci, and *Candida* are common causes of subacute endocarditis.

What is this condition called when it occurs with systemic lupus erythematosus?

Libman-Sacks endocarditis, or "sterile endocarditis," occurs with systemic lupus erythematosus. This condition is believed to result from autoimmune damage to cardiac valves.

What characteristic of this microbe confers resistance antibiotics?

Penicillin resistance by *S aureus* develops through the secretion of penicillinase (a β-lactamase), which inactivates penicillin. Vancomycin resistance develops through the acquisition of a gene that changes the vancomycin binding site from a D-ala D-ala sequence to D-ala D-lac on bacterial cell wall precursors. Loss of the binding site results in resistance to vancomycin.

What are the complications of this condition?

A serious complication of endocarditis is embolization of valvular vegetations. Embolization to the brain, liver, kidneys, and bone may lead to abscess and may have profound neurological and physiological effects. Small pieces of vegetations may embolize peripherally leading to Roth spots (retinal hemorrhages), Janeway lesions (nontender hemorrhagic lesions on palms or soles), and Osler nodes (tender lesions on palms or soles).

What is the most appropriate treatment for this condition?

The best treatment for infective endocarditis is IV antibiotics targeted at the causative agent.

■ CASE 14

A previously healthy 16-year-old boy presents to the emergency department because of difficulty breathing and substernal chest pain radiating to the neck and shoulder while he was playing soccer. He is now feeling much better. He denies any drug or cigarette use and is not aware of any medical problems in his family, except for two uncles who died suddenly in their youth. Physical examination reveals a heart rate of 70/min, blood pressure of 124/80 mm Hg, and respiratory rate of 12/min. Heart sounds are notable for a normal S_1 and normally split S_2, along with a murmur. His point of maximum impulse is enlarged and anteriorly displaced. The precordial tracings from his ECG are shown in Figure 5-11.

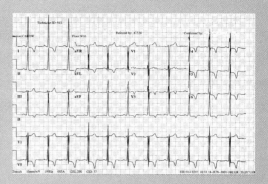

FIGURE 5-11. (Reproduced, with permission, from Fuster V, et al. *Hurst's The Heart*, 12th ed. New York: McGraw-Hill, 2007: Figure 30-9.)

What is the most likely diagnosis?

Hypertrophic cardiomyopathy (HCM) is suggested by the patient's age, symptoms, family history of sudden death (a common presentation in young people with HCM), murmur, and ECG findings. It is characterized by the overgrowth of myocardium with myocardial disarray.

What is the epidemiology of this condition?

HCM is believed to be the most common genetic cardiovascular disorder. Its overall prevalence is estimated to be 1:500 to 1:1000. No gender preference is observed, and clinical manifestation varies by age.

How should the ECG findings in Figure 5-11 be interpreted?

The ECG shows normal sinus rhythm.

These ECG findings suggest significant left ventricular hypertrophy, as indicated by the deep S wave in V_1 and tall R wave in V_5 or V_6 (ie, S wave in V_1 + R wave in V_5 or $V_6 \geq 35$ mm). In athletic young patients, high voltage in the R and S waves may not be abnormal; however, patients with HCM have more marked evidence of left ventricular hypertrophy than healthy individuals.

ST-segment depression with T-wave inversion in V_4 to V_6 may suggest lateral infarction, given their presence only in these lateral leads.

What is the etiology of this condition?

Multiple mutations that affect the cardiac sarcomere have been associated with HCM, many of which are transmitted in an autosomal dominant pattern.

What is the classic murmur associated with this condition?

The classic murmur is due to left ventricular outflow tract obstruction caused by the hypertrophic septum within a shrunken ventricular cavity. A systolic, crescendo-decrescendo murmur most audible at the left sternal border that ends shortly before S_2 is often heard. This murmur decreases with squatting and increases with standing or with low-volume states such as dehydration. The murmur of HCM is enhanced by maneuvers that worsen the obstruction below the aortic value and diminished by maneuvers that increase venous return thus distending the left ventricle and decreasing the degree of stenosis. A mitral valve (MV) regurgitation murmur may also be heard, as the MV leaflets can be pulled into the outflow tract midsystole.

What major classes of pharmacologic agents may benefit this patient?

β-Adrenergic antagonists are used to decrease heart rate, myocardial oxygen consumption, and outflow tract gradient and to increase diastolic filling time.

Calcium channel blockers are used to decrease inotropy and chronotropy and improve diastolic relaxation. Verapamil is preferred because it acts primarily on the heart rather than the blood vessels and so has minimal effects on the afterload.

■ CASE 15

A 51-year-old man comes to the physician's office for a routine physical examination. At his last examination 3 years ago, he was advised to modify his lifestyle because his blood pressure was 144/87 mm Hg. At the current visit, his blood pressure is 150/95 mm Hg. The patient is overweight (body mass index 28 kg/m^2) and he has smoked one pack of cigarettes per day for the past 30 years.

What additional symptoms would indicate an emergent situation?

Blood pressure goals in most patients are < 140/90 mm Hg; the goal is lower in patients with diabetes or other comorbid conditions. Hypertensive urgency is characterized by severely elevated blood pressure (systolic > 180 mm Hg or diastolic > 110 mm Hg) without evidence of end-organ damage. Hypertensive emergencies are characterized by severely elevated blood pressure with signs of end-organ damage including mental status changes, stroke, myocardial infarction, and renal failure.

What is the primary treatment for this condition?

Lifestyle modification is attempted before pharmacologic therapy is undertaken. This includes moderate dietary sodium restriction, weight reduction in obese patients, avoidance of smoking and excess alcohol intake, increased fruit and vegetable intake, and regular aerobic exercise.

What is the initial pharmacologic therapy of choice for this condition?

The initial pharmacologic therapy of choice is a **thiazide diuretic**, which inhibits sodium chloride reabsorption in the distal tubule, thereby promoting diuresis. Compared to other classes of diuretics, these drugs are equally effective and less expensive. Chlorthalidone has the longest half-life and the best evidence to support its use. Hydrochlorothiazide is also frequently used.

What are the mechanism of action and major toxicities of angiotensin-converting enzyme (ACE) inhibitors?

ACE inhibitors, such as captopril and enalapril, are particularly useful when comorbidities such as diabetes mellitus with microalbuminuria and left heart failure coexist with hypertension. These drugs work by inhibiting ACE, thereby reducing levels of angiotensin II and preventing inactivation of bradykinin (a vasodilator). Toxicities include cough, angioedema, taste changes, hypotension, fetal renal damage, rash, and hyperkalemia. Angiotensin II receptor blockers such as losartan have a decreased incidence of cough as an adverse effect.

What are the mechanisms of action and major toxicities of β$_1$-adrenergic blockers?

β$_1$-Selective blockers (acebutolol, betaxolol, esmolol, atenolol, and metoprolol) are particularly useful in decreasing mortality after ischemic events and in patients with congestive heart failure. They work by blocking β-adrenergic receptors, slowing the heart rate, and decreasing blood pressure. Although β$_1$-specific antagonists have fewer respiratory adverse effects than nonspecific β-blockers (such as propranolol), major adverse effects include bradycardia, congestive heart failure, atrioventricular block, sedation, sleep alteration, and impotence.

What are the mechanisms of action and major toxicities of calcium channel blockers?

Calcium channel blockers such as nifedipine (which is more specific for vasculature than verapamil and diltiazem) block voltage-dependent L-type calcium channels of smooth and cardiac muscle, thereby reducing muscle contractility. They are particularly useful when hypertension is not adequately controlled with the above agents. Major toxicities include cardiac depression, peripheral edema, flushing, dizziness, and constipation.

■ CASE 16

A 3-year-old boy is brought to his pediatrician by his mother because he has had a high fever for the past week. Physical examination reveals bilateral injected conjunctivae, palmar erythema, oral mucositis (Figure 5-12), cervical lymphadenopathy, and solar erythema.

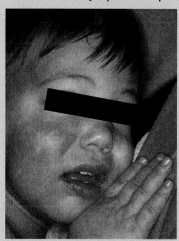

FIGURE 5-12. **Erythema and oral mucositis.** (Reproduced, with permission, from Wolff K, Johnson RA. *Fitzpatrick's Color Atlas and Synopsis of Clinical Dermatology*, 6th ed. New York: McGraw-Hill, 2009: Figure 14-44.)

What is the most likely diagnosis?

Kawasaki disease (mucocutaneous lymph node syndrome). Commonly presents with fever lasting > 5 days, erythematous rash (Figure 5-12), edema in the conjunctivae, lips, and mouth ("strawberry tongue"), palmar and solar erythema, cervical lymphadenitis, and mucositis.

What is the pathophysiology of this disease?

This acute autoimmune disorder is characterized by necrotizing, systemic vasculitis of small and medium-sized vessels as well as veins. Although the exact cause is unknown, it is believed to be triggered by infection evidenced by the fact that Kawasaki disease usually does not occur prior to the age of 6 months, a period of life in which maternal antibodies still circulate in the infant.

Which patients are most commonly affected?

Kawasaki disease is most common in children 6 months to 5 years old. Individuals of Asian ancestry are more often affected.

What is the most appropriate treatment for this condition?

High-dose aspirin and intravenous immunoglobulin G are the preferred treatment. Steroids are used only after failure of first-line treatment. Patients should be treated as promptly as possible to prevent acute complications, including coronary aneurysm, myocardial infarction, severe heart failure, and hydrops of the gallbladder.

Which other infectious diseases commonly present as palmar and solar erythema?

Syphilis, Rocky Mountain spotted fever, meningococcemia, and coxsackievirus A infection can also present as palmar and solar erythema.

CASE 17

A 45-year-old man presents to his physician for a routine health maintenance visit. He reports that he has experienced intermittent heart palpitations. He denies any chest pain, dyspnea on exertion, or syncope. On physical examination, the patient is well appearing and in no distress. His blood pressure is 110/79 mm Hg. Auscultation of his chest while sitting reveals a late systolic click associated with a high-pitched, late systolic murmur. The systolic click occurs closer to S_1 with standing. His ECG is normal; a transesophageal echocardiogram shows a thin leaflike structure entering the inferior left atrium during systole.

What is the most likely diagnosis?

Mitral valve prolapse (MVP), a condition found in 0.6%–2.4% of the population, is the most common valvular heart disease. Most cases are asymptomatic and discovered incidentally. However, left atrial enlargement may occur, resulting in occasional benign supraventricular arrhythmia that the patient perceives as palpitations. Men and women are affected equally. MVP is defined by the echocardiographic measurement of the superior displacement of one or both mitral leaflets into the left atrium (LA).

What is the pathogenesis of this condition?

MVP is multifactorial in origin with an autosomal dominant pattern of inheritance in some families. It can occur as a result of changes within the valvular tissue, geometric disparities between the left ventricle and mitral valve, and connective tissue disorders, such as Marfan syndrome (prevalence of 91%) and Ehlers-Danlos syndrome (6%).

How does standing and squatting affect the timing of the systolic click?

In MVP, the systolic click represents the sudden tensing of the mitral valve apparatus as the leaflets prolapse into the left atrium during systole and occurs when the left ventricle reaches a critical volume (CV) during ventricular contraction. Standing decreases the end-diastolic volume (EDV) by reducing systemic afterload and venous return, thereby allowing the CV to be reached earlier. The click therefore is heard closer to S_1. In contrast, squatting increases the EDV. The click is thus heard closer to S_2.

What are the major complications of this condition?

MVP typically has a benign prognosis. A poorer prognosis is more likely in male, elderly patients with a systolic murmur, thickened and redundant mitral leaflets, or left atrial or ventricular hypertrophy. The most common complication is infective endocarditis as the mitral valve is partially damaged and therefore at increased risk for bacterial colonization. Other complications of MVP include severe mitral valve regurgitation, and cerebrovascular ischemic events. Risk stratification by clinical examination and echocardiography is necessary.

■ CASE 18

A 65-year-old man presents to the emergency department complaining of a sudden onset of substernal chest pain that radiates to his shoulder. It began while he was watching TV on his couch. He describes that the paramedics administered nitroglycerin spray, which alleviated his chest pain for about 20 minutes, but then the pain returned. When examined in the emergency department, the patient states that he has had similar pain with exercise in the past, but it always vanished with rest. A troponin test is negative.

What is the most likely diagnosis?

Chest pain that occurs at rest is commonly seen in unstable angina, subendocardial infarction, and transmural infarction. However, only unstable angina presents without damage to the myocardium, and hence does not produce a troponin leak. In this condition, the flow of a coronary vessel is limited to the extent that it cannot meet the metabolic demand of the heart, but it does not cause death of myocardial tissue. Rest and dilation of the coronary vessels (nitroglycerin) improve the pain. Given his history of coronary heart disease, unstable angina is most likely.

What is the mechanism of action of nitroglycerin?

Nitrates undergo denitration that results in the liberation of nitric oxide (NO) in vivo. NO activates guanylyl cyclase, thereby increasing cyclic guanosine monophosphate (cGMP) concentrations and stimulating cGMP-dependent protein kinases. In smooth muscles this results in the dephosphorylation of myosin light chains and inhibition of calcium entry and increases potassium channel activity. This ultimately leads to vasorelaxation. Clinically, this leads to a reduction in preload (venous relaxation) and a reduction in afterload (some arterial relaxation). As the heart operates at lower pressures, myocardial oxygen demand is also reduced. Furthermore, nitroglycerin dilates coronary vessels, improving myocardial oxygenation. If combined with a phosphodiesterase inhibitor such as sildenafil, life-threatening hypotension may result.

How can ECG studies differentiate between ischemia, subendocardial infarction, and transmural infarction?

Inverted T waves and pathologic Q waves occur once the infarction progresses (Figure 5-13A). In the event of a subendocardial infarction, the subtotal occlusion of the feeding artery allows the epicardial side of the myocardium to remain viable while the endocardial side is starved of nutrients. Subendocardial infarctions appear as inverted T waves without ST-segment changes on ECG.

Stable and unstable angina pectoris lead to ST-segment *depression* in at least two contiguous leads (Figure 5-13B). Transmural infarction features ST-segment *elevation* > 1 mm in at least two contiguous leads.

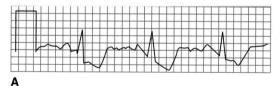
A

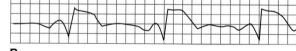
B

FIGURE 5-13. **ECG changes in (A) ischemia and (B) transmural infarction.**

CASE 19

A 56-year-old woman presents to the emergency department complaining of severe pain in her lower jaw and neck that has developed over the past hour. She describes the pain as a pressure that is not relieved by rest or by changes in position. She took ibuprofen at home without relief. She also complains of nausea that began shortly before the onset of jaw and neck pain. On further questioning, she admits to a "heavy" feeling in her chest, which she describes as a squeezing or crushing sensation. She is profusely diaphoretic.

What is the most likely diagnosis?

Acute myocardial infarction (AMI) most often results from a thrombotic event in a coronary artery due to plaque rupture. Myocardial tissue dies (infarction) if perfusion is not reestablished.

How does diabetes affect the presentation of myocardial infarction?

Typical myocardial infarctions feature crushing chest pain that may radiate to the arms, back, or jaw. However, since patients with diabetes are prone to develop neuropathies, pain signals from the heart may not be relayed to the brain effectively, resulting in myocardial infarctions without chest pain or atypical pain patterns. A special instance in all patients regardless of diabetes is the inferior MI, caused by an occlusion of the right coronary artery. It commonly presents with abdominal discomfort but no chest pain.

What serum markers are useful in making this diagnosis?

Serum cardiac markers such as creatinine kinase-MB fraction (CK-MB) and cardiac-specific troponin I (cTnI and cTnT), are released into the blood at varying times in response to cardiac tissue necrosis after AMI. **cTnI**, which is more specific than the other markers for AMI, is used within the first 4 hours, and cTn1 levels may remain elevated for 7–10 days. **CK-MB** levels peak about 20 hours after the onset of coronary artery occlusion and usually return to baseline within 48 hours.

What complications are associated with this condition?

See Table 5-1.

TABLE 5-1   Time and Type of Post-MI Complications

POST-MI COMPLICATION	TIME OF OCCURRENCE
Cardiogenic shock	Immediately
Dressler syndrome, arrhythmia	After 48 hours
Papillary muscle, septal, or free-wall rupture	After 1 week
Ventricular aneurysm with risk of thrombus	After 1 month

CASE 20

A 47-year-old man presents to the emergency department after experiencing substernal chest pain. The pain is worsened with inspiration and is relieved only when he leans forward. He says he recently recovered from an upper respiratory infection. Cardiac examination reveals a leathery friction rub and distant heart sounds. An ECG is shown in Figure 5-14.

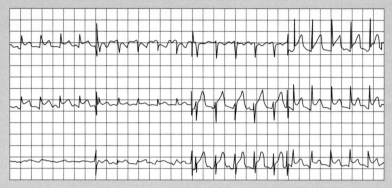

FIGURE 5-14. **ECG strip.** (Reproduced, with permission, from Kasper DL, et al. *Harrison's Principles of Internal Medicine*, 16th ed. New York: McGraw-Hill, 2005: 1318.)

What is the most likely diagnosis?

Pericarditis often presents with diffuse ST-segment elevation, positional chest pain, and friction rub. The latter is due to inflammation of the pericardium, resulting in decreased production of lubrication. The typical friction rub has three phases (atrial contraction, ventricular contraction, and ventricular relaxation).

What is an ECG likely to show?

Classic findings of pericarditis include diffuse ST-segment elevations and PR-segment depression (Figure 5-14). This is in contrast to the ST-segment elevations in some MIs, in which the elevations are limited to ischemic regions (contiguous leads). Likewise, the J point (where the QRS-complex transitions into the ST segment) is usually a smooth curve in pericarditis but abrupt in transmural infarction, allowing distinction when multivessel infarction is suspected.

How is this patient's condition classified?

There are three types of pericarditis: serous, fibrinous and hemorrhagic. Risk factors for the development of **serous pericarditis** include systemic lupus erythematosus, rheumatoid arthritis, and uremia. Preceding viral infection is also possible cause of serous pericarditis, as is the case in this patient. Risk factors for **fibrinous pericarditis** include uremia, myocardial infarction (Dressler syndrome), and rheumatic fever. Risk factors for **hemorrhagic pericarditis** include tuberculosis and malignancy.

Which physical examination and ECG findings would be suspicious for cardiac tamponade in this patient?

Tamponade is the compression of the heart by fluid in the pericardium, which inhibits diastolic filling, reducing the amount of blood available for the heart to pump (reduced cardiac output). This results in systemic hypotension and elevated jugular venous pressure. The fluid around the heart also causes distant, or muffled, heart sounds. **Pulsus paradoxus**, a decrease in arterial blood pressure by > 10 mm Hg during inspiration, is also a sign of tamponade. **Electrical alternans**, a beat-to-beat variation in the amplitude of the QRS complex, may also be noted.

■ CASE 21

A 62-year-old diabetic woman with a 50-pack-year history of smoking and a history of myocardial infarction comes to the emergency department with "excruciating" abdominal pain that began suddenly, awaking her from sleep. For the past several months, she has experienced abdominal pain after eating leading to an unintentional weight loss. She denies surgical history except an appendectomy when she was a teenager. However, she states that she is currently being evaluated for pain in her legs that occurs when she is walking. On physical examination, she appears very uncomfortable, and her abdomen is slightly distended with hypoactive bowel sounds. She has only minimal pain on palpation, in the midepigastric area. She has no rebound or guarding. She denies changes in bowel habits, but her stool is heme positive.

What is the most likely diagnosis?

The patient's severe gastrointestinal symptoms that are out of proportion to the physical signs elicited suggest mesenteric ischemia. Given the sudden onset, this is most likely a thrombotic event. Ischemia affecting the small bowel initially presents with severe pain; peritoneal signs develop later. Ischemia of the large bowel is less painful and typically presents with hematochezia.

What composes the arterial supply of the intestines?

The superior mesenteric artery (SMA) supplies part of the duodenum and part of the head of the pancreas (the territory of inferior pancreaticoduodenal artery), jejunum, ileum, ascending colon, and proximal two-thirds of the transverse colon. The inferior mesenteric artery (IMA) supplies the hindgut, which includes the distal third of the transverse colon, the descending colon, the sigmoid colon, and the rectum. This is schematically shown in Figure 5-15.

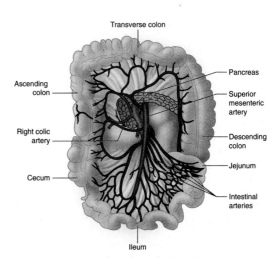

FIGURE 5-15. **Arterial supply to the intestines.**

What is the most appropriate treatment for this patient?

Blood flow must be restored urgently. Thrombolytic medications may resolve the thrombus but also predispose the patient to severe gastrointestinal bleeding upon reperfusion. Hence, a surgical approach is favored (thrombectomy, bypass). In addition, any necrotic segments of the intestine must be surgically removed.

■ CASE 22

A 2-month-old boy is brought to his physician because of poor feeding since discharge from the hospital on his second day of life. The mother reports that he seems to tire easily. His medical history is notable for an uncomplicated 38-week gestation and a normal, spontaneous vaginal delivery. On physical examination, the patient is small for his age but is otherwise well appearing and breathing comfortably without cyanosis. Palpation reveals a hyperdynamic precordium and wide, bounding peripheral pulses. A grade III/VI continuous, "machine-like" murmur that peaks at the second heart sound is audible over the left sternal border and below the left clavicle.

What is the most likely diagnosis?

Patent ductus arteriosus (PDA) is indicated by the characteristic continuous "machine-like" murmur and physical examination.

What is the purpose of the ductus arteriosus?

The ductus arteriosus (DA) typically originates from the origin of the left pulmonary artery to connect to the lower aspect of the aortic arch at the origin of the left subclavian artery. Before birth, it shunts blood away from the pulmonary vasculature (right-to-left shunt), because the lungs are fluid filled and do not provide oxygenation. Patency is maintained during fetal life by the low arterial oxygen tension and circulating prostaglandins produced largely by the placenta. Upon birth, blood pressure in the pulmonary circulation drops because of the lower resistance in the pulmonary vessels, reversing the blood flow through the DA.

What is the pathogenesis of this condition?

The DA typically closes within 2–3 days of birth and becomes the ligamentum arteriosum. This spontaneous closure occurs from a combination of factors, including the increased partial pressure of oxygen secondary to lung-mediated oxygenation, the removal of the vasodilatory effects of prostaglandin E_2 (PGE_2) derived from the placenta, and a decreased number of PGE_2 receptors. Inadequate closure of the DA results in a PDA and permits a left-to-right blood shunt that increases volume load of the left ventricle and the pulmonary arteries.

What is the prognosis of this condition?

The additional stress on the heart and lungs derived from the left-to-right shunt eventually results in left ventricular hypertrophy and ultimately heart failure, vascular damage, and pulmonary hypertension. Regardless of size, a PDA also increases the risk for infective endocarditis. Pharmaceutical closure can often be achieved with a prostaglandin inhibitor, such as indomethacin. Otherwise, a surgical or catheter-based closure may be required.

CASE 23

A 35-year-old woman presents to her physician complaining of fatigue and fever. She has lost 7 kg (15 lbs) over the past 2 months and also reports occasional abdominal pain, headaches, and muscle pain. On physical examination, her blood pressure is 154/92 mm Hg. Retinal examination reveals cotton-wool spots, and skin examination is notable for palpable purpura. Laboratory studies showed an erythrocyte sedimentation rate of 121 mm/h. An enzyme-linked immunosorbent assay (ELISA) is positive for hepatitis B surface antigen antibodies.

What is the most likely diagnosis?

This patient has polyarteritis nodosa with palpable purpura and other common symptoms such as weight loss, inflammatory markers, and evidence of vasculitis in her retina.

What is the pathophysiology of this disease?

Polyarteritis nodosa is an autoimmune disorder characterized by segmental, transmural inflammation of small and medium-sized arteries due to necrotizing immune complexes. Vessels supplying the kidneys, heart, liver, and gastrointestinal tract are most often involved.

What laboratory test can help establish the diagnosis?

The presence of perinuclear antineutrophilic cytoplasmic antibody (P-ANCA) correlates with disease activity. P-ANCAs are more commonly seen in small-artery disease. Furthermore, antibody testing against hepatitis B may strengthen the diagnosis, as approximately 30% of cases of polyarteritis nodosa are associated with this infection.

What other small to medium vasculitides could this patient have?

Churg-Strauss syndrome is a variant of polyarteritis nodosa characterized by eosinophilia and asthma. Autoantibodies mostly target blood vessels in the lungs, but in the late stage other organ systems can become involved (including the skin). Wegener granulomatosis features ANCAs that damage blood vessels in the upper respiratory tract and kidney. However, it can also involve joints, skin, and the gastrointestinal tract.

What complications may be seen in polyarteritis nodosa?

Inflammation of the small and medium-sized arteries induces a local state of hypercoagulability. This may lead to thromboses and subsequent ischemia or infarction of distal tissues. Unfortunate individuals have suffered strokes and heart attacks, but ischemia is possible in any organ system. Damaged arteries are at risk for aneurysms. Treatment with prednisone and cyclophosphamide, however, produces remission or even cure in approximately 85% of affected individuals and prevents these complications.

■ CASE 24

A 33-year-old woman who recently immigrated to the United States from India presents to her physician complaining of profound shortness of breath. Over the past few weeks, she has been progressively unable to walk up a flight of stairs without stopping to catch her breath. For the past few nights, she has been waking up suddenly, gasping for air. She also notes that she has recently been unable to fit into her dress shoes. The patient says she is generally healthy, leads an active lifestyle, and takes no medication except for vitamin supplements. Her past medical history is significant only for a 2-week hospitalization when she was a teenager for fever, sore throat, and joint pain. On physical examination, her blood pressure is 110/80 mm Hg, heart rate is 100/min, and respiratory rate is 24/min. Jugular venous distention is noted, as are diffuse wheezes and rales at both lung bases. There is edema of her ankles bilaterally. Heart auscultation reveals a low-pitched, diastolic murmur with an opening snap, heard best at the apex. X-ray of the chest is normal with the exception of congestion of the pulmonary vasculature.

What is the most likely diagnosis?

This patient has rheumatic heart disease. Mitral stenosis (fish-mouth buttonhole deformity) is often seen in patients with previous rheumatic fever infection. This disease primarily affects the mitral and aortic valves; involvement of tricuspid and pulmonary valves is rare. This condition is not commonly seen in the United States.

What hemodynamic changes occur in the heart in this condition?

Left *atrial* diastolic pressure increases in cases of mitral stenosis because the left atrium must pump against a small, stiff valve. This can increase pulmonary hydrostatic pressure, leading to pulmonary congestions and edema. Eventually, right heart failure ensues.

What pathogen is responsible for the underlying infection in this condition?

Rheumatic heart disease is a result of group A β-hemolytic streptococci infection. Valvular heart disease, as in this patient, often occurs many years after the acute infection. Antistreptolysin O antibodies are often seen in patients long after the acute infection resolves.

What is the appropriate treatment for this condition?

Cautious use of diuretics and sodium restriction to relieve pulmonary congestion is recommended. Surgery for valve replacement may be indicated for patients with severe symptoms. Prophylactic antibiotics for endocarditis are indicated for all invasive procedures, including dental work.

▎CASE 25▐

A 59-year-old woman consults her physician because she recently experienced a brief episode of blurred vision in her right eye when reading the newspaper. The episode resolved spontaneously after approximately 20 minutes. On further questioning, she reports she has recently started to have headaches over her right temple, which worsen at night, especially when she lies on her right side. She also states that she can no longer eat large meals because her jaw muscles tend to get tired; instead, she has to eat frequent small meals.

What is the most likely diagnosis?

Biopsy of the temporal artery reveals temporal arteritis. An elevated erythrocyte sedimentation rate and elevated C-reactive protein levels are nonspecific markers associated with temporal arteritis.

Which histopathologic features are associated with this condition?

Temporal arteritis is a systemic vasculitis of large and medium-sized vessels. It is not restricted to the temporal artery. Mononuclear infiltrates in vessel walls and frequent giant cell formations are expected findings (Figure 5-16).

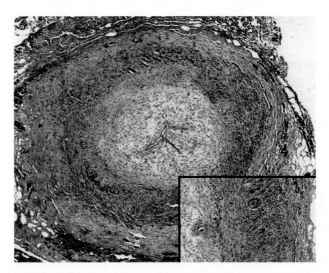

FIGURE 5-16. **Histology of temporal arteritis.** (Reproduced, with permission, from Hellmann DB. Vasculitis. In: Stobo J, et al. *Principles and Practice of Medicine.* Norwalk, CT: Appleton & Lange. Copyright © The McGraw-Hill Companies, Inc., 1996.)

What is the appropriate treatment for this condition?

Corticosteroids should be started as soon as possible. Nonsteroidal anti-inflammatory drugs can be given for pain.

What complications are associated with this condition?

Without treatment, blindness in one or both eyes due to involvement of the ophthalmic artery or posterior ciliary arteries is the most common complication. Patients may also have fever, fatigue, new-onset headache, and jaw or arm claudication. More serious complications, such as thoracic aneurysm, occur less frequently. Additionally, temporal arteritis is often associated with **polymyalgia rheumatica**, a syndrome that features pain and stiffness in muscles and joints of the hips, shoulders, and neck. It is thought to have an autoimmune etiology.

■ CASE 26

A 13-month-old adopted boy is brought to the pediatrician by his mother, who reports that he hyperventilates and becomes blue around his lips and in his fingertips after crying, eating, or any exertion. She has also noticed he tends to squat when he gets these symptoms, which causes him to "pink up" again.

What is the most likely diagnosis?

Tetralogy of Fallot (TOF) (cyanotic congenital heart disease known as "blue baby syndrome") presents as dyspnea on exertion, such as feeding or crying. Exertion results in systemic vasodilation, which lowers left-sided resistance, thereby increasing the right-to-left shunting of blood. Bypass of oxygen exchange in the lungs causes hypoxia and cyanosis. Squatting significantly increases systemic (left-sided) resistance, reducing the amount of blood shunted and alleviates symptoms.

What anatomic findings are characteristic of this condition?

Anatomic findings in TOF are as follows: **P**ulmonary stenosis (1); **R**ight ventricular hypertrophy (2); **O**verriding aorta (deviation of the origin of the aorta to the right) (3); and **V**entricular septal defect (VSD; 4); (mnemonic: PROVe).

Which developmental defect is responsible for this condition?

In TOF, the infundibular septum (the portion of the septum adjacent to the outflow tracts) is anteriorly and superiorly displaced during development, leaving a hole in the ventricular septum (Figure 5-17). This displacement also causes pulmonary stenosis by blocking flow to the pulmonary artery; the result is increased pressure on the right side of the heart and right ventricular hypertrophy.

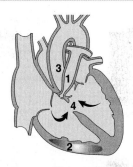

FIGURE 5-17. **Drawing of heart in Tetralogy of Fallot.** (Adapted, with permission, from Chandrasoma P, et al. *Concise Pathology,* 3rd ed. Stamford, CT: Appleton & Lange, 1997: 345. Copyright © The McGraw-Hill Companies, Inc.)

What is the characteristic radiologic finding in this condition?

X-ray of the chest typically shows a boot-shaped heart, due to right ventricular hypertrophy and the absence of a pulmonary artery shadow above the left side of the heart. An echocardiogram with Doppler mode shows the altered pattern of blood flow.

What additional physical finding is commonly associated with this condition?

Clubbing of the fingers may appear in adults (Figure 5-18) secondary to chronic hypoxemia. It is believed that the lungs secrete growth factors in patients with chronic hypoxia, resulting in abnormal tissue growth that first becomes evident in the distal phalanges.

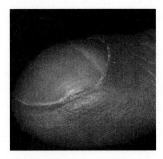

FIGURE 5-18. **Clubbing of the fingers.** (Reproduced, with permission, from Wolff K, et al. *Fitzpatrick's Dermatology in General Medicine,* 7th ed. New York: McGraw-Hill, 2008; Figure 87-31.)

▪ CASE 27

A full-term baby girl presents from the well-baby nursery with bluish discoloration of her lips. Her caretakers report that she becomes sweaty with feeding even though she recently had her cleft palate repaired. Her prenatal history is notable for the lack of prenatal care. Physical examination reveals tachycardia and tachypnea, but she is afebrile. Her S_2 heart sound is single and loud. An early systolic ejection click is audible at the left sternal border. Her hips are maintained in flexion, and her extremities are warm and well perfused.

What is the most likely diagnosis for this condition?

Truncus arteriosus (TA) accounts for 1% of congenital cardiac malformations. It is also associated with DiGeorge syndrome, as is the case in this patient.

What is the characteristic anatomy in this condition?

The TA is the embryologic precursor that normally separates into the aorta and pulmonary artery by formation of the spiral septum. Persistent TA is caused by failure of the spiral septum to develop and thereby failure of aorta and pulmonary artery to septate. Normally, neural crest cells that are present in the TA grow in a spiral formation, separating the two outflow tracts and forming the intertwined aorta and pulmonary artery. If this septum fails to form, a single outflow tract persists (Figure 5-19A). A ventricular septal defect (VSD) is always present; lack of a VSD in the setting of TA is incompatible with life and results in stillbirth. Instead of separate aortic and pulmonary valves, there is one truncal valve with two to six leaflets (leading to the characteristic absence of S_2 splitting). Surgical repair of these defects is required for survival (Figure 5-19B).

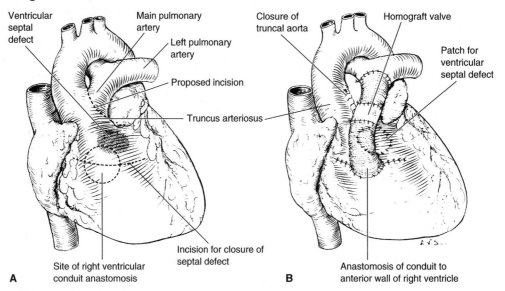

FIGURE 5-19. Truncus arteriosus. (A) The main pulmonary artery derives from the truncus arteriosus. VSD is present. (B) In this method of repair, an artificial conduit connects the right ventricle to the main pulmonary artery that has been separated from the truncus arteriosus. The VSD is closed with a patch and directs blood from the left ventricle to the truncus arteriosus. (Reproduced, with permission, from Doherty GM, et al. *Current Surgical Diagnosis & Treatment*, 12th ed. New York: McGraw-Hill, 2007: 438.)

What are the reasons for this patient's symptoms?

The clinical presentation depends on the amount of pulmonary flow. High pulmonary flow ultimately increases arterial oxygen saturation, reducing risk of cyanosis. However, this patient likely has low pulmonary flow; this results in central cyanosis and earlier presentation with congestive heart failure, which is indicated by the tachycardia and respiratory distress.

■ CASE 28

A 22-year-old man comes to his physician for a routine preemployment physical examination. He is healthy and takes no medications. However, he admits he has recently experienced a few episodes of shortness of breath, dizziness, and palpitations. Physical examination is unremarkable. However, the patient's ECG is notable for a shortened PR interval (< 0.12 sec); a prolonged QRS complex (> 0.12 sec); and a slurred, slow-rising onset of the QRS complex (known as a delta wave; see Figure 5-20).

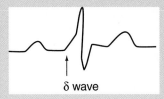

FIGURE 5-20. (Reproduced, with permission, from Le T, et al. *First Aid for the USMLE Step 1: 2011.* New York: McGraw-Hill, 2011: 263.)

What is the most likely diagnosis?
Wolff-Parkinson-White (WPW) syndrome (also known as preexcitation syndrome).

What is the pathophysiology of this condition?
In a normal heart, the only excitatory pathway between the atria and ventricles is the atrioventricular (AV) node. In WPW, the presence of an abnormal band of myocytes creates an accessory conduction pathway, distinct from the AV node, between the atrial and ventricular systems Because the myocytes contain sodium channels, whereas the AV node has calcium channels, excitation often progresses faster through the accessory pathway than the AV node.

Why is the PR interval on ECG shortened in this condition?
The PR interval is the interval between atrial excitation (the P wave) and ventricular excitation (the QRS complex). Thus, it is analogous to the conduction time through the AV node. It is shortened in WPW syndrome because AV conduction occurs via a faster, accessory pathway (frequently, the bundle of Kent), which bypasses the AV node.

What would be the consequence if this patient developed atrial fibrillation?
The consequences would be potentially lethal. Atrial fibrillation has an atrial rate of up to 300 excitations/min. In a normal heart, the AV node is still refractory when subsequent depolarizations arrive and maximally allows a ventricular rate of approximately 150 depolarizations/min. However, the accessory pathway has a short refractory period and may transmit excitatory impulses at their atrial rate. Ventricular contraction at up to 300/min does not allow enough time for ventricular filling and sudden cardiac death occurs.

Why are class II and class IV antiarrhythmic drugs not useful in this condition?
Class II and IV antiarrhythmic agents, the β-blockers and calcium channel blockers, may not be useful in patients with WPW syndrome because they increase AV node refractoriness and decrease AV node conduction velocity. They do **not** slow conduction over accessory pathways, and may even shorten the refractory period for accessory pathways. This may increase ventricular response to atrial fibrillation or flutter, causing hemodynamic collapse. Instead, quinidine, disopyramide, and procainamide may be used to control arrhythmias in this syndrome.

What is the appropriate treatment for this condition?
For most patients with WPW syndrome, electrophysiologic ablation is performed to ablate the accessory pathway. Cure is achieved in 90% of cases with no need for medication.

■ CASE 29

A 61-year-old man with chronic sinusitis and a family history of autoimmune disorders presents to his physician with cough and hemoptysis of 3 weeks' duration. He also complains of frequently becoming short of breath. Laboratory tests show an antibody binding intracellular proteinase-3 diffusely throughout the cytoplasm (antineutrophil cytoplasmic antibodies, C-ANCA). Urinalysis reveals hematuria with RBC casts.

What is the most likely diagnosis?

Wegener granulomatosis. Necrotizing granulomatous vasculitis of small and medium-sized vessels leads to manifestations in the kidney and lungs (Figure 5-21).

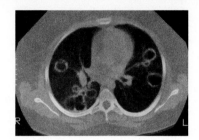

FIGURE 5-21. **Lung findings in Wegener granulomatosis.** (Reproduced, with permission, from Kasper DL, et al. *Harrison's Principles of Internal Medicine*, 16th ed. New York: McGraw-Hill, 2005: 2004.)

What laboratory test can help establish the diagnosis?

The presence of C-ANCA is associated with Wegener granulomatosis, which must be differentiated from **Goodpasture syndrome**, an autoimmune disorder that also presents with hemoptysis and renal disease (Table 5-2). Instead of C-ANCA antibodies, Goodpasture syndrome features anti–glomerular basement membrane antibodies (anti-GBM).

TABLE 5-2	Distinguishing Features of Wegner Granulomatosis and Goodpasture Syndrome	
FEATURE	**WEGENER**	**GOODPASTURE**
Antibody	ANCA	GBM
Renal biopsy	Leukoclastic vasculitis	Liner deposits among basement membrane
Organ involvement	All organs	Lung and kidney

What are the likely findings on gross pathology of the kidney?

Renal involvement in Wegener granulomatosis commonly manifests as a pauci-immune or type III rapidly progressive glomerulonephritis. Immunofluorescence reveals no antibodies or immune complex deposition. By contrast, Goodpasture syndrome shows linear deposition of anti-GBM antibodies.

If this patient also had severe renal dysfunction, which treatment should be avoided?

Methotrexate, although therapeutic, can be nephrotoxic in patients with Wegener granulomatosis. Preferred treatments include other immunosuppressants such as cyclophosphamide and corticosteroids.

What other findings are common in patients with this condition?

Perforation of the nasal septum (the so-called "saddle-nose" deformity; Figure 5-22), chronic sinusitis, mastoiditis, cough, hemoptysis, hematuria, and RBC casts are common findings in patients with Wegener granulomatosis. See Table 5-2 for the distinguishing features of Wegener granulomatosis and Goodpasture syndrome.

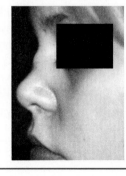

FIGURE 5-22. **Nasal septum perforation in Wegener granulomatosis.** (Reproduced, with permission, from Imboden J, et al. *Current Rheumatology Diagnosis & Treatment*. New York: McGraw-Hill, 2004: 249.)

6

Endocrine

◼ CASE 1

Endocrine

■ CASE 1

A 4-year-old girl with a history of ambiguous genitalia is brought to her pediatrician for a check-up. The child's blood pressure is found to be 130/89 mm Hg. Physical examination is notable for clitoral enlargement, partial labial fusion, and scant pubic hair growth. Laboratory tests reveal the following:

Sodium: 142 mEq/L
Potassium: 3.1 mEq/L
Chloride: 102 mEq/L
Bicarbonate: 25 mEq/L

What enzyme-deficiency is this?

11β-Hydroxylase deficiency is suggested by the constellation of **hyper**tension, masculinization, and **hypo**kalemia.

How is this condition differentiated from a more common, but similar, enzyme deficiency?

21β-Hydroxylase deficiency presents with **hypo**tension and **hyper**kalemia. Both deficiencies present with masculinization of the external genitalia. A review of adrenal steroid synthesis is shown in Figure 6-1.

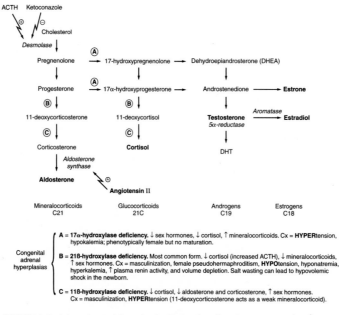

A = 17α-hydroxylase deficiency. ↓ sex hormones, ↓ cortisol, ↑ mineralocorticoids. Cx = **HYPER**tension, hypokalemia; phenotypically female but no maturation.

B = 21β-hydroxylase deficiency. Most common form. ↓ cortisol (increased ACTH), ↓ mineralocorticoids, ↑ sex hormones. Cx = masculinization, female pseudohermaphroditism, **HYPO**tension, hyponatremia, hyperkalemia, ↑ plasma renin activity, and volume depletion. Salt wasting can lead to hypovolemic shock in the newborn.

C = 11β-hydroxylase deficiency. ↓ cortisol, ↓ aldosterone and corticosterone, ↑ sex hormones. Cx = masculinization, **HYPER**tension (11-deoxycorticosterone acts as a weak mineralocorticoid).

Congenital adrenal hyperplasias

FIGURE 6-1. Adrenal steroid synthesis. (Reproduced, with permission, from Le T, et al. *First Aid for the USMLE Step 1: 2011.* New York: McGraw-Hill, 2011: 291.)

How does this enzyme deficiency result in hypertension?

11β-Hydroxylase converts 11-deoxycorticosterone into corticosterone, and 11-deoxycortisol into cortisol. 11β-Hydroxylase deficiency causes a lack of cortisol and aldosterone. However, the precursor 11-deoxycortisone is a weak mineralocorticoid and causes hypertension.

What is the appropriate treatment for this condition?

Dexamethasone or hydrocortisone can be used to replace the missing corticosteroid. The lowest effective dose should be used to avoid the Cushingoid adverse effects of glucocorticoids, including bone demineralization and growth retardation.

What is the mode of inheritance of this condition?

Inheritance is autosomal recessive, with mutations in the *CYP11B1* gene. All of the congenital adrenal hyperplasias are inherited in an autosomal recessive manner.

CASE 2

A baby is born, without complications, to a healthy mother. Physical examination reveals a dangerously hypotensive neonate with ambiguous genitalia, fused labia, and an enlarged and masculinized clitoris. Intravenous fluids are started.

What is the most likely diagnosis?

The patient's ambiguous external genitalia (masculinization) and **hypo**tension suggest congenital adrenal hyperplasia. These signs are caused by lack of cortisol and aldosterone.

What enzyme deficiency is responsible for this condition?

The defective enzyme is 21β-hydroxylase, an enzyme in the pathway that converts cholesterol into aldosterone and cortisol (Figure 6-1). This leads to excess substrates, which are shunted toward synthesis of sex hormones. Decreased cortisol leads to loss of feedback inhibition, increased adrenocorticotropic hormone, and further stimulation of the conversion of cholesterol into sex hormone precursors.

What are the likely findings on laboratory testing?

Hyponatremia and **hyperkalemia** are likely because mineralocorticoids (which are low in these patients) are responsible for the retention of sodium and the excretion of potassium. Salt wasting causes hypotension, which leads to activation of the renin-angiotensin system, resulting in elevated serum renin levels.

Is this an example of hermaphroditism or pseudohermaphroditism?

Pseudohermaphroditism is a condition in which an infant is born with the gonads of one sex and the external genitalia of the opposite sex (eg, normal female gonads but ambiguous, male-like external genitalia). **True hermaphroditism** (rare) occurs when the infant has both male and female gonadal tissue.

What is the appropriate treatment for this condition?

Treatment consists of replacement of the deficient hormones.

■ CASE 3

A 40-year-old woman visits her physician because of fatigue and weakness, which she has experienced for several months. She says she often feels lightheaded when she first gets out of bed in the morning or stands suddenly. Review of symptoms is positive for frequent headaches, nausea, and vomiting. Her vital signs are notable for a blood pressure of 125/75 mm Hg seated and 105/60 mm Hg standing. Physical examination reveals several patches of hyperpigmentation on the skin. Relevant laboratory findings are as follows:

Sodium: 126 mEq/L
Bicarbonate: 19 mEq/L
Potassium: 5.2 mEq/L
Cortisol: 4.3 mg/dL
Chloride: 97 mEq/L

What is the most likely diagnosis?

Addison disease, or primary adrenal insufficiency, is suggested by the clinical history of weakness and orthostatic hypotension and by the signs of hyperpigmentation, hyponatremia, hyperkalemia, and a low serum cortisol level.

What are common etiologies of this disease?

Most cases of Addison disease are idiopathic or autoimmune related. Other causes include the following:
- Disseminated intravascular coagulation.
- **Waterhouse-Friderichsen syndrome** (hemorrhagic necrosis of the adrenal gland, classically due to meningococcemia).
- Granulomatous diseases such as tuberculosis.
- HIV infection.
- Neoplasm.
- Trauma.
- Iatrogenic vascular disorders.

What is the cause of this patient's metabolic abnormalities?

Adrenal insufficiency causes a deficiency of cortisol. Hyponatremia, hyperkalemia, and a low bicarbonate level can result from low aldosterone levels associated with primary adrenal insufficiency.

How would this patient's cortisol level change if she were administered adrenocorticotropic hormone (ACTH)?

The cortisol level should not change appreciably since it is low because of a **primary** adrenal insufficiency (ie, the problem is within the adrenal gland itself). This is suggested by the **hyperpigmentation,** which is due to the attempt of the pituitary gland to overcome the cortisol deficiency by increasing ACTH production. ACTH, in turn, stimulates the release of melanocyte-stimulating hormone, causing hyperpigmentation.

What are the secondary and tertiary forms of this condition?

Secondary adrenal insufficiency is caused by decreased ACTH secretion by the pituitary gland. Administration of ACTH results in a cortisol response. This syndrome does not cause hyperpigmentation. **Tertiary adrenal insufficiency** is caused by a decrease in corticotropin-releasing hormone production by the hypothalamus.

■ CASE 4

A 35-year-old woman presents to her internist complaining of recent episodes of weakness and tingling in her extremities. She also complains of polyuria, nocturia, and polydipsia. Although her blood pressure has been normal in the past, on the day of this visit it is 160/100 mm Hg. Laboratory studies reveal a serum sodium level of 147 mEq/L, a potassium level of 2.8 mEq/L, and very low serum renin activity.

What is the most likely diagnosis?

Primary hyperaldosteronism, also known as Conn syndrome, is suggested by the patient's history and her hypertension, hypernatremia, and hypokalemia. Approximately 30%–60% of cases are due to solitary adrenal adenomas in the zona glomerulosa, the aldosterone-secreting layer of the adrenal cortex. Bilateral hyperplasia of the zona glomerulosa can also cause Conn syndrome.

How is aldosterone regulated?

Renin, produced by the **juxtaglomerular cells** of the kidney, cleaves **angiotensinogen** (produced by the liver) to form **angiotensin I.** Angiotensin I, in turn, is cleaved by angiotensin-converting enzyme to form **angiotensin II.** In response to volume contraction, **angiotensin II** becomes a potent stimulator of aldosterone synthase, a key enzyme in aldosterone synthesis.

Other key stimuli of aldosterone secretion include decreased plasma sodium and increased plasma potassium.

Another patient presents with similar symptoms, but his laboratory tests show increased serum renin activity. What is his most likely diagnosis?

Hypertension has a variety of causes. Approximately 95% of patients with hypertension have primary or "essential" hypertension, which has no identifiable cause. The remaining patients have secondary hypertension, which is caused by an identifiable underlying etiology such as extra-adrenal hyperstimulation of aldosterone secretion (Table 6-1).

TABLE 6-1	Distinguishing Features of Primary vs. Secondary Hypertension	
	PRIMARY HYPERTENSION	SECONDARY HYPERTENSION
Causes	Genetic factors, including conditions such as Bartter syndrome and Gitelman syndrome.	• Vascular disease/renal hypoperfusion (renal artery stenosis, decreased effective circulating volume). • Endocrine disorders (renin-secreting tumors, Conn syndrome, Cushing syndrome, pheochromocytoma). • Intrinsic renal disease (chronic renal failure, glomerulonephritis).
Labs	Decreased renin levels.	Increased renin levels.

Given the patient's serum potassium level, what are the most likely findings on electrocardiogram (ECG)?

Typical ECG findings include prominent U waves, flattened T waves, and ST-segment depression (Figure 6-2).

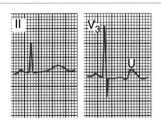

FIGURE 6-2. **ECG in hypokalemia.** (Reproduced, with permission, from Kasper DL, et al. *Harrison's Principles of Internal Medicine,* 16th ed. New York: McGraw-Hill, 2005: 1319.)

What is the appropriate treatment for this condition, and what are the adverse effects?

If a solitary, aldosterone-secreting adrenal adenoma is found, surgical resection (adrenalectomy) is indicated. Bilateral adrenal hyperplasia is treated medically with an aldosterone antagonist such as spironolactone. Major adverse effects of spironolactone are due to its antiandrogen effects, including gynecomastia, loss of libido, menstrual irregularities, and impotence.

■ CASE 5

A 36-year-old woman with no significant medical history presents to her primary care physician with a 6-month history of amenorrhea, weight gain, and excessive facial hair growth. She denies any recent diet or medication changes. Her vital signs are notable for a pulse of 80/min and blood pressure of 148/90 mm Hg. Physical examination reveals a well-developed hirsute female with truncal obesity, abdominal striae, and peripheral edema. She has difficulty arising from a chair during her neurological exam. Relevant laboratory findings are as follows:

Sodium: 140 mEq/L   Chloride: 92 mEq/L
Bicarbonate: 25 mEq/L   Glucose: 225 mg/dL
Potassium: 3.4 mEq/L

What is the most likely diagnosis?

Cushing syndrome results from excess glucocorticoids, either from increased cortisol production or exogenous glucocorticoid therapy. Common causes include the following:

- Iatrogenic (eg, steroid ingestion, most common).
- Pituitary adenoma (Cushing disease).
- Adrenal tumor/hyperplasia.
- Adrenocorticotropic hormone (ACTH)-producing tumor (most commonly secondary to small cell lung cancer).

What laboratory tests can help confirm the diagnosis?

Screening tools for Cushing syndrome or glucocorticoid excess include the following:

- 24-hour urine free cortisol test. Elevated cortisol level indicates hypercortisolism.
- Dexamethasone suppression test. A normal result is a decrease in cortisol after administration of low-dose dexamethasone. In glucocorticoid excess due to Cushing disease, low-dose dexamethasone will not suppress cortisol levels.

After identifying elevated cortisol levels, what diagnostic tests help define the source of the hormonal abnormality?

Serum ACTH levels:

- High ACTH: Pituitary adenoma or an ectopic ACTH-producing neoplasm.
- Low ACTH: Adrenal tumor/hyperplasia or exogenous glucocorticoid administration.
- **A high-dose dexamethasone suppression test** can differentiate between a pituitary adenoma and an ectopic ACTH-producing tumor. Pituitary adenomas are suppressed by high-dose ACTH, whereas ectopic ACTH-producing tumors usually are not.

What are the appropriate treatments for this condition?

The most appropriate treatment for adrenal tumors is surgery. Treatments for nonresectable tumors or hyperplasia are as follows:

- Ketoconazole: Inhibits glucocorticoid production.
- Metyrapone: Inhibits cortisol formation in adrenal pathway.
- Aminoglutethimide: Inhibits the synthesis of steroids.

What is the regular cycle of cortisol levels in the body?

Cortisol levels peak in the early morning (approximately 8 AM) and reach their lowest levels at midnight. Basal body temperature fluctuates with the cortisol cycle (Figure 6-3).

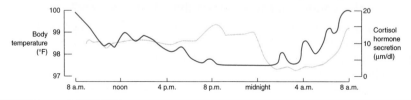

FIGURE 6-3. **Cortisol and basal body temperature.** Light blue line represents temperature. Darker blue line represents cortisol.

▮ CASE 6

A mother brings her 7-year-old son in to see the pediatrician. She says the boy has been less active and has also begun wetting his bed again, something he had stopped doing 2 years ago. Chart review reveals that within the past year the child's weight dropped from the 75th percentile to the 50th percentile even though he has been eating and drinking more than usual, the mother reports. Relevant laboratory findings include the following:

WBC count: 11,400/mm³, normal differential
Chloride: 100 mEq/L
Blood urea nitrogen: 14 mg/dL
Sodium: 132 mEq/L

Creatinine: 1.2 mg/dL
Potassium: 5.0 mEq/L
Glucose: 350 mg/dL

What is the most likely diagnosis?

Autoimmune destruction of pancreatic islet cells results in insulin deficiency (Figure 6-4), leading to type 1 diabetes mellitus (DM). Common presenting symptoms include polydipsia, polyphagia, weight loss, and polyuria (osmotic diuresis secondary to glycosuria).

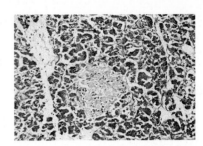

FIGURE 6-4. **Pancreatic islet cells in type 1 diabetes mellitus.** (Reproduced, with permission, from Le T, et al. *First Aid for the USMLE Step 1: 2011.* New York: McGraw-Hill, 2011: Color Image 67B.)

What are the two types of this condition?

Type 1 DM is characterized by absolute insulin deficiency; **type 2 DM** is characterized by insulin resistance and increased insulin levels. Type 1 DM typically presents in thin individuals younger than 30 years of age. Type 2 DM typically affects obese individuals older than 30 years of age (although it is increasingly seen among younger obese individuals). Both types of diabetes can result in retinopathy, nephropathy, and neuropathy.

What is diabetic ketoacidosis (DKA)?

DKA is a life-threatening complication of uncontrolled type 1 DM. In the absence of insulin, increased levels of fatty acids are delivered to the liver, where ketogenesis occurs. This lowers the pH of the blood. Presenting symptoms include **Kussmaul hyperpnea** (deep respirations), abdominal pain, dehydration, and nausea/vomiting. Patients may have a sweet/fruity/alcoholic odor to their breath.

What is the appropriate treatment for DKA?

Acute DKA requires rapid fluid resuscitation with normal saline, followed by the administration of intravenous insulin and repletion of depleted electrolytes, especially potassium. Administration of bicarbonate to correct the acidic blood pH is usually not recommended unless the acidosis is severe.

Following an episode of DKA, lifelong insulin replacement is required for patients diagnosed with type 1 DM. Oral hypoglycemic agents are effective in type 2 DM but not in type 1.

What electrolyte abnormalities are frequently associated with DKA?

DKA is associated with depletion of total body potassium stores through osmotic diuresis. Serum potassium levels may appear normal or elevated even though total body potassium stores are low; this is because intracellular potassium is shifted into the extracellular space in exchange for hydrogen ions to buffer the effects of metabolic acidosis. Treatment of DKA with insulin drives potassium back into cells, and patients undergoing treatment for DKA can thus become profoundly hypokalemic.

■ CASE 7

A worried mother brings her 12-year-old son to the pediatrician with concerns that he is "too tall." Both she and the patient's father are relatively short, as are other members of the family. The patient, an avid Little League player, complains only that his baseball cap, mitt, and shoes do not fit any more. On physical examination, the patient is above the growth curve for his age and has large hands and feet, frontal bossing of the cranium, prominent jaw, and coarse facial features with oily skin.

What is the most likely diagnosis?

Gigantism, which is caused by excess growth hormone (GH). In patients with fused epiphyses (ie, growth plates), the disease is called **acromegaly.** In older patients, physical changes may go unnoticed until hats, gloves, and shoes no longer fit.

What is the pathophysiology of this condition?

Excess GH can arise from pituitary excess, hypothalamic GH-releasing hormone (GHRH) excess, or an ectopic source. A genetic component of the disease is suggested by the high levels of GH seen in **McCune-Albright syndrome** and multiple endocrine neoplasia type I.

How is GH produced?

GH is produced and stored in the acidophilic cells of the anterior pituitary. Basophilic cells in the anterior pituitary can be recalled with the mnemonic **B-FLAT.** Basophils: Follicle-stimulating hormone, Luteinizing hormone, Adrenocorticotropic hormone, and Thyroid-stimulating hormone. Acidophils: GH and prolactin.

How is secretion of GH controlled?

GH is released in a **pulsatile** fashion. Secretion is controlled by the hypothalamus (Figure 6-5). GHRH stimulates GH production. Somatostatin interferes with its effect on the pituitary. Insulin-like growth factor-1 (IGF-1) exerts negative feedback to inhibit GH secretion. At puberty, the frequency and amplitude of GH secretory pulses increase because of gonadal hormones. The combination drives the "growth spurt."

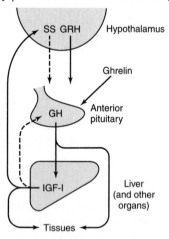

FIGURE 6-5. **Feedback control of growth hormone secretion.** Stimulatory effects (solid line) and inhibitory effects (dashed line). IGF-1 stimulates the secretion of somatostatin (SS) from the hypothalamus, which in turn acts directly on the pituitary to inhibit GH secretion. (Reproduced, with permission, from Ganong WF. *Review of Medical Physiology,* 22nd ed. New York: McGraw-Hill, 2005: 405.)

How is this condition diagnosed?

Excess GH production is diagnosed by physiologic testing and brain imaging.

* **Screening:** The best screening test for excess GH secretion is a measurement of serum **IGF-1 levels.** IGF-1 levels are a more reliable indicator of GH excess than GH levels because IGF-1 remains constant throughout the day whereas GH fluctuates. IGF-1 levels are elevated in acromegaly and gigantism because IGF-1 synthesis is dependent on GH.
* **Confirmatory test:** The diagnosis of GH excess can be confirmed with an **oral glucose suppression test.** In normal patients, GH levels are suppressed after the administration of a glucose load. In patients with gigantism or acromegaly, GH values may rise, remain unchanged, or suppress only partially.
* **Imaging:** MRI of the pituitary gland may reveal adenoma as the source of excess GH secretion.

CASE 8

A previously healthy 30-year-old woman visits her physician complaining of a racing heart, sweating, weight loss, and tremulousness. She appears anxious, and on further questioning reports that her anxiety and restlessness have begun to cause problems at her workplace. Physical examination reveals tachycardia, moist skin, fine body hair, and bilateral bulging of her eyes.

What is the most likely diagnosis?

Graves disease.

What demographic group does this condition typically affect?

Graves disease occurs eight times more frequently in women than men. The prevalence is higher in populations with a high iodine intake. The disease rarely occurs before adolescence and typically affects individuals in the fourth to sixth decades of life.

What is the pathophysiology of this condition?

It is caused by autoimmune-induced hyperthyroidism. Immunoglobulins mimic thyroid-stimulating hormone (TSH) and activate the TSH receptor.

What are other common causes of hyperthyroidism?

- **Iatrogenic:** Excess thyroid hormone medication.
- **Silent thyroiditis:** Inflammation of the thyroid gland, which progresses from hyperthyroidism to hypothyroidism.
- **Struma ovarii:** Ovarian neoplasm (mature teratoma) that contains thyroid tissue.
- **Subacute thyroiditis:** Inflammation of the thyroid gland thought to be secondary to viral infection.
- **Thyroid adenoma:** Benign thyroid neoplasm.
- **Toxic multinodular goiter (Plummer disease):** Enlarged thyroid gland containing multiple active nodules that produce thyroid hormone (called "hot" nodules because of their active appearance on radioactive iodine scans.)

Note: Infiltrative ophthalmopathy and pretibial myxedema is seen only in hyperthyroidism caused by Graves disease.

What are the appropriate treatments for this condition?

Graves disease can remit and recur. Effective treatment includes thyroidectomy, thyroid-inhibiting medications, or radioactive iodine ablation (radioactive iodine is taken up by, and then destroys, hyperfunctioning thyroid tissue).

Medications such as propylthiouracil (PTU) and methimazole inhibit iodine organification and coupling in the thyroid. PTU and steroids also inhibit the peripheral conversion of thyroxine to triiodothyronine.

What is thyroid storm?

Thyroid storm is an acute, life-threatening surge of thyroid hormone in the blood, usually precipitated by surgery, trauma, infection, acute iodine load, or long-standing hyperthyroidism. Manifestations include tachycardia (> 140/min), heart failure, fever, agitation, delirium, psychosis, stupor, and/or coma. Gastrointestinal symptoms can also be present. This condition is treated with methimazole and agents that reduce peripheral conversion of T_4 to triiodothyronine.

CASE 9

A 62-year-old woman presents to her physician with a month-long history of vague abdominal pain, constipation, and nausea and vomiting. She also has experienced diffuse bone pain over the past month, which she attributed to "just getting old." Physical examination reveals diffuse abdominal tenderness. Relevant laboratory findings are as follows:

Sodium: 140 mEq/L
Calcium: 12.3 mg/dL
Chloride: 110 mEq/L
Bicarbonate: 26 mEq/L

Potassium: 4.0 mEq/L
Phosphate: 2.0 mg/dL
Blood urea nitrogen/creatine: 20:1.2 mg/dL

What is the most striking laboratory finding?

Hypercalcemia. Common causes of hypercalcemia are: **M**alignancy, **I**ntoxication with vitamin D, **S**arcoidosis, **H**yperparathyroidism, **A**lkali syndrome, and **P**aget disease of bone (mnemonic: **MISHAP**). In outpatients, hyperparathyroidism is the most common cause of hypercalcemia; in inpatients, malignancy is the most common cause.

How is calcium regulated in the body?

- **Parathyroid hormone (PTH)** stimulates osteoclasts to resorb calcium from bone; increases calcium reabsorption in the distal convoluted tubules of the kidney; increases production of 1,25-$(OH)_2$ vitamin D by the kidney; and decreases renal reabsorption of phosphate.
- **Vitamin D** promotes calcium reabsorption from bone and the small intestine.
- **Calcitonin** inhibits osteoclast activity, thereby decreasing reabsorption of calcium from bone. In normal calcium homeostasis, calcitonin is likely not as significant.

The patient is found to have elevated PTH and normal creatine. How does this help explain her clinical presentation?

The patient has primary **hyperparathyroidism** (Table 6-2), as evidenced by high PTH, high calcium, and normal renal function. To recall the symptoms of hyperparathyroidism (and hypercalcemia in general) use the following mnemonic: "Painful **bones**, renal **stones** (nephrolithiasis), abdominal **groans** (abdominal pain, nausea, vomiting, and anorexia), psychic **moans** (changes in mental status, concentration, and mood), and fatigue **overtones.**"

TABLE 6-2	Types of Hyperparathyroidism		
	PRIMARY	SECONDARY	TERTIARY
Cause	(80%) due to a PTH-producing parathyroid adenoma that is not responsive to normal feedback regulation.	Elevated production of PTH in response to decreased calcium levels (as in renal failure).	Autonomous hyperparathyroidism in the setting of long-standing secondary hyperparathyroidism (end-stage renal failure).

What is the appropriate treatment for acute, severe forms of this condition?

Hydration. If the electrolyte abnormality persists, a loop diuretic can be used (to increase calcium excretion). If needed, calcitonin and bisphosphonates can also be prescribed.

What is the most appropriate long-term treatment for this patient?

Parathyroidectomy. Surgery for primary hyperparathyroidism has cure rates of 96%–98%.

■ CASE 10

A 52-year-old woman presents to the clinic with several months' history of generalized weakness, cold intolerance, and weight gain. Physical examination reveals alopecia, a thick and beefy tongue, myxedema, and delayed deep tendon reflexes. Her heart rate is 55/min and her blood pressure is 100/70 mm Hg. She is not taking any medications. Relevant laboratory findings are as follows:

Free thyroxine (T_4): 4.5 pmol/L (normal: 10.3–35 pmol/L)
Thyroid-stimulating hormone (TSH): 31 µU/mL (normal: 0.8–2 µU/mL)
Cholesterol: 230 mg/dL

What is the most likely diagnosis?

The patient's cold intolerance, weight gain, myxedema, fatigue, prolonged relaxation phase of deep tendon reflexes, and low free T_4 with high TSH suggest primary hypothyroidism.

What is the most common cause of this condition?

Hashimoto thyroiditis (autoimmune destruction of the thyroid gland). Patients are typically positive for **antithyroid peroxidase (antimicrosomal) antibodies.** Additional causes of hypothyroidism include Riedel thyroiditis, subacute thyroiditis, and silent thyroiditis. The prevalence of Hashimoto thyroiditis is increased in patients with other autoimmune disease such as vitiligo.

What endocrine disorder is associated with low free T_4 and low serum TSH levels?

Low T_4 levels in the setting of low or normal TSH levels imply **secondary hypothyroidism,** the most common cause of which is **hypopituitarism.** Other manifestations of hypopituitarism include sexual dysfunction and diabetes insipidus.

What is the appropriate treatment for this condition?

Levothyroxine (synthetic T_4 hormone). Levels of T_4 typically take 4–6 weeks to reach steady state after initiation of therapy.

How are thyroid hormones produced and metabolized?

Iodine is essential for the production of thyroid hormones in the follicular cells of the thyroid gland. Following T_4 production in the thyroid gland, deiodinases in the peripheral tissues convert T_4 to the active form, T_3.

What are the primary functions of thyroid hormones in the peripheral bloodstream?

T_3 has a role in brain maturation, bone growth, β-adrenergic effects, and increasing the basal metabolic rate.

■ CASE 11

A 14-year-old Hispanic-American boy with a family history of obesity and hypertension presents to the pediatrician for a mandatory school physical examination. He has no medical complaints. Social history is notable for a sedentary lifestyle. His diet consists of pizza, sandwiches, potato chips, and 2 cups of soda daily. Physical examination reveals a male with an abdominal circumference > 40 inches. His body mass index is 36 kg/m², pulse is 100/min, and blood pressure is 140/95 mm Hg. Skin examination reveals velvety, darkly pigmented patches in the skin folds at the nape of his neck and axilla (Figure 6-6).

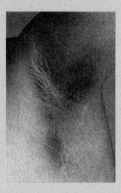

FIGURE 6-6. (Reproduced, with permission, from Wolff K, et al. *Fitzpatrick's Color Atlas & Synopsis of Clinical Dermatology*, 5th ed. New York: McGraw-Hill, 2005: 87.)

What is the most likely diagnosis?

Metabolic syndrome, also known as dysmetabolic syndrome, syndrome X, and insulin resistance syndrome.

What are the diagnostic criteria for this condition?

The National Cholesterol Education Program Adult Treatment Panel III defines metabolic syndrome as the presence of any three of the following five traits:

- Abdominal obesity (male > 40 inches; female > 35 inches).
- Hypertriglyceridemia (≥ 150 mg/dL).
- Low levels of high-density lipoprotein (HDL) cholesterol (male < 40 mg/dL; female < 50 mg/dL).
- Blood pressure ≥ 130/85 mm Hg.
- Fasting glucose ≥ 110 mg/dL.

What do the skin findings represent?

Acanthosis nigricans is a common physical sign of insulin resistance, particularly in Hispanics and African Americans. It may be due to high levels of circulating insulin or insulin-like growth factor receptors in the skin. Other conditions with acanthosis nigricans include **polycystic ovarian syndrome** and some visceral **malignancies.**

What is insulin resistance?

Insulin resistance (IR) is the state in which endogenous or exogenous insulin produces a less-than-expected biological effect. Patients have elevated blood glucose with normal to elevated insulin levels. Today, IR is nearly universal in obese individuals and is correlated with amount of intra-abdominal fat. Several mechanisms of IR in obesity have been proposed:

- Insulin receptor downregulation.
- Intracellular lipid accumulation.
- Increased free fatty acids that impair insulin action.
- Cytokines and "adipokines," which modify the effect of insulin.

Treatment with metformin can be initiated to increase insulin responsiveness.

What class of drugs should be avoided in patients with this condition?

Atypical antipsychotics, such as **clozapine,** are associated with the metabolic syndrome, particularly weight gain and hypertriglyceridemia. Even for patients without weight gain, the effect on serum triglycerides increases the risk for adverse cardiovascular events.

■ CASE 12

A 40-year-old woman presents to her physician with a 2-month history of hoarseness and occasional palpitations and headaches. Her blood pressure is 170/90 mm Hg. Physical examination reveals a lump at the base of her neck. Results of biopsy of the mass are shown in Figure 6-7. Laboratory values are significant for hypercalcemia. Family history is not contributory, as the patient is adopted.

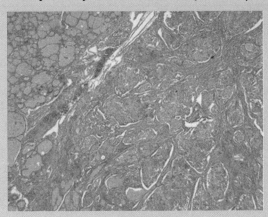

FIGURE 6-7. (Reproduced, with permission, from USMLERx.com.)

What is the most likely diagnosis?

Multiple endocrine neoplasia (MEN) type IIA, or Sipple syndrome, is characterized by medullary carcinoma of the thyroid, pheochromocytoma, and hyperparathyroidism (due to either hyperplasia or tumor). Medullary carcinoma of the thyroid is characterized by nests of cells in amyloid stroma. Figure 6-7 shows the lobular pattern of growth of this tumor. Table 6-3 presents MEN types.

TABLE 6-3	MEN Types		
	TYPE I	TYPE IIA	TYPE IIB
Inheritance	Autosomal dominant	Autosomal dominant	Autosomal dominant
Neoplasms	Pancreatic islet cell tumors (Zollinger-Ellison, insulinoma, VIPoma) Parathyroid hyperplasia Pituitary adenomas	Medullary thyroid cancer Parathyroid hyperplasia Pheochromocytoma	Medullary thyroid cancer Mucosal neuroma Pheochromocytoma
Body habitus			Marfanoid

What genetic screening tests can help confirm the diagnosis?

The presence of the *RET* oncogene mutation in the setting of medullary carcinoma is diagnostic for MEN IIA. A variant of the *RET* mutation is also seen in MEN IIB.

What additional laboratory tests can help confirm the diagnosis?

- Elevated calcitonin and carcinoembryonic antigen levels due to medullary carcinoma.
- Elevated parathyroid hormone and calcium levels from parathyroid hyperplasia or adenoma.
- Elevated urinary levels of catecholamines and catecholamine metabolites (vanillylmandelic acid, metanephrine, and normetanephrines) in pheochromocytoma.
- Elevated plasma levels of metanephrines and normetanephrines in pheochromocytoma.

If this patient has the *RET* mutation, what is the probability that her children will develop this condition?

MEN IIA is an autosomal dominant disease. Therefore, the probability of her children's having the mutation is 50%.

CASE 13

A 50-year-old woman presents to the emergency department complaining of 2 hours of vertigo, headache, palpitations, blurry vision, and diaphoresis. She has a history of occasional tension headaches but no significant cardiac history. She does not smoke and has no history of hypertension. At presentation her blood pressure is 200/140 mm Hg, her heart rate is 120/min, and she is afebrile. Her skin is sweaty and flushed. Noncontrast imaging of the brain is negative for blood or other mass lesions. Her blood pressure is stabilized pharmacologically. Laboratory testing reveals increased plasma metanephrine and normetanephrine levels. Results of a serum thyroid-stimulating hormone test are within normal limits. Twenty-four-hour urine catecholamines and meta/normetanephrines are elevated.

What is the most likely diagnosis?

Pheochromocytoma is a catecholamine-secreting tumor of chromaffin cells of the adrenal medulla.

What are the key steps in epinephrine catabolism?

Catecholamines are substrates for monoamine oxidase (MAO) and catechol-*O*-methyltransferase (COMT) (Figure 6-8). Epinephrine can undergo two paths of catabolism. In the first, COMT converts epinephrine into metanephrine, which MAO then converts into 3-methoxy-4-hydroxymandelic acid. In the second, MAO converts epinephrine into dihydroxymandelic acid, which COMT then converts into 3-methoxy-4-hydroxymandelic acid (the same product as the first pathway).

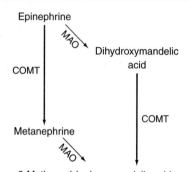

FIGURE 6-8. **Epinephrine catabolism.**

What receptors do catecholamines act on to produce hypertension?

Catecholamines act on α_1 and β_1 receptors. Activation of α_1 receptors contracts vascular smooth muscle, and activation of β_1 receptors in the heart increases heart rate, conduction velocity, and contractility.

During removal of an adrenal gland, the surgeon must secure the adrenal vasculature, especially the adrenal vein. How is the blood supplied to the adrenal gland?

The arterial blood supply to the adrenal gland can be variable, with blood supply from the superior suprarenal artery originating from the inferior phrenic artery; the middle suprarenal artery originating from the aorta; and the inferior suprarenal artery originating from the renal artery. The adrenal gland typically has a dominant vein, which empties into the left renal vein (left adrenal gland) and the inferior vena cava (right adrenal gland).

What is the probability that this patient's condition is malignant?

Approximately 10%. Remember the **"rule of 10's"** for pheochromocytomas: 10% are malignant, 10% bilateral, 10% extra-adrenal, 10% calcify, 10% are pediatric, 10% are familial, and they are 10 times more likely to appear on the boards than in real life!

What is the structure and function of the adrenal gland?

The adrenal gland is composed of the cortex and medulla, each with its own secretory products. The zones of the adrenal cortex can be remembered with the memory trick, "the deeper you go, the sweeter it gets": salt-related hormones (aldosterone) from the zona glomerulosa, sugar-related hormones (cortisol) from the zona fasciculata, and sex-related hormones (testosterone, DHEAS) in the zona reticularis. The adrenal medulla produces catecholamines such as epinephrine and norepinephrine.

CASE 14

A 10-year-old girl is brought to her pediatrician for a workup of new-onset seizures. The patient had been in her usual state of health until 3 months ago, when she developed numbness and tingling in her fingertips and frequent muscle cramps. Last week, she had a grand mal seizure. CT scan of the head at that time revealed no intracranial lesions. Physical examination reveals a well-nourished female with short stature and shortened fourth and fifth digits. Tapping on her cheek and inflation of the blood pressure cuff produces rapid muscle spasms. Relevant laboratory findings include the following:

Calcium: 7 mg/dL
Phosphate: 6 mg/dL
Parathyroid hormone (PTH): 100 pg/dL (normal: 10–60 pg/dL)

What is the most likely diagnosis?

Pseudohypoparathyroidism (type 1a) is characterized by renal unresponsiveness to PTH. A genetic cause of this disorder results from a mutation in the $G_s\text{-}a_1$ protein of adenylyl cyclase. **McCune-Albright hereditary osteodystrophy** is also present in type 1a pseudohypoparathyroidism, and some patients have growth hormone–releasing hormone resistance.

What would hypocalcemia with a low serum PTH level suggest?

Primary hypoparathyroidism, usually caused by accidental removal or injury of the parathyroid glands during thyroid surgery, causes decreased PTH levels, which results in decreased serum calcium levels.

What are Chvostek and Trousseau signs?

Chvostek sign (twitching of ipsilateral facial muscles upon tapping of the facial nerve just anterior to the ear) and **Trousseau sign** (carpal contractions provoked by inflating a blood pressure cuff above systolic blood pressure for more than 3 minutes) are signs of hypocalcemia.

How is the serum calcium level regulated?

Serum calcium is regulated by PTH and vitamin D.

PTH has two major sites of action: bone and kidney. In bone, PTH increases bone turnover, liberating calcium. In the kidney, PTH increases enzymatic formation of $1,25\text{-}(OH)_2$-cholecalciferol from vitamin D, phosphate excretion, and calcium reabsorption.

The active form of **vitamin D** stimulates calcium and phosphate absorption in the gut as well as bone resorption.

Where is PTH synthesized?

PTH is synthesized in the **chief cells** of the parathyroid glands.

What are the other physiologic effects of hypocalcemia?

In addition to muscle cramping, paresthesias, and convulsions, low calcium levels also may prolong the QT interval on ECG. It is important to identify patients with prolonged QT intervals as it is a risk factor for serious cardiac arrhythmias including torsades de pointes. By contrast, patients with hypercalcemia have a shortened QT interval.

■ CASE 15

A 30-year-old African-American woman with a history of hypertension presents to her new primary care physician for a physical examination. She claims to be in good health but has noticed she is urinating more frequently and has had several urinary tract infections in the past year. Her family history is significant for premature coronary artery disease and diabetes in multiple first-degree relatives. Her heart rate is 70/min and her blood pressure is 140/90mm Hg. Physical examination is notable for morbid obesity (body mass index: 48 kg/m²), and a urine dipstick reveals 2+ glycosuria.

What is the most likely diagnosis?

Non-insulin-dependent (type 2) diabetes mellitus (NIDDM).

What are the diagnostic criteria for this condition?

Random plasma glucose > 200 mg/dL with symptoms

or

Fasting plasma glucose > 126 mg/dL on two separate occasions

or

Plasma glucose > 200 mg/dL 2 hours after a glucose tolerance test

What is the production and structure of insulin?

Insulin is originally produced as **pre-proinsulin** in the pancreas. During posttranslational processing, a signal peptide is removed, producing **proinsulin.** Proinsulin contains two polypeptide chains connected by two sulfhydryl bonds (cysteine to cysteine) and a **C-peptide.** In the conversion from proinsulin (the zymogen) to active insulin, the C-peptide is cleaved off (Figure 6-9). Synthetic insulin lacks the C-peptide. Therefore, measuring C-peptide is useful in patients in whom surreptitious insulin injection is suspected (factitious hypoglycemia).

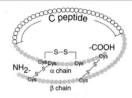

FIGURE 6-9. **Structure of human insulin.** (Reproduced, with permission, from Le T, et al. *First Aid for the USMLE Step 1: 2011.* New York: McGraw-Hill, 2011: 289.)

How does insulin exert its effects on organs?

The insulin receptor is a heterodimer of α and β subunits. The β subunit is a **tyrosine kinase.** When insulin binds, this subunit autophosphorylates itself, leading to activation of downstream signaling cascades. Insulin stimulates glucose storage as glycogen in the liver, triglyceride storage in adipose tissue, and amino acid storage as protein in muscle. It also promotes utilization of glucose in muscle for energy (Figure 6-10).

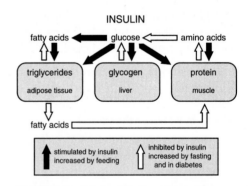

FIGURE 6-10. **Actions of insulin on human tissues.** (Reproduced, with permission, from Brunton LL, et al. *Goodman & Gilman's The Pharmacological Basis of Therapeutics,* 11th ed. New York: McGraw-Hill, 2006: 1621.)

What is the most appropriate treatment for this patient?

The number one reason this patient has NIDDM is her obesity. Therefore, nonpharmacologic treatments such as diet, weight reduction, and exercise must be employed. However, these have limited long-term success. Pharmacologic treatment for type 2 DM includes **oral hypoglycemic agents.** Only in refractory cases is insulin added to the regimen (Table 6-4 lists common drugs for both type 1 and type 2 DM). Tight glucose control markedly reduces microvascular and neurologic complications of DM. The goal is a hemoglobin A$_{1c}$ level of 7%.

TABLE 6-4	Common Pharmacologic Agents for the Treatment of Type 1 and 2 Diabetes Mellitus		
DRUG CLASSES	**ACTION**	**CLINICAL USE**	**TOXICITIES**
Insulin: Lispro (rapid-acting) Aspart (rapid-acting) Regular (rapid-acting) NPH (intermediate) Glargine (long-acting) Detemir (long-acting)	**Bind insulin receptor** (tyrosine kinase activity). Liver: ↑ glucose stored as glycogen. Muscle: ↑ glycogen and protein synthesis, K^+ uptake. Fat: aids TG storage.	Type 1 DM, type 2 DM, gestational diabetes, life-threatening hyperkalemia, and stress-induced hyperglycemia.	Hypoglycemia, hypersensitivity reaction (very rare).
Sulfonylureas: First generation: Tolbutamide Chlorpropamide Second generation: Glyburide Glimepiride Glipizide	Close K+ channel in β-cell membrane, so cell depolarizes → **triggering of insulin release via** ↑ Ca^{2+} influx.	Stimulate release of endogenous insulin in type 2 DM. Require some islet function, so useless in type 1 DM.	First generation: disulfiram-like effects. Second generation: hypoglycemia.
Biguanides: Metformin	Exact mechanism is unknown. **↓ gluconeogenesis,** ↑ glycolysis, ↑ peripheral glucose uptake (insulin sensitivity).	Oral. Can be used in patients without islet function.	Most grave adverse effect is lactic acidosis (contraindicated in renal failure).
Glitazones/ **thiazolidinediones:** Pioglitazone Rosiglitazone	↑ insulin sensitivity in peripheral tissue. Binds to PPAR -γ nuclear transcription regulator.	Used as monotherapy in type 2 DM or combined with above agents.	Weight gain, edema. Hepatotoxicity, CV toxicity.
α-glucosidase inhibitors: Acarbose Miglitol	**Inhibit intestinal brush-border α-glucosidases.** Delayed sugar hydrolysis and glucose absorption lead to ↓ postprandial hyperglycemia.	Used as monotherapy in type 2 DM or in combination with above agents.	GI disturbances.
Mimetics: Pramlintide	↓ glucagon.	Type 2 DM.	Hypoglycemia, nausea, diarrhea.
GLP-1 analogs: Exenatide	↑ insulin, ↓ glucagon release.	Type 2 DM.	Nausea, vomiting; pancreatitis.

(Reproduced, with permission, from Le T, et al. *First Aid for the USMLE Step 1: 2011.* New York: McGraw-Hill, 2011: 304.)

CASE 16

A 32-year-old woman is postpartum day 4 after delivery of her fourth child. The delivery was complicated by massive hemorrhage. She desires to breast-feed, but her breast milk has not come in (normally it begins 24–48 hours postpartum). She breast-fed all of her other children without delay. In addition, she complains of intense fatigue, mental sluggishness, lightheadedness, and a racing heartbeat. On physical examination she is pale, diaphoretic, and weak. Vital signs are as follows: temperature 36.2°C (97.1°F); pulse 100/min supine, 115/min sitting, and 130/min standing; and blood pressure 90/70 mm Hg supine, 80/60 mm Hg sitting, and 70/50 mm Hg standing.

What is the most likely diagnosis?

Sheehan syndrome.

What is the likely cause?

This patient's massive hemorrhage during pregnancy likely led to ischemia and necrosis of the pituitary gland.

What hormones are secreted by the pituitary gland?

The pituitary gland can be separated into anterior and posterior components. The anterior pituitary (adenohypophysis) is derived from ectoderm and produces follicle-stimulating hormone (FSH), luteinizing hormone (LH), adrenocorticotropic hormone (ACTH), growth hormone, thyroid-stimulating hormone, melanotropin, and prolactin. (Know the role of each of these hormones.) The posterior component (neurohypophysis) is derived from neuroectoderm and produces antidiuretic hormone and oxytocin. **Oxytocin** is required for **lactation** and **contraction** of the uterus.

What are the clinical manifestations of this condition?

The presentation can be broken down into deficiencies of each of the pituitary hormones. Severe presentations can present within the first days to weeks of delivery with profound lethargy, anorexia, weight loss, cardiovascular instability, and inability to lactate. Less severe cases may present months to years after the event with hypothyroidism, menstrual irregularities, and other hormonal disturbances.

What is the significance of the patient's vital signs?

The patient displays **orthostatic hypotension**, defined as a systolic blood pressure decrease of at least 20 mm Hg systolic (or a diastolic blood pressure decrease of 10 mm Hg) within 3 minutes of standing. There is a compensatory increase in heart rate to maintain peripheral perfusion. The cause of hypotension in this patient is **loss of cortisol**, which is required for maintenance of peripheral vascular tone. This is a medical emergency, as the patient is at risk for vascular collapse.

What other laboratory abnormalities can be expected in this patient?

Hyponatremia and hyperkalemia, due to loss of ACTH (secondary hypoaldosteronism), hypocortisolism, hypothyroidism, and FSH and LH deficiency are all seen. Lifelong hormone replacement is required.

■ CASE 17

A 13-year-old girl presents to her pediatrician 2 weeks after an upper respiratory infection with a complaint of a "lump in her neck." Physical examination demonstrates a round, freely mobile, slightly tender midline mass that elevates with swallowing. The remainder of the examination is within normal limits. Her birth and developmental history are unremarkable.

What is the most likely diagnosis?
Thyroglossal duct cyst.

What is the differential diagnosis?
The differential for benign midline neck masses is vast, including thyroglossal duct cysts, dermoid cysts, sebaceous cysts, ectopic thyroid tissue, midline branchial cleft cysts (usually are lateral), lipomas, and lymphadenopathy.

Hint: If the question describes a **lateral** neck mass in a patient with a webbed neck, shield chest, short stature, and coarctation of the aorta, think Turner syndrome. The neck mass is likely to be a **cystic hygroma.**

How does the thyroid gland form during development?
The thyroid is derived from **endoderm** at the **foramen cecum,** the junction between the developing anterior and posterior tongue. The thyroid descends to its final position over the trachea by the seventh week of gestation, and its pharyngeal connection forms a stalk called the thyroglossal duct (Figure 6-11).

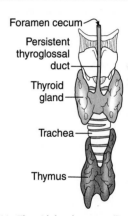

FIGURE 6-11. **Thyroid development.** (Reproduced, with permission, from Le T, et al. *First Aid for the USMLE Step 1: 2011.* New York: McGraw-Hill, 2011: 130.)

What is the pathophysiology of this condition?
The thyroglossal duct should degenerate by the tenth week of gestation. However, in some individuals cystic remnants of the tract remain. Most never become clinically relevant. However, many cysts are detected in patients with recent upper respiratory tract infections, either because infection leads to cyst inflammation, or simply because the cysts are found incidentally on examination of the neck.

What is the most common location of this neck mass?
Thyroglossal duct cysts are in close relation to the hyoid bone and the thyrohyoid membrane. More than 50% are at the level of the hyoid bone within 2 cm of the midline.

What is the most common site of ectopic thyroid tissue?
It is commonly found in the tongue **(lingual thyroid).** If ectopic foci of thyroid tissue will be surgically removed, it must first be confirmed that the ectopic tissue is not the only thyroid tissue the patient has, as thyroid hormone is necessary for survival.

■ CASE 18

As part of Federal Aviation Administration requirements, a 55-year-old pilot presents for a complete checkup. Upon examination of the patient's neck, the physician notes a firm nodule in the right upper lobe of the thyroid that remains fixed with swallowing. Ultrasound-guided fine-needle aspiration (FNA) reveals ground-glass cytoplasm, inclusion bodies, and calcifications.

What is the most likely diagnosis?

Papillary thyroid cancer.

What is the prevalence of this condition?

Thyroid cancer represents approximately 1% of all human cancers. **Papillary** thyroid cancer is the most common type (~ 85%). Other types include **follicular** (~10%), **medullary** (5%), and **anaplastic** (1%). Papillary and follicular types make up the well-differentiated thyroid cancers, whereas the medullary and anaplastic types are considered poorly differentiated.

How is this condition diagnosed?

Careful physical examination, serum thyroid function tests, ultrasound, and FNA of the thyroid.

The first diagnostic step is measuring thyroid-stimulating hormone (TSH) levels. The next step is imaging of the mass with ultrasound and/or radioactive iodine scans. In a patient with a functional nodule that produces thyroid hormone, TSH levels are expected to be suppressed. These functional or "hot" nodules (called "hot" because of their appearance on radioactive iodine scanning) are rarely malignant and thus do not necessitate biopsy. By contrast, a patient with a nonfunctional thyroid mass (called a "cold" nodule) requires biopsy to evaluate for malignancy.

What characteristic features of this condition are likely to be seen on excisional biopsy?

There is no single pathognomonic feature of papillary thyroid cancer. However, the combination of **"ground-glass"** cytoplasm, **"Orphan Annie"** inclusion bodies, prominent nuclei with clefts and grooves, and calcified **psammoma bodies** point to the diagnosis.

What are the risk factors for this condition?

- Male gender (although women are more likely to have thyroid nodules, a thyroid nodule in a man is more likely to be cancerous).
- Age younger than 20 years or older than 60 years.
- Prior **radiation exposure** (eg, acne treatment as a child, victims of Hiroshima, and frequent flyers).
- Medical or family history of thyroid cancer (especially medullary thyroid cancer).

What is the appropriate treatment for this condition?

Total thyroidectomy (with/without lymph node dissection) and postoperative radioactive iodine ablation is indicated. The radioactive iodine is necessary to destroy microsatellites of disease that may have been left behind at surgery. Lumpectomy and lobectomy are no longer recommended in the surgical management of thyroid cancer.

CASE 19

A 55-year-old woman with a history of external neck radiation therapy as a child presents to her physician for her yearly checkup. Physical examination reveals a firm nodule in the neck. Ultrasound confirms several bilateral thyroid nodules; the largest nodule measures 1.5-cm in the left lobe. Biopsy of the nodule confirms the presence of papillary carcinoma. Two weeks later, the patient undergoes total thyroidectomy.

Care must be taken during thyroidectomy not to remove all functioning parathyroid gland tissue. How many parathyroid glands are there?

Most people (85%) have four parathyroid glands. However, 13%–15% of people have more than four glands, and less than 2% of people have fewer than four glands.

What is the embryologic origin of the parathyroid glands?

The superior parathyroid glands are derived from the fourth pharyngeal pouch. The inferior parathyroids are derived from the third pharyngeal pouch. Most ectopic sites are derived along the embryologic descent path (eg, carotid sheath and mediastinum).

What layers of muscle are encountered during a thyroidectomy?

- Platysma (facial nerve innervation).
- Cervical fascia.
- Sternohyoid (a flat, "strap" muscle).
- Sternothyroid (a flat, strap muscle).
- The other two strap muscles (thyrohyoid and omohyoid) are not commonly encountered during routine thyroidectomy.

What nerves in this region are particularly at risk during thyroidectomy?

Damage to the **recurrent laryngeal nerve** in the tracheoesophageal groove results in a hoarse voice. The external laryngeal branch of the superior laryngeal nerve accompanies the superior thyroid artery and therefore can be ligated with the artery in thyroid surgery (Figure 6-12). It is spared by ligating the artery close to the gland. Damage results in changes in pitch and reduction in voice volume.

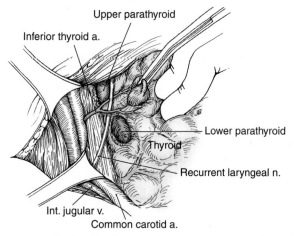

FIGURE 6-12. **Relationship of the parathyroids to the recurrent laryngeal nerve.** (Reproduced, with permission, from Brunicardi FC, et al. *Schwartz's Principles of Surgery*, 8th ed. New York: McGraw-Hill, 2005: 1402.)

After total thyroidectomy, this patient will require lifelong thyroid hormone replacement. What are some other causes of hypothyroidism?

- Autoimmune (Hashimoto thyroiditis)
- Alcohol
- Drugs (amiodarone and lithium)
- Infection

■ CASE 20

A 77-year-old man is brought to the clinic by a concerned neighbor to evaluate a large neck mass. According to the neighbor, the patient lives alone and keeps to himself. The neighbor has noticed that the neck mass has enlarged over several months. Meanwhile, the patient has lost approximately 5.4 kg (12 lb) and has developed noticeable tremor when he reaches for his morning paper or walks his dog. On physical examination, the man is thin with a large goiter containing many palpable nodules. ECG reveals atrial fibrillation. Exophthalmos and pretibial myxedema are absent. Thyroid function tests reveal elevated free thyroxine (T_4) and barely detectable thyroid-stimulating hormone levels.

What is the most likely diagnosis?

Plummer disease (also known as toxic multinodular goiter) is the second most common cause of hyperthyroidism in the Western world after Graves disease and the number one cause among the elderly and in endemic areas of iodine deficiency. This is not to be confused with the uncommon **Plummer-Vinson syndrome** (esophageal web plus iron deficiency anemia).

How does the physical examination help establish a differential diagnosis?

Patients with Graves disease typically have a diffusely enlarged painless goiter rather than a multinodular goiter. Exophthalmos, pretibial myxedema, and acropachy (thickening of peripheral tissues), characteristic of Graves disease, are absent in Plummer disease. Subacute thyroiditis (also known as de Quervain thyroiditis) presents with an enlarged **painful** goiter (Figure 6-13), neck pain, and fever, frequently after a viral illness such as mumps or coxsackievirus. The erythrocyte sedimentation rate is typically elevated, and the condition resolves with time and use of nonsteroidal anti-inflammatory drugs.

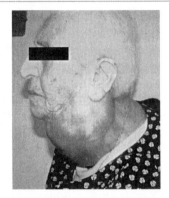

FIGURE 6-13. **A large multinodular goiter.** (Reproduced, with permission, from Brunicardi FC, et al. *Schwartz's Principles of Surgery,* 8th ed. New York: McGraw-Hill, 2005: 1413.)

What are the signs and symptoms of local compression by a neck mass?

- **Symptoms:** Dysphagia (difficulty swallowing), dysphonia (hoarseness), and dyspnea (difficulty breathing).
- **Signs:** Stridor, tracheal deviation, superior vena cava syndrome. (Pemberton sign is engorgement of the facial and neck veins upon simultaneous raising of the arms overhead, secondary to superior vena cava compression at the thoracic inlet.)

What will a radioactive iodine scan likely show?

A thyroid scan with radioactive iodine or Tc^{99m} will likely show **patchy uptake,** with multiple **"hot" nodules** interspersed among areas with decreased uptake. A "hot" nodule means that the activity of the thyroid tissue in that area is elevated. Patients with Graves disease have homogenously high uptake on thyroid scan, whereas patients with thyroiditis (de Quervain or silent lymphocytic thyroiditis) have low uptake on thyroid scan. In general, nodules containing thyroid cancer tend to be "cold" nodules and should be biopsied via fine-needle aspiration.

What is the appropriate treatment for this condition?

Given the size of his goiter, signs of local compression, and symptoms of hyperthyroidism, **thyroidectomy** should be performed. This will alleviate the symptoms of hyperthyroidism in approximately 90% of cases and will rapidly relieve the compression. Preoperatively, the patient should be treated with **antithyroid medication** (such as methimazole) and β-**blockers** to render him euthyroid and to alleviate the atrial fibrillation.

Gastrointestinal

■ CASE 1

A 50-year-old man presents to his physician complaining of problems swallowing for the past several months. Solid foods have been most difficult for him to swallow but recently liquids have also become problematic. He often has chest discomfort after eating and occasionally regurgitates bits of undigested food. His physical examination is unremarkable.

What is the most likely diagnosis?

Achalasia (an esophageal motility disorder that results in dysphagia).

What is the general approach to diagnosing dysphagia?

Refer to Figure 7-1.

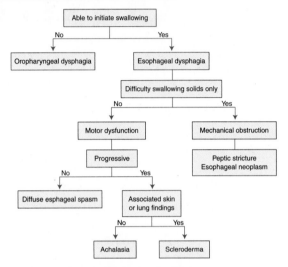

FIGURE 7-1. **Steps in diagnosing dysphagia.**

What condition should be considered in an immigrant patient with this presentation?

Chagas disease, caused by the parasite *Trypanosoma cruzi* (transmitted by the reduviid bug), is indistinguishable from idiopathic forms of achalasia and should be considered in patients from endemic areas (eg, Central and South America).

What is the pathophysiology of this condition?

Achalasia is an idiopathic motility disorder caused by impaired relaxation of the lower esophageal sphincter (LES) and loss of smooth muscle peristalsis in the lower two thirds of the esophagus. It is thought that nitric oxide–producing inhibitory neurons are lost in the myenteric plexus, resulting in the clinical picture described above.

What other imaging or testing can help confirm this diagnosis?

- A barium esophagram demonstrates a "bird's beak" appearance of the esophagus (Figure 7-2).
- Esophageal manometry reveals complete absence of peristalsis and failure of the LES to relax after swallowing to confirm the diagnosis.

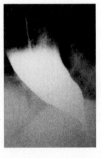

FIGURE 7-2. **"Bird's beak" appearance of the esophagus in achalasia.** (Reproduced, with permission, from Lalwani AK. *Current Diagnosis & Treatment in Otolaryngology—Head & Neck Surgery*, 2nd ed. New York: McGraw-Hill, 2008: 489.)

What is the appropriate treatment for this condition?

Pneumatic dilation of the LES provides effective but temporary relief in most patients and may need to be repeated. Surgical myotomy is also effective. In nonsurgical candidates, trials of calcium channel blockers and multiple injections of botulinum toxin in the LES are also used.

CASE 2

A 50-year-old HIV-positive man presents to his primary care physician with a 1-day history of nausea and vomiting. He also has severe epigastric pain radiating to the back. Review of the patient's medical history reveals that he is taking the reverse transcriptase inhibitor didanosine. Laboratory testing reveals an amylase level five times higher than normal and a lipase level six times higher than normal.

What is the most likely diagnosis?

Acute pancreatitis.

What are the common causes of this condition?

Acute pancreatitis occurs when pancreatic enzymes (trypsinogen, chymotrypsinogen, and phospholipase A) are activated in pancreatic tissue rather than in the lumen of the intestine, resulting in the autodigestion of pancreatic tissue. The most common causes are Gallstones (leading to common bile duct obstruction) and EtOH. Other causes include Trauma, Steroids, Mumps, Autoimmune diseases, Scorpion stings, Hyperlipidemia, and certain Drugs, including antiretrovirals (mnemonic: GET SMASHeD).

What are the top three conditions to consider in the differential diagnosis?

- **Cholelithiasis** refers to the presence of gallstones in the gallbladder that can obstruct the cystic duct. This obstruction can lead to biliary colic (short-term waxing-and-waning pain associated with the ingestion of fatty food) or cholecystitis (more prolonged, constant pain due to inflammation of the gallbladder).
- **Intestinal obstruction** often presents with abdominal pain, nausea, and vomiting but also with changes in bowel habits.
- **Acute coronary syndrome** should be considered in patients 50 years of age or older with abdominal pain and associated risk factors.

In this patient, the significantly elevated amylase and lipase levels are sensitive and specific for acute pancreatitis.

Why is this condition more common in patients with HIV infection?

Patients with HIV and/or AIDS are susceptible to infection with organisms such as cytomegalovirus, *Mycobacterium avium* complex, and *Cryptosporidium,* all of which can cause pancreatitis. Antiretroviral agents such as didanosine, pentamidine, and trimethoprim/sulfamethoxazole can also cause acute pancreatitis.

What is the appropriate treatment for this condition?

Most cases (85%–90%) are self-limited and resolve within 4–7 days of the start of treatment. Typical treatment for acute pancreatitis includes avoiding oral intake, aggressive intravenous fluid resuscitation, pain control, and possibly nasogastric tube placement to decrease gastric secretions in the stomach. Antibiotics are not recommended in uncomplicated pancreatitis but may be of use in severe, necrotizing pancreatitis.

CASE 3

A 42-year-old man presents to his doctor for a checkup after several years without medical care. His medical history is significant for extensive smoking, alcohol, and intravenous drug abuse. On review of systems, the patient reports bleeding gums and increased bruising. Physical examination reveals an overweight white male who appears older than his stated age, mild gynecomastia, palmar erythema, and pitting edema of the lower extremities. Abdominal examination reveals shifting dullness. Relevant laboratory findings are as follows:

WBC count: 3200/mm^3
Hematocrit: 28%
Platelets: 90,000/mm^3
Blood urea nitrogen (BUN): 36 mg/dL
Creatinine (Cr): 1.5 mg/dL
Albumin: 3.3 g/dL
Partial thromboplastin time (PTT): 40 seconds
Prothrombin time (PT): 14 seconds
Alanine aminotransferase (ALT): 60 U/L
Aspartate aminotransferase (AST): 100 U/L

What is the most likely diagnosis?

Alcoholic cirrhosis of the liver. The ascites, palmar erythema, and gynecomastia all suggest liver failure. The moderately elevated transaminase levels suggest a chronic process (too many hepatocytes have already died to cause the dramatic rise seen in an acute process). Further indicators of chronicity include decreased albumin, elevated PT and PTT, thrombocytopenia, and decreased hematocrit. An AST level higher than ALT level suggests an alcoholic, rather than viral, etiology (mnemonic: To**AST**ed).

What are the causes of this patient's gynecomastia and bleeding gums?

The liver normally degrades estrogen. In liver failure, circulating serum levels of estrogen are higher, explaining the gynecomastia and palmer erythema. Bleeding gums are likely due to thrombocytopenia secondary to splenic sequestration and decreased platelet proliferation factor secreted by the damaged liver.

How does ascites form?

Ascites (an abnormal accumulation of serous fluid in the abdominal cavity) is caused by increased intrahepatic sinusoidal pressure secondary to intrahepatic obstruction within the cirrhotic liver, decreased degradation of aldosterone by the liver leading to sodium and water retention, and decreased plasma osmotic pressure due to decreased hepatic production of albumin. Physical signs of ascites include shifting dullness, bulging flanks, and a fluid wave.

What do the laboratory findings reveal about renal function?

Elevated BUN and Cr levels (BUN: Cr ratio > 20) suggest prerenal failure. The kidneys are not perfused appropriately because of decreased intravascular volume (due to ascites). Prolonged intravascular volume depletion in the setting of end-stage liver disease can cause intense renal vasoconstriction and renal failure unresponsive to volume loading; known as hepatorenal syndrome.

CASE 4

A 25-year-old woman presents to her physician with a 3-day history of crampy abdominal pain that started in the epigastrium. She also reports nausea, low-grade fever, and loss of appetite. She denies changes in urination or bowel habits, dysuria, or recent sick contacts. Her last menstrual period was 2 weeks ago. Relevant laboratory findings are as follows:

WBC count: 13,000/mm³
β-Human chorionic gonadotropin (β-hCG): Negative
Urinalysis: Negative for blood, WBCs, leukocyte esterase, and protein

What is the most likely diagnosis?

Appendicitis.

What other conditions should be considered in the differential diagnosis of a 25-year-old female with abdominal pain?

- Genitourinary: Ruptured Graafian follicle, ectopic pregnancy (unlikely with a negative β-hCG), pelvic inflammatory disease, and ovarian torsion (usually moderate to severe pain of acute onset).
- Gastrointestinal: Crohn disease (can initially present without changes in bowel habits), peptic ulcer disease, *Yersinia enterocolitica* infection (known as the great mimicker of appendicitis).
- Renal: Urinary tract infections usually present with increased frequency of urination, dysuria, and abnormal urinalysis. Cystitis can present with abdominal pain and pyelonephritis with classic flank pain.

What is the pathophysiology of this condition?

Obstruction is often implicated as the cause of appendicitis but is not required for disease progression. The appendiceal lumen may become obstructed by a fecalith, mucosal secretions, lymphoid hyperplasia or an **infectious process** resulting in a distended appendix, elevated intraluminal pressure, and subsequent arterial insufficiency and tissue death.

What is the McBurney point?

The **McBurney point** is one-third the distance from the right anterior superior iliac spine to the umbilicus; it is where the pain from acute appendicitis classically localizes once there is peritoneal irritation.

Which antibiotics are effective for coverage of enteric organisms?

Ampicillin and sulbactam are empirically used to treat *Escherichia coli* and *Bacteroides fragilis* infections. Gentamicin, clindamycin, imipenem, second-generation cephalosporins, and piperacillin/tazobactam are also effective.

What is the appropriate treatment for this condition?

Surgery is the preferred treatment, along with supportive intravenous fluids and empiric antibiotics (in case of rupture). The gold standard for diagnosis is CT scan of the abdomen with contrast; Figure 7-3 shows calcified appendicolith.

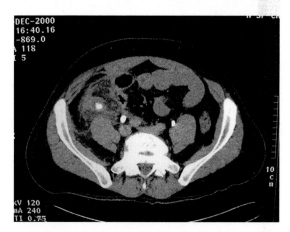

FIGURE 7-3. Contrast-enhanced CT showing a calcified appendolith. (Reproduced, with permission, from Stone CK, Humphries RL. *Current Emergency Diagnosis & Treatment*, 5th ed. New York: McGraw-Hill, 2004: 269.)

CASE 5

A 55-year-old man presents to his physician complaining of burning chest pain that typically occurs after eating and radiates to the neck. Occasionally, the pain and a slight cough awaken him from sleep. He also complains of difficulty swallowing, particularly solid foods. The patient has had these symptoms for several years, but they seem to be worsening.

What is the most likely diagnosis?

Gastroesophageal reflux disease (GERD), complicated by Barrett esophagus (Figure 7-4).

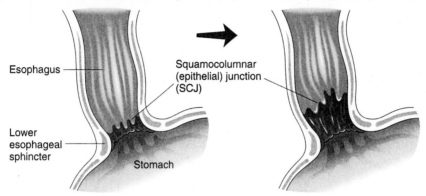

FIGURE 7-4. Barrett esophagus. Note how the columnar epithelium of the stomach has migrated superior to the LES. (Reproduced, with permission, from Le T, et al. *First Aid for the USMLE Step 1: 2008.* New York: McGraw-Hill, 2008: 305.)

What are the expected findings on endoscopy?

Endoscopy reveals an upward shift of the gastroesophageal junction (Z line) due the metaplasia of esophageal nonkeratinized squamous epithelium to gastric columnar epithelium in the setting of recurrent acid exposure.

What are the common treatments for uncomplicated cases of this condition?

- **Proton pump inhibitor (PPI) trial.**
- **Testing for** *Helicobacter pylori* is appropriate in patients not responsive to PPIs. Treatment with triple therapy (PPI, amoxicillin, clarithromycin) is used in *H pylori*–positive cases.
- **Lifestyle modifications** including elevation of the head of the bed, dietary restrictions, and weight loss are often used in conjunction with medical therapy.

Patients with this condition are at greatly increased risk for what other condition?

Compared to the general population, patients with Barrett esophagus are 30 times more likely to develop **esophageal adenocarcinoma** (lifetime risk: ~ 5%).

What factors increase the risk of developing esophageal cancer?

Barrett esophagus is the major risk factor for esophageal adenocarcinoma; alcohol and cigarette smoking are major risk factors for esophageal squamous cell carcinoma. The risk factors for esophageal cancer may be remembered by the mnemonic **ABCDEF:** Achalasia/African American male, Barrett esophagus, Corrosive esophagitis/Cigarettes, Diverticuli (ie, Zenker diverticulum), Esophageal web/EtOH, and Familial.

CASE 6

A 42-year-old obese woman presents to the urgent care facility with a sudden onset of right upper quadrant and epigastric pain that began 8 hours earlier. The pain is steady in nature, worsened by eating, and radiates to the right shoulder. Physical examination reveals inspiratory arrest with deep palpation of the right upper quadrant. Relevant laboratory findings are as follows:

Total bilirubin: 2 mg/dL   AST: 54 U/L
BUN: 16 mg/dL   ALT: 60 U/L
Cr: 1.05 mg/dL

What is the most likely diagnosis?

Choledocholithiasis (a gallstone lodged in the common bile duct). **Note:** The presence of gallstones is termed *cholelithiasis.* Gallbladder disease is common in the United States and manifests as a spectrum of disorders including asymptomatic cholelithiasis, biliary colic, cholecystitis, choledocholithiasis, and cholangitis (infection of the biliary tree). Biliary colic usually resolves within a few hours. The fact that the patient has had unremitting pain for 8 hours and mildly elevated AST and ALT suggests choledocholithiasis.

What physical signs of this condition does the patient exhibit?

- **Boas' sign** is a radiation of pain from the inflamed gallbladder to the right shoulder.
- **Murphy's sign** is the arrest of inspiration with deep palpation in the right upper quadrant.

Infection with which bacteria may result from this condition?

Escherichia coli, Enterobacter cloacae, Enterococcus, and *Klebsiella* are commonly implicated in infection of the gallbladder secondary to obstruction (cholecystitis).

What are the risk factors for this condition?

Cholesterol gallstones are most common in the United States and occur when bile is supersaturated with cholesterol, allowing crystals to form.

Risk factors for gallstones include the 4 F's: Fat, Fertile, Female, and Forty. Other risk factors include oral contraceptive use, spinal cord injury, or diabetes mellitus, all of which cause decreased gallbladder emptying. Intestinal and liver diseases are also risk factors.

Worldwide, **pigmented gallstones** are the most common form and are secondary to bile duct/gallbladder infection, hemolysis, or impaired hepatic synthesis of bilirubin.

What is the pathophysiology of the patient's pain?

Gallstones produce dull, poorly localized visceral pain by obstructing the ampulla of Vater or the cystic duct, causing distention of the gallbladder and irritation of surrounding structures.

Which structures are adjacent to the gallbladder?

The **gallbladder** lies immediately below the liver and above the **right kidney.** The **cystic duct** from the gallbladder joins the common hepatic duct to form the common bile duct. The common bile duct joins with the pancreatic duct and terminates in the **ampulla of Vater,** where bile is excreted into the duodenum.

What is the appropriate treatment for this patient's pain?

Gallstone pain is relieved when the gallstone moves back into the gallbladder, moves into the common bile duct, or passes through the ampulla of Vater. Pain of biliary colic accompanies spasms of the sphincter of Oddi; therefore, **meperidine** should be given for pain, as morphine causes spasms of the sphincter of Oddi.

The hepatoduodenal ligament includes which three structures?

Three structures run through the hepatoduodenal ligament (Figure 7-5):

- The **portal vein** brings blood from the digestive tract to the liver.
- The **hepatic artery** brings oxygen and nutrients to the liver.
- The **common bile duct** connects the liver and gallbladder to the small intestine.

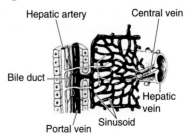

FIGURE 7-5. **Vascular anatomy of the liver lobule.** (Reproduced, with permission, from Doherty GM. *Current Surgical Diagnosis & Treatment,* 12th ed. New York: McGraw-Hill, 2006: 542.)

■ CASE 7

A 6-day-old girl born to Jewish parents is brought to her pediatrician because she "looks yellow," seems weak and floppy, and sleeps all the time. Physical examination reveals a jaundiced infant with scleral icterus, without other obvious abnormalities. Relevant laboratory findings are as follows:

Total bilirubin: 34 mg/dL   AST: 10 U/L
Direct bilirubin: Undetectable   Coombs test: Negative
ALT: 12 U/L

What is the most likely diagnosis?

Crigler-Najjar syndrome.

What is the pathophysiology of this condition?

This is an inherited disorder of bilirubin metabolism, resulting from a mutation in **glucuronyl transferase**, the enzyme that conjugates bilirubin with glucuronic acid. Unconjugated bilirubin is less water soluble than conjugated bilirubin. It is therefore less easily excreted in urine/bile and deposits throughout the body, as evidenced in this patient by jaundice and scleral icterus.

What are the two subtypes of this condition, and how do they differ in severity?

- **Crigler-Najjar type I:** Glucuronyl transferase activity is completely absent, which results in a high likelihood of death in the first year of life.
- **Crigler-Najjar type II:** Glucuronyl transferase activity is present but low. Patients with this form of the disease have a better prognosis than those with type 1 (Table 7-1).

TABLE 7-1	Principal Differential Characteristics of Crigler-Najjar Syndromes	
FEATURE	CRIGLER-NAJJAR SYNDROME	
	TYPE I	TYPE II
Total serum bilirubin, mg/dL	18–45 (usually > 20)	6–25 (usually > 20)
Routine liver tests	Normal	Normal
Response to phenobarbital	None	Decreases bilirubin by > 25%
Kernicterus	Usual	Rare
Hepatic histology	Normal	Normal

Bile characteristics
  Color
  Bilirubin fractions
	Pale or colorless
	> 90% unconjugated
		Pigmented
		Largest fraction (mean: 57%) monoconjugates

Bilirubin UDP-glucuronosyl transferase activity	Typically absent; traces in some patients	Markedly reduced: 0%–10% of normal
Inheritance (both autosomal)	Recessive	Predominantly recessive

(Adapted with permission from Kasper DL, et al. *Harrison's Principles of Internal Medicine*, 16th ed. New York: McGraw-Hill, 2005: 1819.)

This patient is at risk for what life-threatening complication?

Kernicterus is an abnormal accumulation of bile pigment in the basal ganglia of the central nervous system leading to deranged motor function, irreversible brain damage, and even death. Unconjugated bilirubin also penetrates the blood-brain barrier to cause neuronal death.

What is the appropriate treatment for this condition?

In Crigler-Najjar type I, liver transplantation is the only cure. Phototherapy may prevent kernicterus. In type II, hyperbilirubinemia often responds to **phenobarbital**.

■ CASE 8

A 64-year-old woman presents to her physician complaining of gas, constipation, and left lower abdominal discomfort. The pain increases after meals but persists throughout the day. The patient has a history of chronic constipation, but the current symptoms are worse than normal. She denies bloody stools currently but did have a massive gastrointestinal (GI) bleed last year. During that hospitalization she received a barium enema (Figure 7-6). Her only medication is one baby aspirin per day. On physical examination, she is febrile to 38.6°C (101.5°F) with a blood pressure of 110/70 mm Hg, heart rate of 105/min, and respiratory rate of 18/min. Relevant laboratory findings are as follows:

WBC count: 13,400/mm³
Hemoglobin: 13 g/dL
Hematocrit: 38%
Platelets: 250,000/mm³
Chloride: 100 mEq/L

Potassium: 4.3 mEq/L
Bicarbonate: 24 mEq/L
Sodium: 136 mEq/L
Creatinine: 1.2 mg/dL
Stool guaiac test: Negative

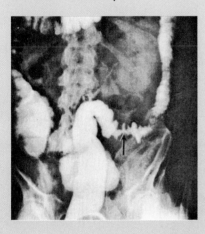

FIGURE 7-6. **Patient's roentgenogram.** (Reproduced, with permission, from Doherty GM, Way LW. *Current Surgical Diagnosis & Treatment*, 12th ed. New York: McGraw-Hill, 2006: 715.)

What is the most likely diagnosis?

Diverticulitis (inflammation of outpouchings involving all layers of the colonic wall). The patient has known diverticula in her distal colon as seen in her roentgenogram. The previous GI bleed was likely secondary to a diverticular bleed.

Which of the clinical signs and symptoms help confirm the diagnosis?

Constipation, flatus, left-sided abdominal pain, tenderness, fever, tachycardia, and elevated WBC count are characteristic of diverticulitis.

What tests can help confirm the diagnosis?

X-ray of the abdomen is needed to rule out free air (a surgical emergency in which upright x-ray of the abdomen shows an area of lucency immediately under the diaphragm caused by diverticular rupture). If there is no surgical emergency, a CT of the abdomen may be ordered. Radiographic findings include bowel wall thickening, fistulas, and/or abscesses. Colonoscopy is contraindicated in acute cases as it may cause perforation but should be completed on follow-up to evaluate for malignancy.

What are the risk factors for this condition, and what steps can prevent recurrence?

Advanced age, chronic constipation, previous diverticulosis, and aspirin use all heighten the risk for diverticular disease. A high-fiber diet and good hydration reduce the risk of developing diverticula and subsequent diverticulitis.

What is the appropriate treatment for this condition?

Treatment includes broad-spectrum antibiotics, such as metronidazole and ciprofloxacin, a clear liquid diet for 1 week, and adequate analgesia. A follow-up colonoscopy should be performed after the acute symptoms resolve.

■ CASE 9

The emergency department triage nurse calls the on-call intern to ask how she should triage a 42-year-old woman with fever, mental status changes, and a history of hereditary spherocytosis. The patient was brought in by her husband after he found her disoriented and sick in bed. She is unable to provide a good history. Vital signs are notable for a temperature of 38.9°C (102°F), heart rate of 125/min, blood pressure of 80/50 mm Hg, and respiratory rate of 24/min. She is overweight, diaphoretic, slightly yellow, and oriented only to person. Physical examination reveals tenderness and guarding in the right upper quadrant (RUQ).

Where should this patient be placed on the triage list?

This patient requires **immediate attention.** Even without laboratory data, her vital signs (fever, tachycardia, hypotension, and tachypnea) and toxic appearance raise suspicion of infection.

What is the most likely diagnosis?

Cholangitis is an infection of the bile ducts secondary to ductal obstruction (Figure 7-7). Most commonly, the common bile duct is obstructed by a gallstone. Other causes include stricture, biliary cancer, and infection (eg, *Clonorchis*).

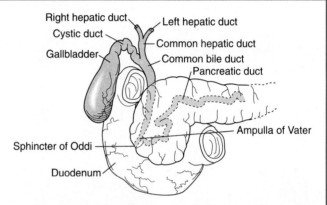

FIGURE 7-7. **Anatomy of the biliary tree.** (Reproduced, with permission, from Le T, et al. *First Aid for the USMLE Step 1: 2008.* New York: McGraw-Hill, 2008: 294.)

How does the physical examination help confirm the diagnosis?

The patient displays **Charcot triad** (RUQ pain, jaundice, and fever) and **Reynolds pentad** (Charcot triad plus hypotension and mental status changes), which are classic for cholangitis.

What risk factors in this patient's history predisposed her to this condition?

The patient likely has underlying cholelithiasis (gallstones). In addition to the **4 F's** (Fat, Fertile, Forty, and Female), the patient also has hereditary spherocytosis (HS). Patients with HS are predisposed to develop **pigment gallstones** due to chronic hemolysis. Pigment gallstones are radiopaque because they are composed of calcium bilirubinate. The high iron content from the hemolyzed red blood cells may also help these stones to be visualized on x-ray.

What laboratory values are expected?

- WBC count will be elevated as a cellular response to infection.
- Hyperbilirubinemia (indirect and direct) will be present. Indirect bilirubin is elevated because of red cell lysis in the setting of hereditary spherocytosis; direct bilirubin is elevated because of inappropriate excretion in the setting of obstruction.
- Alkaline phosphatase, secreted by the mucosal cells of the biliary tree, not specific to biliary obstruction, will be elevated.
- γ-Glutamyl transpeptidase, secreted by the mucosal cells of the biliary tree, will be elevated, specifically as a marker of biliary obstruction.
- Positive blood cultures are consistent with the patient's systemic signs of infection.

What is the appropriate treatment for this condition?

This patient is displaying severe symptoms, so every effort should be made to relieve the obstruction and decompress the biliary tree. Endoscopic retrograde cholangiopancreatography (ERCP) is the tool of choice, as it is both diagnostic and therapeutic.

CASE 10

The mother of a newborn girl complains to the pediatrician that the infant is coughing, drooling excessively, and vomiting immediately after every feeding. The woman's pregnancy was complicated by gestational polyhydramnios. The physician attempts to place a nasogastric tube in the infant, but x-ray of the chest reveals that it cannot pass to the stomach, which is distended with air.

What is the most likely diagnosis?

Esophageal atresia with tracheoesophageal fistula. This variant accounts for 85% of these malformations (Figure 7-8).

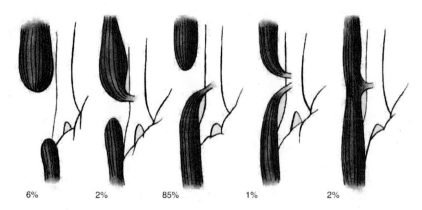

FIGURE 7-8. Variants of esophageal atresia and their prevalence. (Reproduced, with permission, from Brunicardi FC, et al. *Schwartz's Principles of Surgery*, 8th ed. New York: McGraw-Hill, 2005: 1481.)

What is the mechanism of polyhydramnios?

Normally, fetuses swallow amniotic fluid in utero. The fluid is absorbed by the infant's GI tract and returned to the mother via the placenta or eliminated through the urinary system. When a fetus is unable to swallow, amniotic fluid builds up, resulting in polyhydramnios. Polyhydramnios can also result from disorders of the urinary tract, as in neonatal Bartter syndrome.

Lung buds are derived from which embryonic structure?

The lung buds, which will become the bronchial tree, begin as evaginations from the primitive foregut, which also gives rise to the esophagus. Thus, abnormalities anywhere along this developmental pathway can cause a variety of tracheoesophageal fistulae.

Which pathogens are most likely to cause pneumonia in this patient?

Anaerobes are likely to cause pneumonia because of the increased risk of aspiration of GI contents from frequent vomiting and pooling of fluids in the esophageal pouch.

What congenital condition is associated with polyhydramnios and bilious vomiting?

Duodenal atresia, which has an increased incidence in infants with trisomy 21 (Down syndrome). Bilious vomiting indicates gastrointestinal obstruction distal to the opening of the bile duct.

This patient should be screened for what other congenital abnormalities?

The following associations have an unknown genetic link and involve mesoderm-derived structures (mnemonic: **VACTERL**):

- Vertebral anomalies
- Anal atresia
- Cardiovascular anomalies
- Tracheoesophageal fistula
- Esophageal atresia
- Renal anomalies
- Limb defects

■ CASE 11

A 66-year-old woman presents to her physician with left lower quadrant pain; a 3-week history of nausea, vomiting, and diarrhea; and an unintentional 15.9-kg (35-lb) weight loss over the past month. Her medical history is complicated by type 2 diabetes, hypertension, breast cancer, erosive esophagitis, and chronic peptic ulcer disease. She takes several medications, including a β-blocker. CT of the abdomen reveals a 5×5-cm mass in the head of the pancreas. Relevant laboratory findings are as follows:

Gastric pH: < 2.0
Gastrin: 1500 pg/mL (normal: < 90 pg/mL)
Hematocrit: 26%
Basal gastric acid output: > 15 mEq/h (normal: < 15 mEq/h)

What is the most likely diagnosis?

Gastrinoma, a gastrin-secreting, non–β islet cell tumor of the pancreas or duodenum. These tumors cause gastric hypersecretion of hydrochloric acid, which results in disseminated gastrointestinal ulcers.

What test can further support the diagnosis?

The secretin stimulation test elicits increased gastrin secretion by the cells in a gastrinoma, whereas normal gastric G cells are inhibited by secretin. The test therefore differentiates between the presence of a gastrinoma and other causes of hypergastrinemia.

What are the two most common neuroendocrine tumors?

Gastrinoma (two-thirds are malignant) and insulinoma (usually benign) are the most common neuroendocrine tumors.

What are the signs and symptoms of this condition?

- Increased fasting gastrin level.
- Ulcers in unusual locations such as the proximal jejunum.
- Gastroesophageal reflux disease.
- Nausea/vomiting.
- Epigastric pain.
- Weight loss.

With what syndromes is this condition commonly associated?

Zollinger-Ellison (ZE) syndrome is characterized by a classical triad of symptoms: increased gastric acid secretion, peptic ulcer disease, and diarrhea.

Multiple endocrine neoplasia type I (MENI) is a genetic syndrome with an increased risk of parathyroid, pituitary, and pancreatic (such as gastrin-secreting) adenomas.

What is the appropriate treatment for this condition?

Surgical treatment involves resection of the tumor, surrounding pancreatic tissue, regional lymph nodes, and other structures in cases of metastasis (60%).

Medical treatments include proton pump inhibitors and somatostatin. Octreotide is a somatostatin analog with a longer half-life. Both somatostatin and octreotide act by inhibiting release of somatotropin, insulin, gastrin, glucagon, and vasoactive intestinal peptide.

CASE 12

A 35-year-old man presents to his physician with erectile dysfunction, decreased libido, achy joints, increased thirst, and frequency of urination. His wife also notes that he looks like he has a tan, despite being January. On physical examination, his skin appears bronze in color. Relevant laboratory studies are as follows:

Blood glucose: 242 mg/dL
Serum iron: 1200 mg/dL
Transferrin saturation: 99%

What is the most likely diagnosis?

Symptoms suggest hemochromatosis, which has a classic triad of features:

- Micronodular pigment cirrhosis.
- Diabetes mellitus.
- Skin pigmentation.

The last two symptoms give this disease the nickname **"bronze diabetes."**

How is this condition inherited?

Hereditary (primary) hemochromatosis is an **autosomal recessive** disease caused by a defect in the *Hfe* gene of chromosome 6.

What is the pathophysiology of this condition?

In the primary disorder, the mutant *Hfe* gene alters transferrin regulation, leading to excess storage of iron in the parenchymal cells of visceral organs. The organs most affected are as follows:

- Liver, leading to **cirrhosis.** Liver biopsy typically shows extensive hemosiderin deposits within the hepatocytes and Kupffer cells (specialized macrophages). Hemosiderin and other iron-containing compounds stain with **Prussian blue.**
- Pancreas, leading to **diabetes mellitus.**
- Heart, leading to restrictive **cardiomyopathy** and congestive heart failure.
- Joints, leading to arthritis and **arthralgias.**
- Gonads, leading to **testicular atrophy.**

What is the appropriate treatment for this condition?

Treatment involves repeated phlebotomy and an iron chelator such as deferoxamine.

How is this condition differentiated from Wilson disease?

In Wilson disease, a decrease in circulating ceruloplasmin causes copper to accumulate in the liver, brain, and cornea (eg, hepatolenticular degeneration). Like hemochromatosis, patients are at risk for developing hepatocellular carcinoma. Wilson disease is characterized by **ABCD:**

- Asterixis.
- Basal ganglia degeneration (parkinsonian features, choreiform movements, and hemiballismus).
- Corneal deposits in Descemet membrane and cirrhosis.
- Dementia and other mental status disturbances.

Wilson disease is treated with penicillamine.

■ CASE 13

A 34-year-old man with a history of alcohol and drug abuse comes to the emergency department complaining of nausea and vomiting. He notes no recent change in diet or lifestyle and has been in a monogamous relationship for the past year. Physical examination reveals a fever of 38.3°C (101°F), a heart rate of 80/min, and a respiratory rate of 18/min. Scleral icterus is present and there is tenderness in the right upper quadrant and midepigastric region. Workup is negative for gonorrhea and chlamydia. Relevant laboratory findings are as follows:

ALT: 1310 U/L
AST: 1200 U/L
Alkaline phosphatase: 98 U/L
HBsAg: Negative
HBeAg: Negative
Anti-HBeAg antibody: Positive
Anti-HBcAg antibody: Positive
Anti-HBsAg antibody: Negative

What is the most likely diagnosis?

Hepatitis B virus (HBV) infection.

What laboratory findings support the diagnosis?

Hepatitis can be caused by alcohol, viral infection, ischemia, congestive heart failure, or toxins such as acetaminophen or aflatoxin. The history and the roughly equivalent increases of serum transaminases (by > 1000 U/L) here suggest a viral etiology. By contrast, in alcoholic hepatitis, AST is typically elevated more than ALT but does not often rise above 1000 U/L.

The patient is in the "**window phase**" of HBV infection, which occurs after HBsAg has disappeared but before anti-HBsAg antibody is detectable. This conclusion is supported by the presence of anti-HBeAg and anti-HBcAg antibodies. The patient is not a chronic carrier as he is negative for HBsAg. He is also not highly infective because he is negative for HBeAg. In a vaccinated or immune patient, anti-HBsAg would be positive with a negative HBsAg (Table 7-2).

TABLE 7-2	Serologic Responses to Hepatitis B Virus Infections			
TEST	ACUTE DISEASE	WINDOW PHASE	COMPLETE RECOVERY	CHRONIC CARRIER
HBsAg	+	−	−	+
HBsAb	−	−	+	−[b]
HBcAb	+[a]	+	+	+

[a] IgM in acute stage; IgG in chronic or recovered stage.
[b] Patient has surface antibody but available antibody is bound to HBsAg.
(Modified, with permission, from Le T, et al. *First Aid for the USMLE Step 1: 2011.* New York: McGraw-Hill, 2011: 172.)

What percentage of patients with an acute form of this condition progress to a chronic form?

Approximately 10% of adults with acute HBV infection develop chronic hepatitis, whereas 90% of affected neonates develop the chronic disease.

What are the appropriate treatments for this condition?

- Lamivudine (3TC) is phosphorylated into a nucleotide analog and leads to DNA chain termination.
- α-Interferon, an endogenous cytokine, has a high efficacy but can be expensive and has side effects (headache, nausea/vomiting, liver/renal toxicity with chronic use).
- Adefovir is a nucleotide analog of adenosine monophosphate and therefore stops DNA replication. It is often used in cases of lamivudine-resistant chronic hepatitis.

■ CASE 14

A medical student accidently sticks himself while attempting to recap a needle. The patient he was treating is known to have chronic, active hepatitis C virus (HCV) infection. The student has blood drawn for antibody testing, which is found to be negative for anti-HCV antibody. Four weeks later, the medical student is still negative for anti-HCV antibody, but at 13 weeks, results of antibody testing are positive.

Was the third antibody test falsely positive? Why or why not?

No, this student has acute HCV infection. It takes weeks to months for the body to develop an antibody response to HCV (Figure 7-9). The two prior negative tests indicated only that he did not have a pre-existing HCV infection or prior exposure.

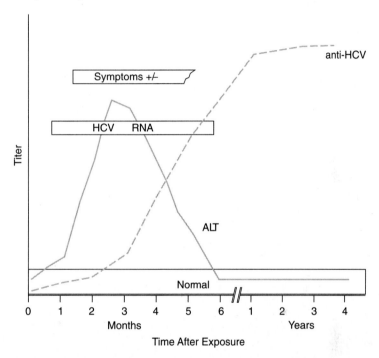

FIGURE 7-9. Serologic pattern of acute hepatitis C virus infection with recovery. (Reproduced, with permission, from South-Paul JE, et al. *Current Diagnosis & Treatment in Family Medicine.* New York: McGraw-Hill, 2004.)

What other laboratory findings are typically found in patients with this condition?

Transaminitis (elevated AST and ALT) secondary to damaged liver cells releasing intracellular enzymes is common. HCV RNA may also be detectable in the serum by reverse transcriptase–polymerase chain reaction.

What is the course of this condition?

The majority of patients with acute HCV infection are asymptomatic. Approximately 25% of patients will become jaundiced. The patient may have flulike symptoms lasting 2–12 weeks. Although only a small percentage of people exposed to HCV by needlestick will develop acute hepatitis, 60%–80% of those who develop acute hepatitis will develop chronic infection. **Chronic infection** has a variable but slowly progressive course; approximately 20% of patients develop cirrhosis. Excessive alcohol consumption further increases the risk of cirrhosis in this patient population.

What are the appropriate treatments for this condition?

A combination of ribavirin and pegylated α-interferon induces remission in approximately 40% of chronic, active HCV cases. Ribavirin is a guanosine analog that inhibits viral mRNA synthesis. Pegylated α-interferon is an endogenous cytokine that induces antiviral host enzymes and causes significant flulike symptoms.

■ CASE 15

A 55-year-old alcoholic male with known chronic liver disease evidenced by cirrhosis presents with increasing weight loss and ascites. Physical examination reveals spider angiomas, palmar erythema, shrunken scrotum, and hemorrhoids. The liver edge is nonpalpable. Axial CT scan shows a round homogeneous and hypervascular mass in the right lobe of the liver (Figure 7-10).

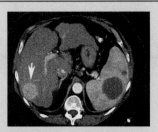

FIGURE 7-10. CT scan showing mass in the right lobe of the liver. (Reproduced, with permission, from Greenberger NJ, et al. *Current Diagnosis & Treatment: Gastroenterology, Hepatology, & Endoscopy.* New York: McGraw-Hill, 2009: Figure 9-28.)

What is the likely diagnosis?

Hepatocellular carcinoma (HCC), also known as hepatoma. (Do not let the "oma" fool you into thinking that this tumor is benign.)

What risk factors are associated with this condition?

- Chronic hepatitis B and C infection.
- Cirrhosis.
- Aflatoxin (produced by *Aspergillus flavus*).
- Heavy metal disorders with liver deposition (Wilson disease, hemochromatosis).
- α_1-Antitrypsin deficiency.

What serum marker may help diagnose this condition?

α-Fetoprotein (AFP). This is not specific for HCC, as elevated serum AFP also occurs in pregnancy, germ cell tumors, and other liver diseases; however, for Step 1, hepatic tumor + AFP = hepatoma.

How can the physical examination findings be explained?

The patient has functional **hyperestrogenemia.** The liver is responsible for the degradation of estrogen, so alcoholics have higher circulating estrogens, leading to:

- Spider angiomata.
- Palmar erythema.
- Testicular atrophy.
- Gynecomastia.

The patient also has **portal hypertension,** which leads to the opening of collateral vessels to bypass the obstructed liver, resulting in:

- Esophageal varices.
- Caput medusae.
- Hemorrhoids.

What nutritional deficiencies are likely to be present in this patient?

Alcoholics may be deficient in several vital nutrients, but the following deficiencies are very common:

- Thiamine (vitamin B_1).
- Vitamin B_{12}.
- Folate.
- Calcium.
- Magnesium.

In addition to the substitution of alcohol for nutrient-containing foods, abusers' gastrointestinal tracts are altered by alcohol, which further reduces absorption.

What role does thiamine play in the metabolism of carbohydrates and amino acids?

Thiamine is present in cells as thiamine pyrophosphate (TPP), which is necessary for the metabolism of pyruvate to acetyl-CoA, and α-Ketoglutarate to succinyl-CoA in the process of aerobic cellular respiration. Thiamine is also used for the oxidative decarboxylation of branched-chain amino acids (leucine, isoleucine, and valine) and the pentose-phosphate shunt.

Why must alcoholics receive thiamine whenever glucose-containing intravenous fluids are given?

This is done to prevent **Wernicke encephalopathy.** Thiamine is necessary for the metabolism of glucose. There is a high level of TPP in the mammillary bodies. If glucose is administered, the remaining thiamine in the mammillary bodies is consumed, leading to irreversible damage. The triad of Wernicke encephalopathy is **confusion, ataxia,** and **ophthalmoplegia (nystagmus). Korsakoff syndrome** is a permanent condition with an etiology similar to Wernicke encephalopathy and characterized by both retrograde and anterograde amnesia with confabulation.

■ CASE 16

An otherwise healthy 36-hour-old boy born at 37 weeks' gestation to a G3P2 mother is noted to have yellowed skin over his entire body. A complete blood count reveals a slightly low hematocrit but normal WBC and platelet counts. Other relevant laboratory findings are as follows:

Direct bilirubin: 0 mg/dL
Serum total bilirubin: 19 mg/dL (elevated even considering age)
Direct Coombs test: Weakly positive
Mother's blood type: O+
Infant's blood type: B+

What is the most likely diagnosis?

Hyperbilirubinemia due to red cell lysis caused by maternal anti-B antibodies (immunoglobulin G) in the infant's blood.

Is this patient's condition likely due to biliary obstruction?

No; it is not likely to be caused by biliary obstruction because the infant's direct bilirubin level is 0 mg/dL, indicating that conjugated bilirubin is being excreted properly.

The patient is given phototherapy. Why is this effective?

Phototherapy irreversibly converts unconjugated bilirubin into **lumirubin,** which is similar to conjugated bilirubin in that it is soluble and able to be excreted in bile and urine.

The patient is given a blood transfusion for his anemia. What ABO blood types should the packed RBC donor and the plasma donor be to minimize hemolysis upon transfusion?

The RBC donor should be type O to avoid hemolysis of donor cells by maternal anti-B antibodies in the infant's blood. The plasma donor should be type B or AB, so that the plasma will not contain anti-B antibodies, which would be incompatible with the infant's blood.

Which drugs, when ingested by the mother, increase the baby's risk of kernicterus?

Drugs that are highly bound to albumin—such as aspirin, ceftriaxone, and sulfa-based drugs—may displace bilirubin from albumin, thus increasing the level of neurotoxic free bilirubin in the blood and leading to the development kernicterus.

Despite phototherapy, the infant's total serum bilirubin climbs to 26 mg/dL. An infusion of albumin followed by an exchange transfusion is ordered. Why is this treatment effective?

Infused albumin binds free bilirubin, helping to draw extravascular bilirubin from tissues into the blood, which will then be removed by the exchange transfusion.

■ CASE 17

An 18-year-old man presents with a 2-year history of abdominal pain and increasingly frequent bloody diarrhea. He has unintentionally lost 5.4 kg (12 lb) over 6 months and now complains of joint and lower back pain. He reports that several relatives have had similar complaints, and recently his 40-year-old uncle was diagnosed with colon cancer. Physical examination reveals diffuse voluntary guarding, no rebound tenderness, no masses, and no rectal fistulas. Colonoscopy reveals inflamed mucosa with friable pseudopolyps from the rectum to the splenic flexure.

What is the most likely diagnosis?

An inflammatory bowel disease. In this case, ulcerative colitis (UC) is more likely than Crohn disease (CD) because of the genetic component, associated joint/lower back pain, and gross appearance.

How can these two conditions be differentiated from one another?

Features of **UC**:

- Bimodal age distribution.
- Possibly autoimmune in origin.
- Males > females.
- Involvement of the rectum in all cases.
- **Continuous lesions** confined to the **mucosa.**
- Friable mucosal **pseudopolyps** on gross morphology and crypt abscesses and ulcers on microscopic morphology.
- No strictures or fistulas, but possibly a **"lead pipe"** colon without haustra and colon shortening.
- Colectomy is curative.

Features of **CD**:

- Involvement of the entire gastrointestinal tract, including the mouth (oral ulcers) and anus (bloody diarrhea or constipation).
- Distal ileum is often affected.
- **Transmural** inflammation and thickening ("string sign" on x-ray), **cobblestone** mucosa, **skip lesions,** and creeping fat.
- Frequently causes strictures, fistulas, and perianal disease.
- **Noncaseating granulomas** on histology.
- Surgery is not curative, as disease may develop anywhere along the gastrointestinal tract.

What extraintestinal manifestations are possible in this patient?

Extraintestinal manifestations in UC relate to its association with **HLA-B27:** ankylosing spondylitis, reactive arthritis (ie, arthritis, uveitis, urethritis), primary sclerosing cholangitis, and pyoderma gangrenosum. Patients with primary sclerosing cholangitis have an even greater risk of colorectal cancer (CRC).

What further screening is recommended for the future?

There is a significantly increased risk of CRC among patients with UC. The risk depends on duration and extent of disease, especially at 8–10 years after onset of symptoms. Patients should undergo colonoscopy and biopsy approximately 8 years after first diagnosis and, if negative, undergo a repeat examination every 1–3 years thereafter.

CASE 18

A 75-year-old woman presents to the emergency department (ED) after passing two bright red, plum-sized clots of blood per rectum. There was no stool passed with the clots. The patient denies any abdominal discomfort or cramping but states she becomes lightheaded upon standing. She also reports being very constipated over the past few months. She takes one 81-mg aspirin per day. In the ED, her hematocrit is 28%, and her blood pressure is 110/70 mm Hg supine and 80/50 mm Hg standing.

Where is the likely origin of the blood?

The blood is most likely from the lower gastrointestinal (GI) tract. **Hematochezia** (maroon or bright red blood/clots per rectum) is a hallmark of a lower GI bleed. **Hematemesis** (vomiting of blood or coffee grounds–like material) and/or **melena** (black, tarry stools) are characteristic of an upper GI bleed. While this distinction is not absolute, it is a good rule of thumb.

What are the top three conditions that should be considered in the differential diagnosis?

- **Diverticulosis** (characterized by outpouchings of the colonic mucosa with bleeding due to vessel wall weakness).
- **Neoplasm** (polyp, carcinoma).
- **Angiodysplasia** (small vascular malformation).

What is the most likely cause of this patient's bleeding?

Diverticulosis. The most common causes of acute lower GI bleeding are diverticulosis (33%), cancers/polyps (19%), colitis/ulcers (18%), angiodysplasia (8%), and anorectal/hemorrhoids (4%). By 85 years of age, approximately 65% of the population has diverticula. Hemorrhoids should be suspected in a younger patient.

What is the pathophysiology of this condition?

Diverticulosis occurs when **diverticula** form, exposing the surrounding arterial vasculature to injury and causing thinning of the media. This predisposes to rupture, arterial bleeding, and rapid loss of blood per rectum. This is in contrast to **angiodysplasia,** which can cause venous intestinal bleeding. Although most diverticula form in the left colon, right-sided diverticula are more likely to bleed. Risk factors for diverticular formation include nonsteroidal anti-inflammatory drugs, lack of dietary fiber, older age, and constipation.

What is the initial diagnostic test for this condition?

Colonoscopy can be both diagnostic and therapeutic. The urgency of colonoscopy is based on the amount of blood produced and surrogate markers of the briskness of the bleed such as blood pressure and orthostatic hypotension. Additional tests include radionuclide imaging (radiologic monitoring of radionuclide tagged red blood cells to determine site of bleeding) and mesenteric angiography.

■ CASE 19

A worried mother rushes her 2-year-old son to the clinic after finding a large amount of bright red blood in his diaper. She notes that over the past week the child has been intermittently extremely irritable, curling into a ball with his legs pulled to his chest. His irritability resolves after vomiting (bilious) or passing a small stool. On examination, the child's vital signs are within normal limits, and he is in no apparent distress. Dried blood is noted at the anus. He is slightly uncomfortable with abdominal palpation, although no masses are appreciated.

What is the most likely diagnosis?

Intussusception is the telescoping of one portion of the bowel (often at the ileocecal junction) into another. This process can lead to luminal obstruction and vascular compromise.

What are the common causes of this condition?

- Anatomical causes include Meckel diverticulum or polyp/tumor.
- Infectious causes include adenovirus, rotavirus vaccine, enteric bacteria.
- Vasculitic causes include Henoch-Schönlein purpura.

What is the embryonic origin of a Meckel diverticulum?

A Meckel diverticulum is the most common congenital abnormality of the small intestine, resulting from failure of the **vitelline duct** to close. The role of the vitelline duct is to connect the developing midgut to the yolk sac. Normally, the duct closes and obliterates by approximately 7 weeks' gestation.

What are the classic characteristics of a Meckel diverticulum?

Meckel diverticulum classically follows the **"rule of 2's"**:

- Occurs in 2% of the population, the majority of which are < 2 years of age.
- Complications develop in 2%.
- Male: ratio is 2:1.
- Found within 2 feet of the ileocecal valve.
- Length is 2 inches long.

What explains the patient's temperament on presentation?

Intussusception makes the child irritable. The classic presentation on the boards will be an inconsolable child with a sausage-like palpable abdominal mass and "currant-jelly" stools. Children may appear completely well between episodes of obstruction. Patients often curl into a ball in an effort to reduce the intussusception. A barium enema can be both diagnostic and therapeutic.

What is the cause of the bright red rectal bleeding?

The two most common tissue types found in a Meckel diverticulum are gastric (80%) or pancreatic (~ 20%). The heterotopic gastric tissue releases gastric enzymes into the surrounding sensitive intestinal mucosa, which can lead to ulceration, pain, and bleeding.

Is a Meckel diverticulum a true or false diverticulum?

This is a true diverticulum, in that it involves all layers of the intestinal wall (Figure 7-11).

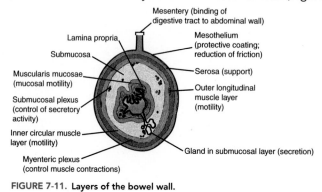

FIGURE 7-11. Layers of the bowel wall.

CASE 20

A 53-year-old man with a history of hepatitis C virus (HCV) infection and cirrhosis presents to his physician with increasing jaundice, increased abdominal girth, weight loss, and early satiety. He says he is often fatigued and feels lightheaded when he stands. Laboratory testing reveals anemia, hyperbilirubinemia, and an increased serum α-fetoprotein level.

What is the most likely diagnosis?

Primary hepatocellular carcinoma (HCC). Incidence of HCC is increased in patients with HCV who develop cirrhosis. By contrast, patients who are infected with hepatitis B virus may develop HCC without cirrhosis.

What is the blood supply to the liver?

The liver is supplied by the portal vein (75% of blood flow) and hepatic artery. Branches of these vessels divide the liver into the left and right lobes. Efferent blood is carried from the hepatic vein to the inferior vena cava. Portal hypertension occurs when blood flow through the liver is obstructed, often due to cirrhosis.

How does the fetal blood supply to the liver differ from the adult blood supply?

The umbilical vein is the major blood supply to the fetal liver and provides nutrients to the developing fetus. The umbilical vein enters the fetus via the umbilicus and then joins the left portal vein. A small amount of placental blood perfuses the liver. Most placental blood, however, bypasses the liver via the ductus venosus and joins the left hepatic vein. The left hepatic vein then empties into the inferior vena cava and ultimately the right atrium. The umbilical vein and ductus venosus disappear 2–5 days after birth, becoming the **ligamentum teres** and **ligamentum venosum**, respectively.

What is the falciform ligament and where is it located?

During development, the **falciform ligament** connects the portion of the primitive foregut that will form the liver to the anterior abdomen at the umbilicus. This connection enables the umbilical vein from the placenta to enter its free border at the umbilicus and reach the portal vein at the porta hepatis. The falciform ligament on the anterior surface of the liver divides the liver into the left and right anatomic lobes.

Why does this patient have increased abdominal girth?

The increased abdominal girth is likely due to ascites, or excess peritoneal fluid, resulting from portal hypertension and a failing liver. In liver failure, albumin production falls, decreasing oncotic pressure within vessels. Transudative fluid leaves vessels as a result of the relative increase in hydrostatic pressure (Starling forces).

What calculation can differentiate transudative from exudative causes of ascites?

The serum-ascites albumin gradient (SAAG) = serum albumin minus albumin in ascites.

SAAG value > 1.1 g/dL = transudative cause; diagnosing portal hypertension with 97% accuracy.
SAAG value < 1.1 g/dL, exudative causes (eg, nephrotic syndrome, tuberculosis, and various cancers).

■ CASE 21

A 47-year-old white man is brought to the emergency department by a policeman after being found wandering and incoherent on the streets. He has multiple watery bowel movements on arrival. Physical examination reveals a pigmented, scaling rash on his neck, arms, and hands as well as glossitis.

What is the most likely diagnosis?

Vitamin B$_3$ (niacin) deficiency. This is commonly known as **pellagra** and is characterized by the **3 D's:** dementia, diarrhea, dermatitis.

What is the function of vitamin B$_3$?

Niacin is a precursor for oxidized nicotinamide adenine dinucleotide (NAD+) and reduced nicotinamide adenine dinucleotide phosphate (NADPH). **NAD** helps carry reducing equivalents away from catabolic processes, such as oxidative phosphorylation. **NADPH** is used as a supply of reducing equivalents in anabolic reactions, such as the biosynthesis of steroids and fatty acids to maintain reduced glutathione, and in the oxygen-dependent respiratory burst of macrophages.

From what amino acid is vitamin B$_3$ derived?

Tryptophan.

What are the most likely causes of this presentation?

In developed nations, pellagra is seen most commonly in alcoholics (due to malnutrition). It can also be seen in patients with **Hartnup disease** (a disorder of tryptophan absorption) and carcinoid syndrome (in which there is increased conversion of tryptophan to serotonin). Isoniazid inhibits the conversion of tryptophan to niacin; therefore, patients receiving isoniazid are often prescribed niacin replacement.

What are the symptoms of overdose of vitamin B$_3$?

Prostaglandin-mediated **flushing** is a symptom seen in overdose. Patients receiving niacin as a treatment for hypertriglyceridemia may experience this adverse effect. Prophylaxis with aspirin often prevents this reaction.

■ CASE 22

A 56-year-old woman presents to her primary care physician complaining of significant pruritus of her skin. She has tried multiple over-the-counter skin lotions and creams with no effect. On physical examination, extensive excoriations on her extremities, slight scleral icterus, and xanthelasma are found. Initial laboratory tests reveal the following:

AST: 40 IU/L
ALT: 40 IU/L
Direct bilirubin: 1 mg/dL
Total bilirubin: 2 mg/dL
Alkaline phosphatase: 540 U/L (normal < 230 U/L)
γ-Glutamyl transferase (GGT): 80 U/L (normal < 50 U/L)

What is the most likely diagnosis?

Primary biliary cirrhosis (PBC) is a presumed autoimmune disease with destruction (inflammation and necrosis) of the **intrahepatic** bile ducts.

What are the signs and symptoms of this condition?

The most common symptoms are fatigue (65%) and pruritus (55%) in a woman 40–60 years of age. Jaundice and xanthelasma are fairly rare (~ 10%).

What laboratory tests support the diagnosis?

Most patients are diagnosed by routine laboratory tests: increased alkaline phosphatase, GGT, and bilirubin (total and direct). AST and ALT are characteristically normal.

What additional laboratory tests should be ordered?

Antimitochondrial antibodies should also be ordered. There may also be an increase in the erythrocyte sedimentation rate and serum **immunoglobulin M** levels.

What other conditions may be present in patients with this condition?

Other autoimmune diseases, such as **scleroderma, Sjögren syndrome,** and **rheumatoid arthritis** may coexist with PBC. Up to 50%–75% of patients with PBC present with sicca syndrome—dry eyes (xerophthalmia) and dry mouth (xerostomia)—commonly seen among Sjögren patients.

What is the appropriate treatment for the patient's pruritus?

Antihistamines.

What is the appropriate treatment for the patient's underlying condition?

Ursodeoxycholic acid (ursodiol). Methotrexate may be added in severe cases.

How is this condition distinguished from primary sclerosing cholangitis?

Primary sclerosing cholangitis is more likely in males; affects both intrahepatic **and** extrahepatic bile ducts; shows negative anti-mitochondrial antibodies; and is associated with ulcerative colitis.

The classic description of endoscopic retrograde cholangiopancreatography findings of the bile ducts is "pearls on a string" or "bile lakes."

■ CASE 23

An 84-year-old man is hospitalized for a course of intravenous clindamycin to treat an abscess. One week later, he develops profuse heme-positive diarrhea, nausea, and malaise. The patient's temperature is 38.8°C (101.8°F). Physical examination reveals abdominal tenderness and distention. The WBC count is 19,000/mm³ with a differential of 91% neutrophils, 7% monocytes, and 2% lymphocytes. Sigmoidoscopy reveals 0.2–2-cm raised, adherent, yellow plaques.

What is the most likely diagnosis?

This is a typical presentation of pseudomembranous colitis, which is notorious among hospitalized patients who receive **clindamycin.** Confirmatory findings include the presence of fecal leukocytes, anorexia, and dehydration.

What is the causative organism of this condition?

Clostridium difficile. This anaerobic gram-positive rod becomes predominant in the bowel after normal flora have been killed off by broad-spectrum antibiotics, such as clindamycin, penicillins (especially ampicillin), and cephalosporins.

What is the underlying pathophysiology of this condition?

C difficile releases two exotoxins *(proteins A and B)* that bind to receptors on intestinal epithelial cells. These toxins cause sloughing of epithelial cells into the lumen and mucosal ulceration. A **pseudomembrane** forms, composed of inflammatory cells, proteins, and mucus (Figure 7-12).

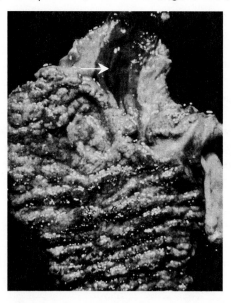

FIGURE 7-12. Autopsy specimen showing confluent pseudomembranes covering the cecum of a patient with pseudomembranous colitis. (Reproduced, with permission, from Kasper DL, et al. *Harrison's Principles of Internal Medicine,* 16th ed. New York: McGraw-Hill, 2005: 760.)

What are other manifestations of infections with this organism?

Infection with *C difficile* can result in a broad spectrum of symptoms, ranging from asymptomatic to fulminant colitis. Antibiotic-associated diarrhea can be mild or profuse and can occur with or without colitis. The colitis itself can appear pathologically nonspecific or can demonstrate pseudomembranes. Fulminant colitis can result in **toxic megacolon (potentially lethal nonobstructive colonic dilation)** or even perforation.

What are the appropriate treatments for this condition?

First-line therapy for pseudomembranous colitis is oral metronidazole. Intravenous metronidazole can be used in serious cases. Oral vancomycin can also be used to treat severe *C difficile* enterocolitis, as it predominantly remains in the gut; however, both vancomycin and metronidazole have also been implicated as causes of pseudomembranous colitis.

CASE 24

A 3-week-old Caucasian boy is brought to your clinic by his mother, who complains that the baby has intermittent bouts of projectile vomiting after meals. The mother also states that the child has been more lethargic than usual. On physical examination, the patient appears weak and has sunken eyes and poor skin turgor. He has fallen to the 25th percentile for weight. An olive-shaped mass is palpated in the right upper quadrant.

What is the most likely diagnosis?

Hypertrophic pyloric stenosis (Figure 7-13).

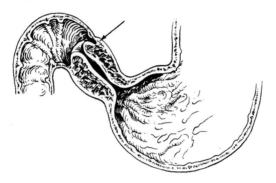

FIGURE 7-13. Hypertrophic pyloric stenosis. (Reproduced, with permission, from Doherty GM, Way LW. *Current Surgical Diagnosis & Treatment*, 12th ed. New York: McGraw-Hill, 2006: 1294.)

What findings support this diagnosis?

This patient demonstrates the classic presentation of pyloric stenosis with immediate postprandial, **nonbilious,** often projectile vomiting ("the hungry vomiter") and a palpable olive-like mass in the epigastrium. **Firstborn white males** are more at risk than other populations.

What are the typical laboratory findings in this condition?

Hypochloremic metabolic alkalosis from the loss of large amounts of gastric **hydrochloric acid** is seen with pyloric stenosis. Unconjugated hyperbilirubinemia may also be seen.

How is the diagnosis confirmed?

Diagnosis is straightforward when the "olive" is palpable. Otherwise, it may be difficult to distinguish this condition from gastroesophageal reflux without an ultrasound or upper gastrointestinal series. The latter may demonstrate an elongated pylorus ("**string sign**") with a tapered end ("**beak sign**").

What is the appropriate management for this condition?

The definitive management is surgery (pyloromyotomy).

Given appropriate management, what is the prognosis?

Patients can be expected to make a complete recovery, including return to normal weight and growth.

What other conditions are commonly associated with this condition?

Associated conditions include hiatal hernia, midgut volvulus, gastroesophageal reflux, and esophageal atresia.

◼ CASE 25

A worried 24-year-old mother brings her 4-year-old daughter to the emergency department (ED). She states the daughter has been ill for the past week with flulike symptoms, including rhinorrhea, cough, headache, and nausea, which she has attempted to treat at home. The child has been increasingly lethargic, and the mother found her barely responsive this morning. The child displays diminished consciousness and sluggish pupils. Kernig and Brudzinski signs are negative. She vomits multiple times in the ED and is admitted to the intensive care unit (ICU).

What is the most likely diagnosis?

Reye syndrome. Although extremely rare, this diagnosis is devastating if missed (and is a board favorite).

What drug did the mother likely administer to the patient?

Aspirin. Always suspect Reye syndrome in a child who has altered mental status, vomiting, and has suffered a recent viral illness.

What other laboratory findings are expected in this patient?

This patient is at risk for developing hepatic failure, cerebral edema, and death. Characteristic laboratory findings include the following:

- Severe transaminitis (aspartate aminotransferase and alanine aminotransferase > 3000 U/L).
- Normal or slightly elevated bilirubin.
- Hypoglycemia.
- Hyperammonemia.
- Prolonged prothrombin time and International Normalized Ratio.
- Anion gap metabolic acidosis with mixed respiratory alkalosis.

What is the pathophysiology of this condition?

It is thought that salicylate metabolites during viral infection damage mitochondria and/or that susceptible individuals have an underlying polymorphism in mitochondrial function. **Mitochondrial dysfunction** leads to increased short-chain fatty acids, hyperammonemia, and cerebral edema, although the exact mechanism is unclear.

What is the association between the patient's recent flulike symptoms and the current presentation?

Although the etiology of Reye syndrome is unknown, the condition typically occurs after a viral infection, particularly an upper respiratory tract infection, influenza, varicella, or gastroenteritis, and is associated with aspirin use during the illness.

What is a possible explanation for the child's change in mental status?

Cerebral edema is the likely cause. If cerebral edema can be controlled, the liver usually makes a full recovery. Therefore, ICU management is essential.

Options for controlling cerebral edema include the following:
- Mannitol (acts as an osmotic diuretic).
- Hyperventilation (reduces systemic carbon dioxide and leads to constriction of the cerebral vasculature).
- Barbiturates (reduce brain stem metabolism and therefore cerebral blood flow).
- Ventricular drainage (shunts cerebrospinal fluid).

Despite treatment, the patient dies. What pathologic findings are expected?

Microvesicular fatty change (**steatosis**) of the liver, kidneys, and brain may be seen on autopsy.

■ CASE 26

A 3-month-old girl born prematurely has been maintained on parenteral nutrition since a length of her bowel was resected secondary to necrotizing enterocolitis when she was 2 weeks of age. The resected bowel included the ascending colon, ileum, and distal portion of the jejunum. She is unable to thrive on enteral feeding alone.

What condition explains the patient's inability to thrive solely on enteral feeding?

Short bowel syndrome due to extensive bowel resection leading to malabsorption.

After resection of the ileum, which specific molecules will be malabsorbed?

Vitamin B$_{12}$ and **bile salts** are absorbed exclusively in the ileum and thus are deficient in short bowel syndrome.

The remainder of the patient's jejunum has adapted by increasing the number of cells in the villi, thereby lengthening the villi. What term describes this type of adaptation?

Adaptation that increases the number of cells within a tissue is known as **hyperplasia.** This is in contrast to **hypertrophy,** in which the cells increase not in number but in size.

During bowel transplantation, which branch(es) of the aorta must be identified and anastomosed to supply blood to the jejunum, ileum, and ascending colon?

- The **superior mesenteric artery** supplies blood to the intestine from the proximal jejunum to the proximal transverse colon.
- The **celiac trunk** supplies the stomach, liver, spleen, and duodenum.
- The **inferior mesenteric artery** supplies the distal transverse colon, descending colon, and sigmoid colon.

How might octreotide be used in this patient?

As a **somatostatin analog,** octreotide inhibits the release of gastrin. This reduces gastric secretions that would otherwise be in excess compared to the length of bowel and further impede absorption.

How will malabsorption of bile salts affect this patient's prothrombin time (PT) and partial thromboplastin time (PTT)?

Malabsorption of bile salts leads to an inability to properly absorb fat and fat-soluble vitamins (ADEK). PT and PTT both increase secondary to a lack of vitamin K, which is a necessary cofactor in the γ-carboxylation of multiple clotting factor glutamate residues.

CASE 27

A 65-year-old immigrant woman from Japan presents with fatigue, weight loss, early satiety, and a gnawing stomach pain. She has been seen by multiple physicians, all of whom diagnosed her with peptic ulcer disease and treated her with antacids. However, the pain has not improved for 8 months. She has lost 16 kg (35 lb) and now complains of painful intercourse (dyspareunia) and painful defecation (dyschezia).

What is the most likely diagnosis?

Gastric cancer. Because of symptoms similar to peptic ulcer disease and gastritis, gastric cancer is frequently misdiagnosed. Hence, patients are typically diagnosed at a late stage and prognosis is therefore poor (5% survival at 5 years).

What risk factors are associated with this condition?

- Infection with *Helicobacter pylori*.
- Chronic gastritis.
- Smoking.
- Diets high in nitrosamines (ie, smoked, cured, or pickled foods) commonly found in East Asia, the Andes, Scandinavia, and eastern Europe.
- Pernicious anemia and type A blood (associated with gastritis).
- Family history.
- Previous gastric surgery.

What will the biopsy findings reveal?

Adenocarcinoma is the most common type of gastric cancer, and its hallmark is **signet-ring cells** on histopathology (Figure 7-14). Other signs include **linitis plastica**, or "leather-bottle stomach," which is a diffusely infiltrative cancer and portends a worse prognosis. It is also important to rule out **gastric lymphoma**, which is frequently associated with *H pylori* and may regress without surgery if the bacteria can be eradicated.

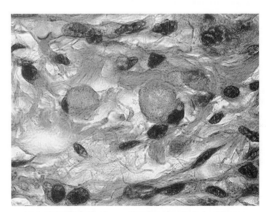

FIGURE 7-14. Signet-ring appearance of cells. Image shows the fairly uniform tumor cells with abundant intracytoplasmic mucin, which pushes the nuclei to the side, giving the cells their typical signet-ring appearance. (Reproduced, with permission, from USMLERx.com.)

How does this condition spread?

Gastric cancer metastasizes by direct extension through the gastric wall and the lymphatic system and via peritoneal spread.

Why does this patient suffer from dyspareunia and dyschezia?

These symptoms result from metastasis via peritoneal spread to the **pouch of Douglas** (the rectouterine cul-de-sac). This may be felt on rectal examination as an anterior rectal wall mass or a "**Blumer shelf.**" Gastric carcinoma metastasis to the ovary is called a **Krukenberg tumor**.

What is a Virchow node?

A Virchow node is an enlarged left supraclavicular lymph node. If it is found on physical examination, likelihood of metastatic disease is increased. Additional signs of lymphatic metastasis include a **Sister Mary Joseph node** (periumbilical nodule) and an **Irish node** (left axillary node).

CASE 28

A 45-year-old man presents to the emergency department after vomiting approximately one-half cup of blood. Two days earlier, he began having nausea and colicky, nonradiating abdominal pain. He has an extensive history of alcohol abuse, and currently drinks 8–10 beers a day. He has a past medical history of pancreatitis and hematemesis, and he currently takes no medications. Digital rectal examination reveals dark, heme-positive stool.

What is the most likely diagnosis, and what are the potential causes of this condition in this patient?

Upper gastrointestinal (GI) bleed. Potential causes in the setting of chronic alcohol abuse include the following:

- **Esophagogastric varices** (collateral circulation in the case of portal hypertension).
- **Mallory-Weiss tears** of the esophageal mucosa (usually with a history of extensive retching before the onset of hematemesis).
- **Boerhaave syndrome** (complete rupture of the esophagus usually with preceding retching).
- **Peptic ulcer disease** (cause of 55% of upper GI bleeds in all adults).
- Tumors.

What anatomic structure distinguishes an upper GI bleed from a lower GI bleed?

The **ligament of Treitz** marks the junction between the duodenum and the jejunum. Bleeding proximal to the ligament of Treitz is defined as an upper GI bleed.

If this patient had presented with bright red blood per rectum rather than dark stool, would the diagnosis change?

Not necessarily: A brisk upper GI bleed may also present with bright red blood per rectum, in which case there is insufficient transit time for breakdown of heme.

If the patient was previously diagnosed with esophageal varices, what medication may have been prescribed to prevent an upper GI bleed?

Nonselective β-blockers such as propranolol reduce blood flow in the portal system by creating unopposed α-adrenergic vasoconstriction of the mesenteric vessels. Because of the side effect of bronchoconstriction, patients with asthma, chronic obstructive pulmonary disease, and other pulmonary conditions must be carefully evaluated before use.

What is the appropriate management for this condition?

In cases of massive hematemesis, the first goal is intravenous fluid resuscitation and stabilization. **Nasogastric tube lavage** is indicated to prevent aspiration. It is also used to distinguish between upper and lower sources of GI bleeding and to identify high-risk lesions as sources of bleeding. Depending on the patient's condition, the next step could be either a diagnostic or therapeutic endoscopy.

■ CASE 29

A 37-year-old woman with a 20-year history of Crohn disease presents to her primary care physician complaining of fatigue. Physical examination reveals tachycardia (heart rate: 106/min), pale conjunctivae, angular cheilitis, and a beefy red tongue. Relevant laboratory findings include a hematocrit of 21% and an elevated mean corpuscular volume.

What is the most likely diagnosis?

Vitamin B_{12} deficiency.

What are the functions of the vitamin implicated in this condition, and how does its deficiency result in this presentation?

Vitamin B_{12} is a cofactor for methionine synthase, which catalyzes the transfer of a methyl group from *N*-methyltetrahydrofolate to homocysteine, producing tetrahydrofolate (TH_4) and methionine. Decreased production of TH_4 interferes with DNA synthesis required for hematopoiesis (Figure 7-15A), resulting in megaloblastic anemia. Vitamin B_{12} is also a cofactor for methylmalonyl CoA mutase (Figure 7-15B), an enzyme involved in the catabolism of odd-numbered fatty acid chains.

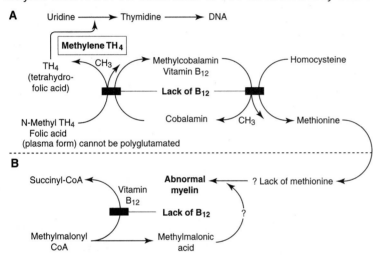

FIGURE 7-15. Role of cobalamin (vitamin B_{12}) and folic acid in nucleic acid and myelin metabolism. (A) As cofactor for methionine synthase. (B) As cofactor for methylmalonic CoA mutase. (Image A reproduced with permission from Tierney LM, et al. *Current Medical Diagnosis & Treatment Online.* New York: McGraw-Hill, 2006. Image B adapted with permission from Chandrasoma P, Taylor CR. *Concise Pathology,* 3rd ed. Stamford, CT: Appleton & Lange, 1997. Copyright © The McGraw-Hill Companies, Inc.)

What are the possible causes of this patient's condition?

The most common cause of vitamin B_{12} deficiency is **pernicious anemia,** an autoimmune disorder in which **intrinsic factor**–producing gastric parietal cells are destroyed. Intrinsic factor is necessary for vitamin B_{12} absorption.

Other causes include malabsorption (eg, celiac sprue, enteritis, or *Diphyllobothrium latum* infection) and absence of the terminal ileum (as in Crohn disease or surgical resection). Vitamin B_{12} deficiency is rarely due to insufficient dietary intake. However, after several years, strict vegetarians are at risk, because the nutrient is found only in animal products.

For what other condition is this patient at risk?

B_{12} deficiency leads to subacute combined degeneration of the spinal cord, mostly affecting the posterior columns. Neurologic problems often manifest as paresthesias and ataxia. Over time, symptoms such as spasticity and paraplegia can develop. The exact role of vitamin B_{12} deficiency in this pathology is unclear. Neurologic symptoms are often irreversible.

What other vitamin deficiency can cause megaloblastic anemia?

Folic acid deficiency. Although there is an elevated level of serum homocysteine as in vitamin B_{12} deficiency, accumulation of methylmalonic acid (Figure 7-15) and neurologic symptoms are not associated with folic acid deficiency.

CASE 30

A 35-year-old woman presents to her physician complaining of several days of severe, gnawing epigastric pain. The pain is worse between meals and is somewhat relieved with milk, food, and antacids. She has had three peptic ulcers in the past 2 years. The pain is occasionally accompanied by diarrhea. She denies bloody stools or hematuria and does not use alcohol or tobacco. Upper endoscopy reveals prominent gastric folds and an erosion in the first portion of the duodenum. The patient's fasting gastrin level is 700 pg/dL.

What is the most likely diagnosis?

A history of recurrent peptic ulcers suggests Zollinger-Ellison (ZE) syndrome, in which there is hypersecretion of gastrin from a gastrinoma, resulting in high gastric acid output.

What are the common risk factors for peptic ulcer disease?

- *Helicobacter pylori* infection.
- Nonsteroidal anti-inflammatory drugs.
- Smoking.

With what endocrine disorder is this condition associated?

Approximately 20% of patients with ZE syndrome also have **multiple endocrine neoplasia** type I (Wermer syndrome). Such patients will also have parathyroid adenomas, resulting in hyperparathyroidism, and/or anterior pituitary tumors.

How is secretion of gastric acid normally regulated?

Gastric acid is secreted by **parietal cells** of the stomach in response to gastrin, acetylcholine (vagal input), and histamine (Figure 7-16). Acid secretion is inhibited by somatostatin.

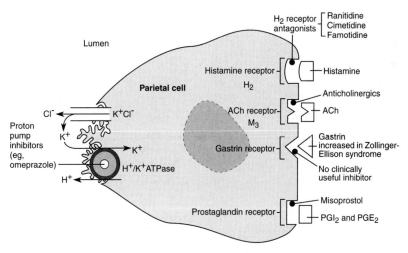

FIGURE 7-16. **Regulation of gastric acid secretion.** ACh = acetylcholine; PGE_2 = prostaglandin E_2; PGI_2 = prostaglandin I_2. (Reproduced, with permission, from Le T, et al. *First Aid for the USMLE Step 1: 2008.* New York: McGraw-Hill, 2008: 303.)

What is the pathophysiology of this patient's diarrhea?

The voluminous acid secretion overwhelms the buffering capacity of pancreatic bicarbonate. Thus, pancreatic enzymes are inactivated in this acidic environment, impeding digestion. Excess acid also interferes with the emulsification of fats, leading to steatorrhea.

What are the appropriate treatments for this condition?

Surgical treatment involves resection of the gastrinoma (typically at the head of pancreas).
Medical treatment uses proton pump inhibitors to suppress gastric acid secretion.

Hematology and Oncology

CASE 1

A 27-year-old woman comes to her physician complaining of severe abdominal pain of 3 days' duration. She has had similar attacks in the past, which she thought were due to menstruation. Review of systems reveals a history of depression and insomnia. On physical examination, the patient has lower extremity hyporeflexia and generalized weakness, which is worse in the lower extremities. Urinalysis reveals urine that is initially light but darkens on exposure to air and light. The porphobilinogen level is 110 mg/24 h (normal 0.0–1.5 mg/24 h).

What is the most likely diagnosis?

Acute intermittent porphyria (AIP).

What biochemical defect is responsible for this condition?

AIP is caused by a deficiency in **porphobilinogen deaminase (also known as hydroxymethylbilane synthase)**, an enzyme required for hemoglobin production. Typically, patients have accumulation of porphobilinogen and present with neuropathy and attacks of abdominal pain caused by precipitants that increase α-aminolevulinic acid (ALA) synthase activity. ALA production from glycine and succinyl CoA by ALA synthase is the rate-limiting step of heme production. As a result, any increase in ALA production leads to more AIP symptoms (Figure 8-1).

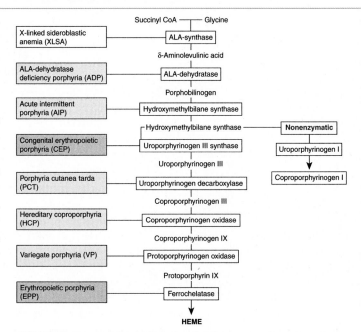

FIGURE 8-1. Heme synthesis. (Reproduced, with permission, from Fauci AS, et al. *Harrison's Principles of Internal Medicine,* 17th ed. New York: McGraw-Hill, 2008: Figure 352-1.)

What are the most likely precipitants of this patient's attacks?

Precipitants that increase ALA synthase activity include the following:

- Endogenous/exogenous gonadal steroids.
- Drugs (sulfonamides, antiepileptic agents).
- Alcohol.
- Low-calorie diets.
- Stress.

What other condition should be considered if the patient has neurologic manifestations but no abdominal pain?

Ascending muscle weakness with hyporeflexia or areflexia is the classic presentation of **Guillain-Barré syndrome**. However, the high level of porphobilinogen in the urine of this patient is essentially pathognomonic for AIP. If the diagnosis is unclear, a lumbar puncture can be performed. Albuminocytologic dissociation is seen in the cerebrospinal fluid of patients with Guillain-Barré syndrome. Other possible causes of peripheral muscle weakness include muscle atrophy, leprosy, myeloma, lead poisoning, and diabetes.

What is the appropriate treatment for this condition?

Heme, as the end product of the biosynthetic pathway, is a repressor of ALA synthase. Therefore, an intravenous injection of hemin (IV heme) decreases synthesis of ALA synthase via negative feedback and often reduces the severity of symptoms. Intravenous infusion of dextrose solution can also help abate acute attacks. Hemin is used for refractory cases after failure of carbohydrate loading. Treatment of pain and monitoring for neurologic and respiratory compromise are essential.

CASE 2

The parents of a 4-year-old girl bring their daughter to the pediatrician because they are concerned about her fever, which has lasted for more than a week. Her parents have also noticed that she is less energetic and now walks with a limp. Physical examination is significant for hepatomegaly, scattered petechiae, and bruising over many surfaces of her body. Relevant laboratory findings include the following:

Hemoglobin: 6 g/dL
White blood cell (WBC) count: 25,000/mm³
Platelet count: 39,000/mm³
Peripheral smear: Many immature white cells with condensed chromatin, absent nucleoli, and scant agranular cytoplasm (Figure 8-2)

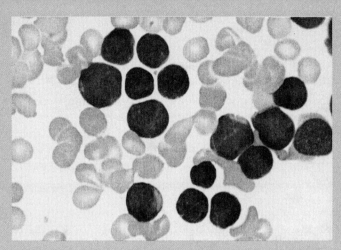

FIGURE 8-2. (Reproduced, with permission, from Lichtman MA, et al. *Williams Hematology*, 7th ed. New York: McGraw-Hill, 2005: Figure 91-4.)

What is the most likely diagnosis?

Acute lymphoblastic leukemia (ALL) is the most common malignancy of childhood. The classic presentation and laboratory findings include fever (the most common sign), fatigue, lethargy, bone pain, arthralgia, and elevated serum lactate dehydrogenase (LDH). Less common symptoms include headache, vomiting, altered mental function, oliguria, and anuria.

What conditions should be considered in the differential diagnosis?

All of the following conditions feature anemia, low platelet count, and/or symptoms similar to this patient's:
- Idiopathic thrombocytopenic purpura.
- Aplastic anemia.
- Infectious mononucleosis.
- *Bordetella pertussis.*
- Epstein-Barr virus.
- Small, round, blue-cell tumors.

However, the markedly elevated WBC and blood smear in this patient make a form of leukemia, in this case ALL, the most likely diagnosis.

What is the etiology of the physical examination findings?

Most findings derive from leukemic expansion and crowding out of the normal marrow. This causes anemia and thrombocytopenia as well as bone or joint pain from invasion into the periosteum. Fever results from pyrogenic cytokines released from leukemic cells. Elevated LDH is a consequence of increased cellular turnover. Painless enlargement of the scrotum and central nervous system symptoms may also be signs of more extensive extramedullary invasion.

What is the appropriate treatment for this condition?

Complex chemotherapy regimens are standard and divided into induction, consolidation, and maintenance phases. Most regimens involve combinations of cyclophosphamide, doxorubicin, vincristine, dexamethasone/prednisone, methotrexate, asparaginase, and cytarabine. Recent advances in treatment have resulted in complete remission rates as high as 80% in children with ALL.

CASE 3

A 67-year-old man presents to his physician with a 10-day history of fatigue, bleeding gums, cellulitis, and a recent weight loss of 9 kg (20 lb). On physical examination, the patient is pale but has no evidence of lymphadenopathy or hepatosplenomegaly. Results of a complete blood count are as follows:

WBC count: 18,300/mm³ (75% blastocytes, 20% lymphocytes)
Hemoglobin: 9.1 g/dL
Hematocrit: 29%
Platelet count: 98,000/mm³

What is the most likely diagnosis?

Acute myelogenous leukemia (AML) is the most common acute leukemia in adults. The median age of diagnosis in the United States is 65 years.

What other symptoms are common at presentation in this condition?

- Epistaxis, skin rash, petechiae, bone pain, and shortness of breath.
- Gingival hyperplasia (leukemic invasion).
- Leukemia cutis (skin infiltrates).
- Neurologic deficits.
- Disseminated intravascular coagulation (often seen with the **acute promyelocytic leukemia** variant of AML).

What are the likely bone marrow biopsy findings in this condition?

The proliferation of myeloblasts with characteristic eosinophilic, needle-like cytoplasmic inclusions, or **Auer rods,** is pathognomonic for AML (Figure 8-3).

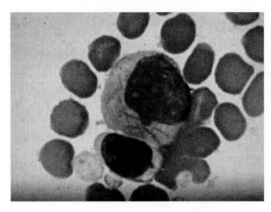

FIGURE 8-3. **Auer rods in acute myelogenous leukemia.** (Reproduced, with permission, from Lichtman MA, et al. *Williams Hematology,* 7th ed. New York: McGraw-Hill, 2007: Figure VI.A.21.)

What cells are affected in this condition?

AML is a neoplasm of myelogenous progenitor cells. The progenitor cells may appear as granulocyte precursors, monoblasts, megakaryoblasts, or erythroblasts.

How can genetic testing influence treatment?

Genetic abnormalities are critical in the diagnosis and treatment of AML. For example, t(15;17) chromosomal translocation indicates acute promyelocytic leukemia (M3 variant) as the specific diagnosis. This can be treated with targeted drugs such as all-*trans* retinoic acid, which differentiates promyelocytes into mature neutrophils, thereby inducing apoptosis of the leukemic promyelocytes. This results in a high likelihood of remission and cure.

Why is cellulitis commonly associated with this condition?

Neutropenia caused by replacement of mature WBCs with leukemic cells increases susceptibility to infection.

CASE 4

A 14-year-old boy presents to his pediatrician with a laceration on his hand that has become badly infected. Upon questioning, the boy says he has felt fatigued for some time. Physical examination reveals pallor of the mucous membranes in addition to bleeding on the inside of his cheeks. Petechiae cover his body, and patches of purpura are present on his thighs, trunk, and arms. Relevant laboratory findings are as follows:

WBC count: 2000/mm^3
Hematocrit: 22%
Platelet count: 48,000/mm^3

What is the most likely diagnosis?

Aplastic anemia results from bone marrow failure or autoimmune destruction of myeloid stem cells, which leads to pancytopenia. Pancytopenia affects all cell lines, resulting in neutropenia, anemia, and thrombocytopenia, all of which are seen on a complete blood count.

What is the most likely cause of this patient's condition?

Most cases of aplastic anemia are **idiopathic** (autoimmune). Other possible causes include the following:

- **Viral** agents (eg, parvovirus B19, hepatitis viruses, HIV, Epstein-Barr virus).
- **Drugs** and **chemicals** (eg, alkylating and antimetabolite agents, chloramphenicol, insecticides, arsenic, and benzene).
- **Radiation.**
- Immune disorders (eg, systemic lupus erythematosus, graft versus host disease).
- Pregnancy.
- **Hereditary transmission** (eg, Fanconi anemia).

Note: The diagnosis is not aplastic anemia if tumor, fibrosis, or myelodysplasia are present.

What other test can help confirm the diagnosis?

Bone marrow biopsy reveals hypocellular bone marrow (< 30% cellularity) with a fatty infiltrate. Figure 8-4A shows a normal bone marrow biopsy; Figure 8-4B shows a biopsy sample from a patient with aplastic anemia.

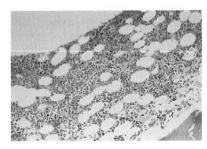
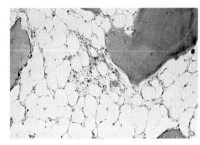

A   **B**

FIGURE 8-4. (A) Normal bone marrow biopsy. (B) Bone marrow biopsy in aplastic anemia. (Reproduced, with permission, from Kasper DL, et al. *Harrison's Principles of Internal Medicine*, 16th ed. New York: McGraw-Hill, 2005: 620.)

What is the appropriate treatment for this condition?

Initial treatment is to withdraw any possible toxic agent causing the condition. Supportive care, including antibiotics for infection and blood transfusion if symptoms develop, is also important. If testing reveals severe depression of one or several cell lines, definitive therapy, including stem cell transplantation or immunosuppression, is appropriate. If possible, transfusion should be avoided before bone marrow transplantation because of the risks of alloimmunization and graft rejection.

CASE 5

A 7-month-old Greek boy is brought to his pediatrician by his parents, who have noticed that the baby has been jaundiced and dyspneic for about 2 weeks. The mother denies any previous health problems with her son. Physical examination reveals tachycardia. Laboratory tests reveal a mean corpuscular volume of 60 fL and a reticulocyte count of 0.3%. The serum iron concentration is within normal limits.

What is the most likely diagnosis?

β-Thalassemia major is the homozygous form of the genetically transmitted disease β-thalassemia, where the β-globin gene of hemoglobin is mutated, resulting in microcytic anemia. It is prevalent in Mediterranean populations.

By contrast, in α-thalassemia, α-globin genes in hemoglobin are deleted; this condition is most commonly present in Southeast Asians and blacks.

What mutations are present in α-thalassemia and in this condition?

Humans have two α-globin genes on chromosome 16, resulting in four alpha alleles. α-Thalassemia results in four types of thalassemia, depending on the number of alpha allele deletions that occur. Increasing severity results from increasing numbers of deletions. These deletions result from unequal meiotic crossover between adjacent alpha genes.

Humans have one β-globin gene on chromosome 11, resulting in two beta alleles. In β-thalassemia, beta allele mutations, rather than deletions, occur. These mutations can occur in the promoter, exon, intron, or polyadenylation sites. Some mutations may produce no β-globin, whereas others may produce a small amount.

What are the symptoms and signs of this condition?

Symptoms of β-thalassemia major emerge after approximately 6 months of life and are due to the decline in γ-hemoglobin production without a rise in β-hemoglobin production. The early signs and symptoms include pallor, growth retardation, hepatosplenomegaly, and jaundice.

How is this condition diagnosed?

Definitive laboratory testing using gel electrophoresis is used for diagnosis, as it can distinguish mutated and normal forms of hemoglobin. An increased concentration of fetal haemoglobin (HbF) may also be seen on electrophoresis. Notably, an increase in HBA_2 is seen in β-thalassemia minor.

What is the appropriate treatment for this condition?

β-Thalassemia major causes severe anemia. HbF induction may be used. Treatment with repeated blood transfusions may also be required. Subsequently, iron chelation for overload is important. Splenectomy may be necessary to treat the resulting hypersplenism. Stem cell transplantation may also be used in selected cases. β-Thalassemia minor is usually asymptomatic and its treatment requires only avoidance of oxidative stressors of RBCs.

■ CASE 6

A 32-year-old woman with systemic lupus erythematosus (SLE) presents to the emergency department reporting increased fatigue and lethargy that has lasted for 3 months. On physical examination, she is afebrile and has mild splenomegaly. Laboratory studies are significant for a hemoglobin concentration of 10.1 g/dL and a hematocrit of 30.6%. The peripheral blood smear (PBS) shows spherocytes and reticulocytes. The direct and indirect Coombs test are positive at 37°C (98.6°F) but not at 4°C (39.2°F).

What is the most likely diagnosis?

Warm autoimmune hemolytic anemia (WAIHA) secondary to SLE. Most cases of this condition are idiopathic or associated with autoimmune processes, lymphoproliferative disorders, or drugs.

What does the positive Coombs test indicate?

The positive Coombs test indicates the presence of antibodies against RBCs, which can cause hemolysis.

What is the difference between a direct and indirect Coombs test?

The difference between the direct and indirect Coombs test is where the antibodies against RBCs are detected. In a positive direct Coombs test, antibodies are detected directly on RBCs. This occurs in WAIHA, called such because a positive agglutination test will be present at 37°C (98.6°F). In a positive indirect Coombs test, antibodies are detected in the serum. This occurs at 4°C (39.2°F), which is why this is referred to as cold hemolytic anemia.

What are other causes of this condition?

The two most common causes are primary (idiopathic) and secondary due to such underlying conditions as autoimmune disorders, such as SLE. Medications (methyldopa), lymphomas, and leukemias are also common triggers.

What is the pathogenesis of this condition?

This is typically an **IgG**-mediated process. IgG coats RBCs and acts as an opsonin, such that the RBCs are phagocytized by monocytes and splenic macrophages.

When medications are the underlying cause, the hapten model has been suggested. RBC-bound drugs are recognized by antibodies and targeted for destruction.

What is the other form of this condition?

Cold agglutinin hemolytic anemia is the other form, and it occurs when **IgM** antibodies bind, fix complement, and agglutinate RBCs at low temperatures. These antibodies typically appear acutely following certain infections such as **mononucleosis** and *Mycoplasma.* This disease is usually self-limited but treatment-resistant forms exist. Clinical manifestations include pallor and cyanosis of distal extremities exposed to cold temperatures; this is secondary to vascular obstruction from complement deposition.

■ CASE 7

A 57-year-old nulliparous woman presents to her general practitioner concerned about a painless lump she has found in the right upper quadrant of her right breast. Her mother died of breast cancer at 60 years of age. Her medical history is significant for mild obesity, an early onset of menarche, and a late onset of menopause 3 years previously. She has noted some unilateral pain and dimpling of her right breast but has been scared to make an appointment with her physician. Laboratory tests show a serum calcium level of 9.7 mg/dL.

What is the likely diagnosis?

Breast cancer is the leading cause of cancer death in women. Most tumors develop in the upper/outer quadrants (Table 8-1).

TABLE 8-1	Types of Breast Cancer
TYPE	**CHARACTERISTICS**
Ductal carcinoma in situ.	Noninvasive, premalignant condition.
Invasive ductal carcinoma.	75% of invasive breast cancers.
Medullary, mucinous, and tubular breast cancer.	15% of invasive breast cancers.
Invasive lobular carcinoma.	10% of invasive breast cancers.
Phyllodes tumors, lymphomas, and sarcomas.	Rare invasive breast cancers.
Inflammatory carcinoma or Paget disease of the breast.	Not specific histologic types of cancer; rather, these are morphologic characteristics of breast cancer (induration, skin puckering, and erythema of the breast).

What is the pathophysiology of this patient's condition?

Breast cancer results from a transforming, or oncogenic, event that leads to clonal proliferation and survival of breast cancer cells. There are two general types of breast cancer: sporadic and hereditary. The events that trigger sporadic breast cancer are often unknown, but abnormalities in cell-cycle pathways, including HER-2, estrogen, and progesterone signaling, have been implicated. *BRCA1* and *BRCA2* genes have been linked to hereditary breast and ovarian cancer and are linked to defects in DNA mismatch repair. Notably, hereditary breast cancer only accounts for 5%–10% of all breast cancers diagnosed in the United States. This patient appears to have the sporadic type, supported by the late onset of diagnosis, increased hormone exposure from early menarche, late menopause, and obesity.

What risk factors are associated with an increased incidence of this condition?

- Female gender.
- Alcohol intake.
- Breast density.
- Early menarche or late menopause.
- Age.
- Family history (50%–70% of women carrying the *BRCA1* or *BRCA2* mutations develop breast cancer).
- Hormone replacement therapy (estrogen and progesterone).
- Nulliparity or late first pregnancy.
- Obesity (in postmenopausal women).
- Prior breast biopsy, particularly for lesions with atypia.
- Radiation exposure to the chest.

■ CASE 8

A 35-year-old man presents to his primary care physician complaining of several months' history of watery diarrhea. He reports that the diarrhea is often "greasy looking" but never bloody. On physical examination, the man's face is flushed, and his neck is covered by a blotchy, violaceous erythema. When asked about this flushing, the man says it has happened several times a day over the past few years, often while he is feeling stressed at work.

What is the most likely diagnosis?
Carcinoid syndrome (secretory) is the most likely diagnosis. Approximately 75%–80% of carcinoid syndrome cases arise from a small bowel carcinoid tumor. However, only approximately 10% of carcinoid tumors result in carcinoid syndrome (see Table 8-2 for signs and symptoms).

TABLE 8-2	Clinical Characteristics in Patients with Carcinoid Syndrome	
SYMPTOMS/SIGNS	AT PRESENTATION	DURING COURSE OF DISEASE
Diarrhea	32%–73%	68%–84%
Flushing	23%–65%	63%–74%
Pain	10%	34%
Asthma/wheezing	4%–8%	3%–18%
Pellagra	2%	5%
None	12%	22%

(Adapted, with permission, from Kasper DL, et al. *Harrison's Principles of Internal Medicine*, 16th ed. New York: McGraw-Hill, 2005: 2224.)

What laboratory test can help confirm the diagnosis?
Many conditions, such as menopause, as well as reactions to alcohol, glutamate, and calcium channel blockers, may cause flushing. However, flushing in conjunction with an increase in **5-hydroxyindoleacetic acid** on urinalysis occurs only in carcinoid syndrome.

What is the pathophysiology of this condition?
Carcinoid syndrome occurs only when sufficient concentrations of substances secreted by carcinoid tumors (derived from neuroendocrine cells) reach the circulation. Carcinoid tumors secrete a variety of gastrointestinal peptides, including gastrin, somatostatin, substance P, vasoactive intestinal polypeptide, pancreatic polypeptide, histamine, chromogranin A, and serotonin. Carcinoid syndrome is unlikely to occur in intestinal carcinoid tumors unless liver metastases are present.

What type of cardiac involvement is typically seen in patients with this condition?
Right-sided valvular involvement occurs in 11% of patients initially and up to 41% during the course of the disease. Cardiac disease results from serotonin-mediated fibrosis in the endocardium, most commonly in the tricuspid valve. Up to 80% of patients with cardiac involvement develop heart failure.

What is the appropriate treatment for this condition?
If localization of a discrete carcinoid tumor is possible, surgical resection is the optimal therapy. For other cases, symptomatic management with octreotide is most beneficial.

CASE 9

A 13-year-old boy is brought to his physician for increasing abdominal distention and pain that has lasted 7 days. Physical examination reveals decreased bowel sounds, tympany, and lower abdominal tenderness. CT scan of the abdomen shows a 6-cm mass involving the distal ileum. A biopsy of the mass is taken under radiographic guidance. The histologic sample shows sheets of intermediate-sized lymphoid cells with nonconvoluted nuclei and coarse chromatin along with many macrophages (Figure 8-5).

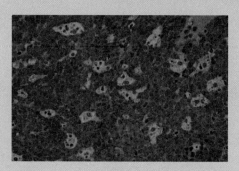

FIGURE 8-5. (Reproduced, with permission, from Lichtman MA, et al. *Williams Hematology*. New York, NY: McGraw-Hill, 2006: Plate XIV-7.)

What is the most likely diagnosis?

Burkitt lymphoma, a highly aggressive B-cell non-Hodgkin lymphoma. The **"starry-sky"** pattern on histology (Figure 8-5) is classic for this condition. Burkitt lymphoma of the gastrointestinal tract typically involves the ileocecum and peritoneum.

What are the three forms of this condition?

- The **sporadic** form, as described in this vignette, is the most common form in the developed world and appears in children and young adults.
- The **African/endemic** form, which is closely associated with Epstein-Barr virus (EBV) infection, is another type. In this type, the lymphoma typically presents as a maxillary or mandibular mass.
- The **HIV-associated** form is the final type and may stem from reactivation of latent EBV virus in immunosuppressed patients. It typically arises in lymph nodes.

What is the typical cytogenetic change in this condition and what gene does it involve?

All forms of Burkitt lymphoma involve the **c-MYC** gene found on chromosome 8. The characteristic translocation is t(8;14), which places the **c-MYC** proto-oncogene adjacent to the immunoglobulin heavy-chain locus on chromosome 14. This results in overexpression of c-MYC, a transcription factor that controls cellular metabolism, leading to increased cell growth. The tumor cells are typically CD20, CD10, and BCL-6 positive.

What is the appropriate treatment for this condition?

Endemic Burkitt lymphoma is treated with chemotherapy, but HIV-associated and sporadic Burkitt are not necessarily as readily treatable. Both HIV-associated and sporadic cases also commonly metastasize to the central nervous system, requiring CNS radiation and intrathecal chemotherapy for control.

What is tumor lysis syndrome?

Tumor lysis syndrome is due to the large amount of neoplastic cell death during treatment with chemotherapy, typically seen in the most rapidly growing cancers, such as Burkitt lymphoma. Laboratory analysis shows multiple metabolic complications including hyperphosphatemia, hypocalcemia, hyperuricemia, and hyperkalemia leading to acute renal failure. Allopurinol or rasburicase, aggressive hydration, and diuresis can be used to prevent these consequences.

■ CASE 10

A 55-year-old woman presents to her primary care physician for a routine physical. She reports an unintentional 14-kg (30-lb) weight loss and chronic fatigue. Abdominal examination reveals an enlarged spleen. Relevant laboratory findings are as follows:

Hemoglobin: 12.9 g/dL
Hematocrit: 38.1%
Mean corpuscular volume: 92 fL
WBC count: 167, 000/mm³
Platelet count: 625, 000/mm³

Blood smear: Many late granulocytic
  precursor cells, eosinophils, and basophils;
  relatively few metamyelocytes
Cytogenetic analysis: t(9;22) translocation

What is the most likely diagnosis?

Chronic myelogenous leukemia (CML) is likely given the t(9;22) translocation coupled with the uncontrolled production of maturing granulocytes (neutrophils, eosinophils, and basophils), platelets, and mild anemia (Figure 8-6). This marked leukocytosis leads to **splenic enlargement.** There are approximately 5000 new cases of CML in the United States annually.

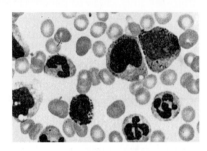

FIGURE 8-6. Chronic myelogenous leukemia. Blood film. Leukemic promyelocytes, a basophilic myelocyte, and segmented neutrophils with increased nuclear material. (Reproduced, with permission, from Lichtman MA, et al. *Williams Hematology,* 7th ed. New York, NY: McGraw-Hill, 2006: Plate XIX.)

What is this chromosomal abnormality called and what is its product?

The translocation of the *BCR* gene on chromosome 22 with the *ABL* gene on chromosome 9 leads to the Bcr-Abl fusion product. This abnormality is called the **Philadelphia chromosome,** and it is considered pathognomonic for CML.

What is the pathophysiology of this condition?

This Bcr-Abl fusion protein results in a constitutively active Abl **tyrosine kinase** in the Ras/Raf/MEK/MAPK pathway. This leads to inhibition of apoptosis and unregulated cell division (Figure 8-7).

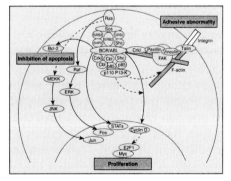

FIGURE 8-7. Cell signaling in chronic myelogenous leukemia. (Reproduced, with permission, from Lichtman MA, et al. *Williams Hematology,* 8th ed. New York: McGraw-Hill, 2010: Figure 90-5.)

What is the targeted drug treatment for this condition?

Imatinib, a highly specific Bcr-Abl tyrosine kinase competitive inhibitor, has been the agent of choice and has radically changed the prognosis for CML patients. Dasatinib is a second-line treatment. Either treatment has shown a 90% cytologic remission rate. Historically, allogeneic bone marrow transplantation has been used for potential cure (with cure rates in the 40%–50% range). However, it is now used in only selected patients who fail to achieve cytogenetic remission with tyrosine kinase inhibitors.

What is a blast crisis?

Untreated CML inevitably progresses, usually in 3–5 years, to an accelerated phase and then a blast crisis in which additional genetic abnormalities accumulate and lead to acute myeloid (or 20% of the time lymphoid) leukemia. Peripheral smears will show a large percentage (> 20%) of blast cells.

■ CASE 11

A 70-year-old man visits his primary care physician complaining of constant vague abdominal pain that has been increasing over the past month. He has noted recent weakness and weight loss, which he attributes to a decreased appetite. His father was diagnosed with colorectal cancer in his late fifties. The patient admits never having a colonoscopy and eats a diet high in fat and low in fiber. Rectal exam reveals a palpable mass and occult blood. Laboratory tests reveal that the patient's hematocrit is 28%.

What is the most likely diagnosis?

Colorectal cancer (CRC) is suggested by the symptoms of abdominal pain, anorexia, weight loss, palpable rectal mass, and anemia. Likewise, he has a family history of CRC at a relatively young age. CRC is the third-leading cause of cancer death in men (after lung and prostate cancer).

What risk factors are associated with this condition?

- Age > 50 years.
- Lifestyle (alcohol, obesity, low-fiber and high-fat diet).
- Family history/syndromes (hereditary nonpolyposis CRC ([HNPCC]), familial adenomatous polyposis ([FAP]).
- Diabetes.
- Inflammatory bowel disease.
- Tumor suppressor gene and proto-oncogene changes.

What are the guidelines for primary screening of this condition?

Screening for CRC includes the following modalities:

- Fecal occult blood testing for individuals older than 40 years of age (controversial).
- Colonoscopy every 10 years in patients aged 50–75 years.
- More frequent screening for patients with genetic risk factors (eg, familial adenomatous polyposis, hereditary nonpolyposis colorectal cancer), family history, and/or history of colorectal neoplasia.

What signs and symptoms are commonly associated with this condition?

Signs and symptoms of colorectal cancer include abdominal pain, anemia with low mean corpuscular volume (MCV), bleeding/mucus per rectum, changes in bowel habits, weight loss, and tenesmus (the feeling of needing to pass stool with an empty rectal vault).

What are the appropriate treatments for this condition?

Surgical treatment is usually the initial treatment of choice. Adjuvant therapy will depend on TNM staging, with adjuvant chemotherapy providing a survival advantage for stage 3 (node-positive) colon cancer. Stage 2 and 3 rectal cancers should be treated with combination chemotherapy and radiation, either before surgery or afterward. In the metastatic setting, radiation can be used for palliation, and current chemotherapy agents can provide disease control for 20–24 months on average. If there are only a few metastatic foci in the liver, resection can be considered, with a 25% chance for long-term control. Carcinoembryonic antigen (CEA) can be a useful tumor marker to monitor for the recurrence of disease.

■ CASE 12

A 56-year-old man presents to the emergency department complaining of a 1-day history of nausea and vomiting, with a 13.6-kg (30-lb) unintentional weight loss over the past few months. He noticed black specks in his emesis, resembling coffee grounds. He reports early satiety with a decreased appetite, specifically for meat. He has no diarrhea, constipation, known sick contacts, or recent travel history but notes occasional fevers and chills with recent night sweats. Physical examination reveals that the patient is afebrile with a nontender, nondistended, soft abdomen with a firm epigastric mass. Relevant laboratory findings are as follows:

Hematocrit: 28%
Hemoglobin: 9 g/dL
WBC count: 9000/mm^3
Stool test: Guaiac positive; negative for ova and parasites

What is the most likely diagnosis?

Gastric cancer. Diagnosis is determined by esophagogastroduodenoscopy and biopsy.

What risk factors are associated with this condition?

Risk factors for gastric cancer are as follows:

- *Helicobacter pylori* infection (causes intestinal metaplasia).
- Barrett esophagus (gastroesophageal junction adenocarcinoma).
- Diet (nitroso compounds and high salt intake).
- Smoking.
- Low socioeconomic status.
- Male gender (female reproductive hormones protective).
- Obesity.
- Previous gastric surgery.
- Epstein-Barr virus infection (causing gastric lymphoma).

What signs and symptoms are commonly associated with this condition?

- Anorexia (especially for meat).
- Dysphagia (caused by lesions at the cardia of the stomach).
- Coffee ground emesis (if bleeding tumor).
- Palpable epigastric mass.
- Postprandial heaviness.
- Vomiting (in cases of pyloric obstruction).
- Weight loss.

If disease has metastasized:

- Intra-abdominal masses.
- Virchow's node (left supraclavicular node).

What are the typical laboratory findings in this condition?

Anemia is present in 50% of patients. CEA levels are elevated in two-thirds of patients.

What is the appropriate treatment for this condition?

Surgical resection for early local disease. A combination of radiation and chemotherapy is often used along with resection in situations where the lesion is initially unresectable, or as adjuvant therapy postsurgery for node-positive disease.

■ CASE 13

A 33-year-old African-American woman has been in the intensive care unit for 2 days after being admitted for treatment of a severe bacteremia. Her medical history is noncontributory. Physical examination reveals mucosal bleeding, oozing from intravenous access sites, and petechiae on her trunk and extremities. Laboratory tests reveal a prolonged prothrombin time (PT) and activated partial thromboplastin time (aPTT).

What is the most likely diagnosis?

Disseminated intravascular coagulation (DIC).

What is the pathophysiology of this condition?

DIC is a systemic process in which widespread activation of hemostasis causes thrombosis and hemorrhage. Systemic, rather than localized, clotting depletes coagulation factors (Figure 8-8).

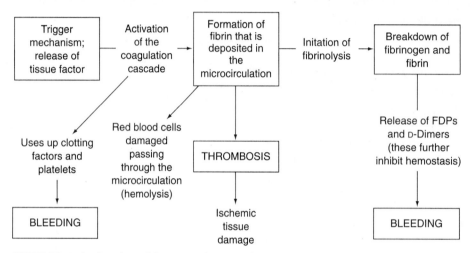

FIGURE 8-8. Pathophysiology of disseminated intravascular coagulation. (Reproduced, with permission, from Tintinalli JE, et al. *Tintinalli's Emergency Medicine: A Comprehensive Study Guide,* 6th ed. New York: McGraw-Hill, 2004: 1328.)

What are common possible causes of this condition?

- Infectious causes include sepsis.
- Malignant causes include acute leukemia (especially acute myeloid leukemia) and other cancers (eg, prostate, causing a chronic DIC).
- Other causes include trauma, obstetric complications (eg, abruptio placentae, amniotic fluid embolism), and snake venom.

Which clotting factors are involved in the intrinsic, extrinsic, and common pathways?

The **intrinsic pathway** involves factors VIII, IX, XI, and XII, prekallikrein, and high-molecular weight-kininogen. The **extrinsic pathway** involves factor VII. The **common pathway** involves factors II, V, and X and fibrinogen (Figure 8-9).

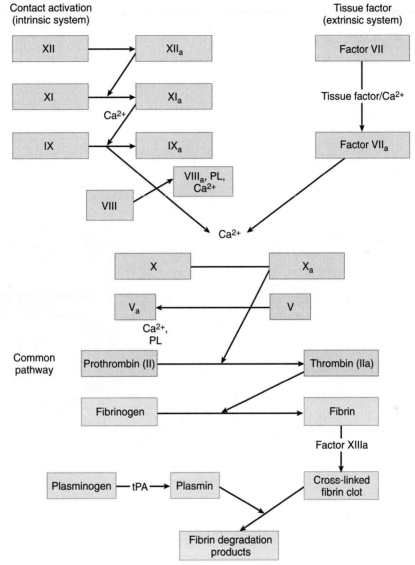

FIGURE 8-9. The clotting cascade. (Reproduced, with permission, from Tintinalli JE, et al. *Tintinalli's Emergency Medicine: A Comprehensive Study Guide,* 7th ed. New York: McGraw-Hill, 2011: Figure 136-1.)

Which laboratory tests help differentiate this condition from thrombocytopenia?

DIC is classically diagnosed from an elevated PT, elevated PTT, low fibrinogen, and high D-dimer. Thrombocytopenia would not show elevated coagulation tests.

What is the prognosis and treatment of this condition?

DIC mortality ranges from 40%–80% if it is associated with sepsis, burns, or trauma. Treatment of the underlying condition causing DIC is essential. Hemodynamic support is the mainstay of treatment, but correction of coagulopathy with platelet or coagulation factor replacement may be necessary if there is a serious risk of bleeding (eg, recent surgery or fibrinogen < 100). Fresh frozen plasma can be used to correct the PT/PTT while cryoprecipitate is used if the fibrinogen < 100.

CASE 14

A 56-year-old man who was previously in excellent health is brought to the emergency department after a rapid decline in mental status that began 3 days earlier. This morning, his wife found him unresponsive and extremely agitated. Currently, the patient is flailing his limbs and is unresponsive to stimuli or to verbal commands. His pupils are equal and reactive. The patient is sedated, and a CT of the head demonstrates a large lesion in the right frontal lobe. MRI establishes the likely diagnosis.

What is the differential diagnosis of a brain lesion?

Neoplastic causes:

- The most common brain tumor is a metastatic lesion (secondary tumor—lung, breast, melanoma, etc).
- Primary brain tumors include gliomas, meningiomas, pituitary adenomas, vestibular schwannomas, and primary central nervous system lymphomas.

Nonneoplastic causes:

- Infectious (eg, abscess, viral, progressive multifocal leukoencephalopathy, toxoplasmosis, or cysticercosis).
- Vascular (cerebral hemorrhage or infarct).
- Inflammatory (associated with multiple sclerosis or postinfectious encephalopathy).

What is the most likely diagnosis?

Glioblastoma multiforme (GBM). MRI is the definitive test for a brain mass. Gliomas appear hypointense on T1-weighted imaging (Figure 8-10) and hyperintense on T2-weighted imaging. They also heterogeneously enhance with contrast and can be distinguished from the surrounding edema. The rapidity of onset of this patient's symptoms without signs of infarct suggests a malignant process.

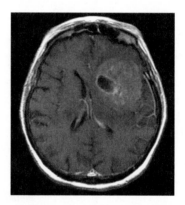

FIGURE 8-10. **Glioblastoma multiforme.** (Reproduced, with permission, from Ropper, AH, Samuels MA. *Adam's and Victor's Principles of Neurology*, 9th ed. New York: McGraw-Hill, 2009: Figure 31-2.)

What are some characteristics of this condition?

GBM is the most commonly diagnosed primary brain tumor. It is a grade IV astrocytoma that is most commonly found in adults, in contrast to the peak childhood prevalence of low-grade (pilocytic) astrocytoma. GBM is typically found in the cerebral hemispheres and can cross the corpus callosum to form the characteristic "butterfly glioma."

What are the most common signs and symptoms associated with this condition?

- Symptoms of GBM include headache (73%–86% of cases) and seizures (26%–32% of cases).
- Signs of GBM include paraparesis, papilledema, confusion, and aphasia.

What is the appropriate treatment for this condition?

The prognosis for GBM is poor; most patients do not survive beyond 1 year of diagnosis. The initial treatment is resection. Adjuvant radiation therapy with chemotherapy (with nitrosoureas and temozolomide) is the current standard of care. Dexamethasone is used to alleviate the vasogenic edema that that is caused by blood-brain barrier disruption that occurs in the area around many brain tumors. Dexamethasone is preferred over other steroids because its relative lack of mineralocorticoid activity decreases the risk of fluid retention.

■ CASE 15

A 42-year-old African-American man presents to the emergency department with sudden-onset shortness of breath. He complains of fatigue and weakness and says he saw blood in his urine for the first time this morning. He denies chest pain or palpitations and has no history of hypertension, coronary artery disease, or ischemic heart disease. He is being treated with trimethoprim-sulfamethoxazole for a urinary tract infection but has no other significant medical history. He denies alcohol or drug abuse. Physical examination reveals hepatosplenomegaly, mild scleral icterus, and tachycardia.

What is the most likely diagnosis?

Glucose-6-phospate dehydrogenase (G6PD) deficiency.

What are the typical PBS findings in this condition?

PBS will likely reveal bite cells and ghost cells, implying **intravascular** hemolytic anemia.

What is the pathophysiology of this condition?

G6PD protects cells from oxidative damage by converting nicotinamide adenine dinucleotide phosphate (NADP+) to its reduced form (NADPH). Patients with a deficiency in this enzyme are less able to cope with oxidative stresses, such as those that are caused by ingestion of a sulfa drug (ie, trimethoprim-sulfamethoxazole).

How is this condition acquired?

G6PD deficiency is an X-linked recessive trait and affects males predominantly. Heterozygous females are usually normal. Patients with G6PD deficiency are normal in the absence of oxidative stress. However, exposure to oxidative stress triggers the disease. G6PD in Mediterranean pedigrees results in favism, or hemolysis induced by the ingestion of fava beans.

How are anemias classified in terms of cell volume?

- **Microcytic anemia** (MCV < 80 fL) is caused by iron deficiency, thalassemia, or lead poisoning.
- **Normocytic anemia** (MCV 80–100 fL) is caused by enzyme deficiency (such as G6PD or pyruvate kinase), blood loss (as from trauma), anemia of chronic disease, renal failure, or bone marrow aplasia.
- **Macrocytic anemia** (MCV >100 fL) can be caused by vitamin B_{12}/folate deficiency, warm or cold hemolysis, myeloma, liver disease, drugs that inhibit DNA synthesis, alcohol, and myelodysplasia.

What is the appropriate treatment for this condition?

Treatment is generally supportive with removal of the offending agent.

CASE 16

A 67-year-old man presents to his physician with pain on swallowing and hoarseness. He has noted some swelling of the right side of his neck. The patient has smoked one pack of cigarettes per day since he was 15 years of age and drinks two beers nightly. Physical examination reveals a palpable neck mass and white plaques in his mouth.

What conditions should be considered in the differential diagnosis of a neck mass?

- **Congenital** causes of a neck mass include torticollis, thyroglossal duct cyst, brachial cleft cyst, cystic hygroma, dermoid cyst, and carotid body tumor.
- **Acquired** causes of neck mass include lymphoma, mononucleosis (Epstein-Barr virus), other causes of lymphadenopathy, and cervical lymphadenitis.
- **Thyroid** causes include goiter (midline).
- **Malignant** causes include thyroid cancer (eg, papillary, medullary, follicular, or anaplastic types), lymphoma, and head or neck malignancy (eg, squamous cell or adenocarcinoma).

What is the most likely diagnosis?
Squamous cell tumor of the head and neck.

What risk factors increase this patient's likelihood of disease?
Tobacco and alcohol use are risk factors for both squamous cell tumors and adenocarcinoma of the head and neck. Human papillomavirus (HPV) infection is now becoming a more common risk factor in head and neck cancers, particularly in association with nonsmokers.

Which procedures can help confirm the diagnosis?
Diagnostic procedures include biopsy via fine-needle aspiration of the mass, and CT and/or MRI to determine the stage and possible vascular involvement and resectability. If lymphoma is suspected, excisional biopsy should be performed (Figure 8-11).

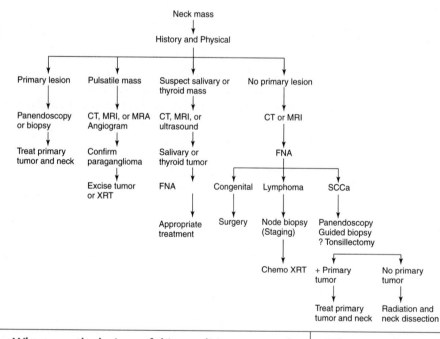

FIGURE 8-11. **Algorithm for neck mass management.** FNA, fine-needle aspiration; MRA, MR angiogram; SCCa, squamous cell carcinoma XRT, radiation therapy. (Reproduced, with permission, from Lalwani AK. *Current Diagnosis and Treatment in Otolaryngology–Head and Neck Surgery,* 2nd ed. New York: McGraw-Hill, 2008: Figure 26-2.)

Where are the lesions of this condition commonly located?
Head and neck cancers are typically found in the oral cavity, nasopharynx, larynx, oropharynx, and salivary glands.

What are the appropriate treatments for this condition?
Localized lesions are removed surgically or by radiotherapy. Palliative radiation is used for larger, more complex lesions. Combined chemotherapy and radiotherapy is the standard of care for advanced lesions.

CASE 17

A 55-year-old Caucasian man is brought to the emergency department after collapsing in a restaurant. He is conscious on arrival and claims he has not seen a doctor for many years. On physical examination, the patient appears jaundiced. An electrocardiogram (ECG) shows atrial fibrillation. Laboratory studies reveal an elevated serum glucose level and the following iron parameters:

Serum iron: 400 μg/dL   Iron saturation: 85%
Transferrin: 150 μg/dL   Ferritin: 2100 ng/mL

What is the most likely diagnosis?

Hereditary hemochromatosis (HH) is an autosomal recessive disease (with variable penetrance), resulting in excessive iron absorption. Excess iron gradually accumulates at a rate of approximately 0.5–1.0 g/year. Normal body iron content is approximately 3–4 g, and symptoms are noticeable at a body iron content exceeding 20 g. As a result, most men are not diagnosed until after 40 years of age, and women are not diagnosed until after cessation of their menstrual periods. Normal iron loss is 1 mg/day in men and 1.5 mg/day in menstruating women.

What is the pathophysiology of this condition?

Normally, iron homeostasis is achieved by regulating iron intake to compensate for losses through the skin, menses, pregnancy, and other processes. However, in HH, an autosomal recessive mutation in chromosome 6 (*HFE* gene) causes excessive iron to be absorbed through the intestine. This iron gradually deposits as hemosiderin throughout the body, particularly in the liver, skin, pancreas, joints, gonads, heart, and pituitary, which eventually leads to oxidative damage to these organs.

What signs and symptoms are commonly associated with this condition?

- Classic triad: cirrhosis, diabetes mellitus, and skin pigmentation ("bronze diabetes").
- Arthropathy (pseudogout, often of the second and third digits).
- Impotence in men.
- Cardiac enlargement.
- Cardiac conduction defects.
- Weakness/lethargy (due to pituitary involvement).

What are the typical laboratory findings in this condition?

Iron saturation of > 60% in men and > 50% in women suggests HH 90% of the time. A cutoff of 45% for both men and women is typically used for simplicity. If you suspect hemochromatosis, genetic testing (a simple blood test) for the HH gene should be performed (see Figure 8-12 for screening algorithm). Other typical laboratory findings include hyperglycemia, elevated liver enzyme levels, elevated serum iron levels, **decreased total iron binding capacity**, and **elevated ferritin levels**.

What is the appropriate treatment for this condition?

Treatment for HH includes serial phlebotomy with the possible use of deferoxamine, an iron-binding agent, especially for patients with homozygous *HFE* mutations (C282Y) and iron overload. Compound heterozygotes with iron overload should also be treated. Deferoxamine, an iron-binding agent, can be used for severe iron overload or in those patients who cannot tolerate phlebotomy (eg, anemia or cardiac disease).

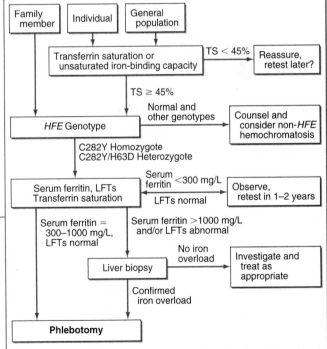

FIGURE 8-12. Hemochromatosis gene screening algorithm. (Reproduced, with permission, from Fauci AS, et al. *Harrison's Principles of Internal Medicine,* 17th ed. New York: McGraw-Hill, 2008: Figure 351-3.)

CASE 18

A 25-year-old man visits his primary care physician for a routine screening evaluation. He explains that he has been having fevers and drenching night sweats for the past 6 months. Additionally, he has been feeling increasingly tired and itchy over his entire body with no obvious explanation. On physical examination, the patient has lost 11 kg (25 lbs) since his last visit and has a markedly enlarged nontender lymph node in his anterior cervical chain. A biopsy of this node is taken (Figure 8-13).

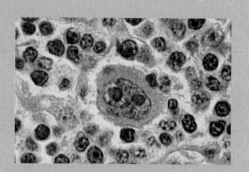

FIGURE 8-13. (Reproduced, with permission, from Lichtman MA, et al. *Williams Hematology*, 7th ed. New York: McGraw-Hill, 2006: Plate XXII-32.)

What type of cell is depicted in Figure 8-13?

This is the classic Reed-Sternberg cell, characterized by large size, bilobed nucleus, and nucleolar inclusion bodies ("owl's eyes"). Classically, these cells, formed from germinal B cell centers, also display a common set of markers, including **CD15+** and **CD30+**.

What is the most likely diagnosis?

Hodgkin lymphoma. Most patients present with nontender asymptomatic palpable lymphadenopathy, often in the neck and supraclavicular area. Alternatively, many patients will present with a fairly large asymptomatic mediastinal mass on routine x-ray of the chest. Approximately one-third of patients experience fever, night sweats, weight loss, fatigue, and pruritus. There are five main classes of Hodgkin lymphoma (Table 8-3).

TABLE 8-3	Five Main Types of Hodgkin Lymphoma	
TYPE OF HODGKIN	**RELATIVE PREVALENCE**	**HISTOLOGY, ASSOCIATIONS, AND PROGNOSIS**
Nodular sclerosis	Most common, especially among younger women	Fibrous bands dividing a lymph node into nodules; lacunar cells; carries a good prognosis
Lymphocyte predominance	Uncommon	Lymphohistiocytic "popcorn cells"
Lymphocyte-rich	Uncommon	Reactive lymphocytes that comprise infiltrate; 40% of cases associated with Epstein-Barr virus
Lymphocyte-depleted	Least common	Very few lymphocytes, relatively plentiful Reed-Sternberg cells; associated with Epstein-Barr virus and HIV; poor prognosis
Mixed cellularity	Uncommon	Polymorphic infiltrate with plentiful Reed-Sternberg cells; 70% of cases associated with Epstein-Barr virus; associated with older age

What are B symptoms?

Classic B symptoms are unexplained weight loss, persistent or recurrent fevers, and drenching night sweats. These symptoms generally correlate with an advanced stage of disease and tumor burden and a slightly worse prognosis independent of stage.

What is the appropriate treatment for this condition?

More than 90% of patients with early-stage localized disease are cured with excision and localized radiotherapy. Patients with more advanced disease typically undergo the ABVD chemotherapy regimen consisting of doxorubicin (adriamycin), bleomycin, vinblastine, and dacarbazine. Cure rates are very high, even with advanced, stage 4 disease.

CASE 17

A 55-year-old Caucasian man is brought to the emergency department after collapsing in a restaurant. He is conscious on arrival and claims he has not seen a doctor for many years. On physical examination, the patient appears jaundiced. An electrocardiogram (ECG) shows atrial fibrillation. Laboratory studies reveal an elevated serum glucose level and the following iron parameters:

Serum iron: 400 μg/dL   Iron saturation: 85%
Transferrin: 150 μg/dL   Ferritin: 2100 ng/mL

What is the most likely diagnosis?

Hereditary hemochromatosis (HH) is an autosomal recessive disease (with variable penetrance), resulting in excessive iron absorption. Excess iron gradually accumulates at a rate of approximately 0.5–1.0 g/year. Normal body iron content is approximately 3–4 g, and symptoms are noticeable at a body iron content exceeding 20 g. As a result, most men are not diagnosed until after 40 years of age, and women are not diagnosed until after cessation of their menstrual periods. Normal iron loss is 1 mg/day in men and 1.5 mg/day in menstruating women.

What is the pathophysiology of this condition?

Normally, iron homeostasis is achieved by regulating iron intake to compensate for losses through the skin, menses, pregnancy, and other processes. However, in HH, an autosomal recessive mutation in chromosome 6 (*HFE* gene) causes excessive iron to be absorbed through the intestine. This iron gradually deposits as hemosiderin throughout the body, particularly in the liver, skin, pancreas, joints, gonads, heart, and pituitary, which eventually leads to oxidative damage to these organs.

What signs and symptoms are commonly associated with this condition?

- Classic triad: cirrhosis, diabetes mellitus, and skin pigmentation ("bronze diabetes").
- Arthropathy (pseudogout, often of the second and third digits).
- Impotence in men.
- Cardiac enlargement.
- Cardiac conduction defects.
- Weakness/lethargy (due to pituitary involvement).

What are the typical laboratory findings in this condition?

Iron saturation of > 60% in men and > 50% in women suggests HH 90% of the time. A cutoff of 45% for both men and women is typically used for simplicity. If you suspect hemochromatosis, genetic testing (a simple blood test) for the HH gene should be performed (see Figure 8-12 for screening algorithm). Other typical laboratory findings include hyperglycemia, elevated liver enzyme levels, elevated serum iron levels, **decreased total iron binding capacity**, and elevated ferritin levels.

What is the appropriate treatment for this condition?

Treatment for HH includes serial phlebotomy with the possible use of deferoxamine, an iron-binding agent, especially for patients with homozygous *HFE* mutations (C282Y) and iron overload. Compound heterozygotes with iron overload should also be treated. Deferoxamine, an iron-binding agent, can be used for severe iron overload or in those patients who cannot tolerate phlebotomy (eg, anemia or cardiac disease).

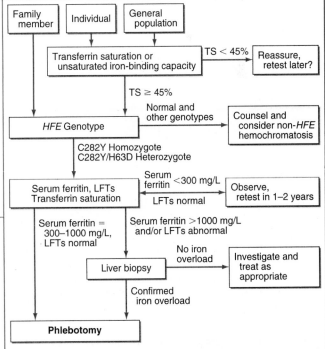

FIGURE 8-12. Hemochromatosis gene screening algorithm. (Reproduced, with permission, from Fauci AS, et al. *Harrison's Principles of Internal Medicine*, 17th ed. New York: McGraw-Hill, 2008: Figure 351-3.)

CASE 18

A 25-year-old man visits his primary care physician for a routine screening evaluation. He explains that he has been having fevers and drenching night sweats for the past 6 months. Additionally, he has been feeling increasingly tired and itchy over his entire body with no obvious explanation. On physical examination, the patient has lost 11 kg (25 lbs) since his last visit and has a markedly enlarged nontender lymph node in his anterior cervical chain. A biopsy of this node is taken (Figure 8-13).

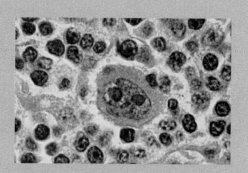

FIGURE 8-13. (Reproduced, with permission, from Lichtman MA, et al. *Williams Hematology*, 7th ed. New York: McGraw-Hill, 2006: Plate XXII-32.)

What type of cell is depicted in Figure 8-13?

This is the classic Reed-Sternberg cell, characterized by large size, bilobed nucleus, and nucleolar inclusion bodies ("owl's eyes"). Classically, these cells, formed from germinal B cell centers, also display a common set of markers, including **CD15+** and **CD30+**.

What is the most likely diagnosis?

Hodgkin lymphoma. Most patients present with nontender asymptomatic palpable lymphadenopathy, often in the neck and supraclavicular area. Alternatively, many patients will present with a fairly large asymptomatic mediastinal mass on routine x-ray of the chest. Approximately one-third of patients experience fever, night sweats, weight loss, fatigue, and pruritus. There are five main classes of Hodgkin lymphoma (Table 8-3).

TABLE 8-3   Five Main Types of Hodgkin Lymphoma

TYPE OF HODGKIN	RELATIVE PREVALENCE	HISTOLOGY, ASSOCIATIONS, AND PROGNOSIS
Nodular sclerosis	Most common, especially among younger women	Fibrous bands dividing a lymph node into nodules; lacunar cells; carries a good prognosis
Lymphocyte predominance	Uncommon	Lymphohistiocytic "popcorn cells"
Lymphocyte-rich	Uncommon	Reactive lymphocytes that comprise infiltrate; 40% of cases associated with Epstein-Barr virus
Lymphocyte-depleted	Least common	Very few lymphocytes, relatively plentiful Reed-Sternberg cells; associated with Epstein-Barr virus and HIV; poor prognosis
Mixed cellularity	Uncommon	Polymorphic infiltrate with plentiful Reed-Sternberg cells; 70% of cases associated with Epstein-Barr virus; associated with older age

What are B symptoms?

Classic B symptoms are unexplained weight loss, persistent or recurrent fevers, and drenching night sweats. These symptoms generally correlate with an advanced stage of disease and tumor burden and a slightly worse prognosis independent of stage.

What is the appropriate treatment for this condition?

More than 90% of patients with early-stage localized disease are cured with excision and localized radiotherapy. Patients with more advanced disease typically undergo the ABVD chemotherapy regimen consisting of doxorubicin (adriamycin), bleomycin, vinblastine, and dacarbazine. Cure rates are very high, even with advanced, stage 4 disease.

■ CASE 19

An 8-month-old boy is brought to the pediatrician by his foster parents for a checkup. They become concerned when he continues to bleed after the heel-stick. They report that during his circumcision, he seemed to bleed for an extended amount of time as well. Physical examination is significant for multiple bruises on the child's knees and elbows. Relevant laboratory findings include a platelet count of 250,000/mm^3, a normal bleeding time, a PT of 12 seconds, and a PTT of > 120 seconds.

What is the most likely diagnosis?

Hemophilia is due to deficiencies in the intrinsic coagulation pathway (factor VIII in hemophilia A and factor IX in hemophilia B). Therefore, this disease is characterized by normal bleeding time, platelet count, and prothrombin time but an **elevated PTT.**

Von Willebrand disease is the most common hereditary bleeding disorder. It is distinguished from hemophilia by its prolonged bleeding time and usually a modest prolongation of the PTT.

What are the variants of this condition?

- Hemophilia A is due to a marked deficiency of factor VIII.
- Hemophilia B (Christmas disease) is due to a marked deficiency of factor IX.

Hemophilia B is clinically indistinguishable from hemophilia A. However, hemophilia A is 5–10 times more prevalent.

How is this condition inherited?

Both disease variants are X-linked recessive.

What are the possible complications of this condition?

- Complications include deep and delayed bleeding into joints (hemarthrosis), muscles (hematoma), and the gastrointestinal tract. The most concerning complications are bleeds in the central nervous system and oropharynx.
- Mucosal or cutaneous bleeding is uncommon and more characteristic of platelet dysfunction or von Willebrand disease.
- Transmission of blood-borne infection (specifically HIV and hepatitis C) through transfusion has been significantly reduced through modern screening technology and recombinant factors.

What are the appropriate treatments for this condition?

- Clotting factor concentrate replacements can be used to prevent bleeding and limit existing hemorrhage. Both monoclonal purified and recombinant factor VIII and IX exist.
- Fresh frozen plasma and whole blood transfusions are used in the acute setting (but they carry the risk of encouraging the development of inhibitor antibodies to factor VIII).
- In mild cases of hemophilia A, desmopressin transiently increases the factor VIII level.

◾ CASE 20

A 19-year-old African-American woman presents to her primary care physician with pelvic pain and discomfort of a few months' duration. A bimanual pelvic examination reveals a large left adnexal mass. A subsequent CT scan confirms a 16-cm well-demarcated solid mass in this area. A stereotactic biopsy reveals primitive mesenchymal cells along with tissue suggestive of glands, bone, cartilage, muscle, and neuroepithelial cells (Figure 8-14).

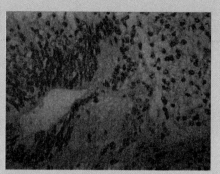

FIGURE 8-14. (Reproduced, with permission, from Kantarjian HM, et al. *MD Anderson Manual of Medical Oncology*. New York: McGraw-Hill, 2006.)

What is the most likely diagnosis?

Teratoma, the most common type of germ cell tumor. The component tissues in a teratoma arise from all three germ layers and vary from immature to well differentiated. Additionally, these tissues are foreign to the anatomic site in which they are found.

What are the three types of this condition?

- **Mature (benign dermoid cysts)** tumors compose 95% of all ovarian teratomata and are typically lined by epidermis and contain hair, bone, or teeth. These lesions can also be bilateral.
- **Immature (malignant)** tumors are usually large, rapidly growing tumors with tissue resembling the fetus or embryo rather than the adult. Due to their rapid growth, these tumors also show necrosis and hemorrhage and present in younger women.
- **Monodermal/highly** specialized tumors are a rare subset that consist of a predominantly mature histologic cell type, the most common of which are struma ovarii and carcinoid.

Most teratomata are benign in women.

What are the typical imaging findings in this condition?

Ultrasound is the most common modality for pelvic imaging, especially for suspected teratomata. Mixed cystic and solid lesions with fat-fluid and hair-fluid levels are commonly found.

How are these masses graded?

Only malignant teratomata are graded, and the grade of differentiation is based upon the proportion of tissue containing immature neuroepithelium. This is an important prognostic indicator of extra-ovarian spread.

What is the appropriate treatment for this condition?

Complete surgical excision is the standard of care. Higher-grade malignant teratomata are additionally managed with chemotherapy such as methotrexate, with a high rate of cure.

CASE 21

An 11-year-old girl is brought to her physician because of frequent epistaxis and "purple spots" on her body. She reports no recent history of trauma. Physical examination reveals petechiae and purpura on her arms, outer thighs, and legs (Figure 8-15). A PBS shows large platelets, but no helmet cells or schistocytes. Results of a Coombs test are positive. Relevant laboratory findings are as follows:

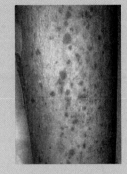

FIGURE 8-15. (Reproduced, with permission, from Bondi EE, et al. *Dermatology: Diagnosis & Treatment*. Norwalk, CT: Appleton & Lange, 1991. Copyright © The McGraw-Hill Companies, Inc.)

Hemoglobin: 12.5 g/dL
Hematocrit: 36%
WBC count: 5000/mm³
Platelet count: 11,000/mm³

Bleeding time: 12 minutes
PT: 13 seconds
PTT: 25 seconds

What is the most likely diagnosis?

Idiopathic thrombocytopenic purpura (ITP), a disease that is associated with antiplatelet antibodies, is the most likely diagnosis. The patient presents with isolated thrombocytopenia (normal WBC and Hct), no coagulopathy, and given her age, ITP is the most common cause of thrombocytopenia.

What are the three main mechanisms of low platelet counts?

Thrombocytopenia may be caused by:

- Splenic sequestration.
- Decreased production (stem cell failure, leukemia, aplastic anemia, EtOH, aspirin, clopidogrel).
- Increased destruction (ITP, thrombotic thrombocytopenic purpura, heparin, quinidine).

What clinical findings are commonly associated with this condition?

- ITP presents with mucous membrane bleeding, petechiae, and purpura (Figure 8-15).
- Epistaxis (nosebleed) and easy bruising are characteristic of bleeding disorders in general.
- ITP in childhood usually develops after a viral infection or immunization and is self-limited.
- Adult ITP, in contrast, is often a chronic disease.

How is the etiology of this condition determined?

Thrombocytopenia can have a number of etiologies, which can be differentiated according to Figure 8-16.

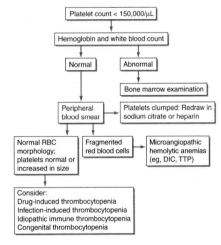

FIGURE 8-16. **Algorithm for thrombocytopenia evaluation.** (Reproduced, with permission, from Fauci AS, et al. *Harrison's Principles of Internal Medicine*, 17th ed. New York: McGraw-Hill, 2008: Figure 109-2.)

What are the appropriate treatments for this condition?

First-line treatment is high-dose steroids. Second-line treatment includes intravenous IgG, anti-Rh, splenectomy, or rituximab (anti-CD20). Thrombopoietin receptor agonists (romiplostim) have been shown to be highly effective in raising platelets counts for long-term control, but long-term safety data and cost of therapy are limiting factors in using these modalities as first-line therapy. Acute bleeding in ITP is treated with intravenous IgG followed by platelets and pulse methylprednisolone.

■ CASE 22

A 60-year-old woman presents to her primary care physician for her annual physical examination. She says she has been feeling "down" and tired lately. Upon questioning, she also admits to some constipation, abdominal pain, joint pain, and muscle aches. Physical examination reveals blue pigmentation in her gum-tooth line. A PBS reveals coarse basophilic stippling. Relevant laboratory findings are as follows:

Hemoglobin: 9.0 g/dL   Mean corpuscular volume: 76 fL
Hematocrit: 26%   WBC count: 5000/mm³

What conditions can cause basophilic stippling?

Basophilic stippling may be caused by lead poisoning, hemolysis, or thalassemia. Laboratory tests, including a Coombs test, reticulocyte count, and hemoglobin electrophoresis, can help differentiate these conditions, as follows:

- In lead poisoning, Coombs test is negative, reticulocyte count is low and hemoglobin electrophoresis is normal.
- In hemolysis, Coombs test is positive, reticulocyte count is elevated, and hemoglobin electrophoresis is normal.
- In thalassemia, Coombs test is negative, reticulocyte count is elevated, and hemoglobin electrophoresis is abnormal.

What is the most likely diagnosis?

Lead poisoning is suggested by the blue pigmentation of the gums (**Burton lines**), microcytic anemia, and characteristic basophilic stippling.

What are other common signs and symptoms of this condition?

Common signs and symptoms of lead poisoning include: colicky abdominal pain; constipation; irritability; difficulty concentrating; depression/psychosis; decreased short-term memory; arthralgias and myalgias; headache; decreased libido; and peripheral neuropathy, often presenting as extensor weakness (eg, wrist drop) due to segmental demyelination and degeneration of motor axons.

What is the most likely cause of the patient's anemia?

Lead poisoning is an environmental cause of porphyria through inhibition of aminolevulinate dehydratase, which converts δ-aminolevulinic acid to porphobilinogen in one of the first steps of heme synthesis. It also inhibits ferrochelatase to inhibit the conversion of protoporphyrin IX to heme in the last step of synthesis (Figure 8-17). This impairment results in decreased hemoglobin production and a microcytic, hypochromic anemia.

What do increased serum lead levels and increased free erythrocyte protoporphyrin (FEP) levels indicate about the duration of this condition?

Increased serum lead levels indicate lead exposure within the past 3 weeks. FEP levels are a measure of intoxication in the past 120 days (the average lifetime of an RBC). Chelation therapy with **succimer** can be useful in severe cases after removing the source of the lead.

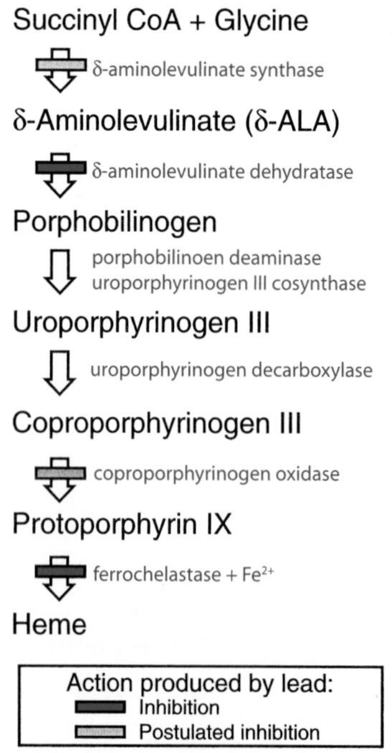

Succinyl CoA + Glycine
⬇ δ-aminolevulinate synthase
δ-Aminolevulinate (δ-ALA)
⬇ δ-aminolevulinate dehydratase
Porphobilinogen
⬇ porphobilinoen deaminase
  uroporphyrinogen III cosynthase
Uroporphyrinogen III
⬇ uroporphyrinogen decarboxylase
Coproporphyrinogen III
⬇ coproporphyrinogen oxidase
Protoporphyrin IX
⬇ ferrochelastase + Fe²⁺
Heme

Action produced by lead:
▬ Inhibition
▭ Postulated inhibition

FIGURE 8-17. Heme synthesis and lead poisoning. (Reproduced, with permission, from Brunton LL, et al. *Goodman & Gilman's The Pharmacological Basis of Therapeutics*, 11th ed. New York: McGraw-Hill, 2006: Figure 65-1.)

CASE 23

A 65-year-old woman presents to her physician with cough, hemoptysis, wheezing, and pain in her shoulder running down her arm. She has noted increased vocal hoarseness and weight loss over the past few months. She also has noted worsening shortness of breath when ascending or descending one flight of stairs. Sputum analysis reveals atypical cells. A complete blood count reveals her hematocrit is 25% and her WBC count is 12,000/mm^3.

What is the most likely diagnosis?

Lung cancer (with Pancoast syndrome). This condition is caused by a tumor of the upper lobe of the lung, which causes pain in the ipsilateral arm and Horner syndrome (ptosis, miosis, and ipsilateral anhidrosis). The tumor is often accompanied by ipsilateral pain or weakness/numbness in the ulnar distribution.

What are the major clinical features of this condition?

- Hoarseness (recurrent laryngeal nerve involvement).
- Neck or facial swelling (superior vena cava obstruction).
- Diaphragmatic paralysis (phrenic nerve involvement).
- Dyspnea (airway obstruction).
- Metastasis.
- Paraneoplastic syndromes (Cushing syndrome, hypercalcemia, the syndrome of inappropriate secretion of antidiuretic hormone, clubbing [hypertrophic osteoarthropathy], and Lambert-Eaton syndrome).

What are the typical laboratory and imaging findings in this condition?

- Sputum analysis reveals atypical cells (not sensitive).
- Anemia of chronic disease.
- Radiograph and CT typically reveal lung nodules.
- Positron emission tomography may be useful to evaluate lymph node involvement; this is critical for staging.

What are the primary pathologic types of this condition?

- **Non–small cell lung cancer** (which is the most common type) includes the following:
  - **Squamous cell carcinoma** accounts for 30% of lung cancers. It occurs centrally near the hilum; slower growth and cavitation are frequently seen.
  - **Adenocarcinoma** accounts for 30% of lung cancers. These tumors may be mucus-secreting as in acinar adenocarcinoma.
  - **Bronchoalveolar carcinoma** occurs more often in nonsmokers and is often multifocal.
  - **Large cell carcinoma,** which is rare.
- **Small cell carcinoma** accounts for 25% of lung cancers. These tumors occur centrally and are early to metastasize. They are sensitive to chemotherapy but frequently relapse.

What are the appropriate treatments for this condition?

Surgery is considered for lesions without distant metastasis if the patient has sufficient cardiopulmonary reserve. Radiotherapy is used to treat unresectable tumors. Adjuvant chemotherapy is also used with some patients undergoing surgery. For patients with metastatic disease, palliative chemotherapy is often used.

CASE 24

A 45-year-old man presents to his physician for a regular checkup. He has no previous medical or surgical history. The patient is complaining of a sense of imbalance and that his legs feel slightly numb. The patient has been eating a well-balanced diet and denies alcohol intake. As part of the checkup, the physician orders routine laboratory tests; relevant findings are as follows:

Hemoglobin: 11 g/dL
Hematocrit: 33%
Reticulocyte count: 0.2%
MCV: 120 fL

What is the most likely diagnosis?

The tests indicate a macrocytic anemia. However, macrocytic anemia is not a diagnosis in itself, and a cause for the anemia must be determined.

What other laboratory test could be used to determine the diagnosis?

In this patient we are suspecting B_{12} deficiency (megaloblastic anemias) given the high MCV and neurologic findings. In megaloblastic anemias, a peripheral blood smear reveals the presence of hypersegmented neutrophils (more than five nuclei) (Figure 8-18).

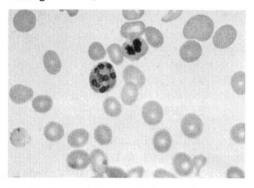

FIGURE 8-18. Multilobed polymorphonuclear leukocytes characteristic of megaloblastic anemias. (Reproduced, with permission, from Kasper DL, et al. *Harrison's Principles of Internal Medicine*, 16th ed. New York: McGraw-Hill, 2005: 605.)

What are some possible etiologies for this condition?

Etiologies of macrocytic anemia include the following:

- Alcoholism
- Folate deficiency.
- Vitamin B_{12} deficiency.
- Hypothyroidism.
- Myelodysplastic syndrome or myeloma.
- Pharmaceutical agents (especially antimetabolites such as methotrexate or chemotherapeutic agents).

What findings distinguish vitamin B_{12} from folate deficiency?

Vitamin B_{12} deficiency results in subacute combined degeneration of the dorsal columns of the spinal cord, causing loss of vibration and position sense. Also, methylmalonic acid is elevated in the urine of patients with B_{12} deficiency.

In folate deficiency, there are no neurologic findings and no rise in methylmalonic acid levels in the urine.

CASE 25

A 66-year-old postmenopausal woman presents to her physician with complaints of fatigue, dyspnea, dizziness, and tachycardia. She says she craves chewing on ice cubes. Physical examination reveals pallor of the mucous membranes of her mouth. The cells on a PBS are microcytic and hypochromic (Figure 8-19). Relevant laboratory findings are as follows:

Hemoglobin: 11 g/dL
Hematocrit: 30%
Reticulocyte count: 0.2%
MCV: 74 fL

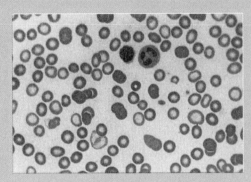

FIGURE 8-19. (Reproduced, with permission, from Le T, et al. *First Aid for the USMLE Step 1: 2008*. New York: McGraw-Hill, 2008: Color Image 20.)

What is the most likely diagnosis?

Iron deficiency anemia. This diagnosis would be supported by laboratory studies demonstrating a **decreased iron concentration, increased total iron binding capacity, and decreased ferritin levels.** The cause for a patient's iron deficiency, however, needs to be further pursued. In addition, comorbid inflammatory conditions can raise serum ferritin, resulting in values within the normal range.

What factors can lead to this condition?

Causes of iron deficiency anemia include the following:

- Chronic blood loss (especially gastrointestinal blood loss secondary to colon cancer).
- Dietary deficiency (increased demand or decreased absorption).
- Intestinal hookworm infection (this is the most common cause worldwide and should be considered in patients who have immigrated from developing countries).

In general, in a postmenopausal woman and all men, one must look for GI blood loss in any newly diagnosed patient with iron deficiency anemia unless the cause of the iron loss is obvious (nose bleeds, recent trauma, etc).

Why are total iron binding capacity (TIBC) measurements important in this condition?

TIBC is high in iron deficiency anemia and low in anemia of chronic disease. Both illnesses have decreased serum iron levels. A low ferritin (< 41 ng/mL) is sensitive and specific for iron deficiency anemia. The normal iron/TIBC ratio is typically 0.25–0.45, and levels < 0.12 indicate iron deficiency. Anemia of chronic disease often has a normal iron/TIBC ratio because of the concomitant decrease of TIBC and serum iron.

What other conditions is this patient at greatly increased risk for developing?

Because of the extreme lack of iron, this patient is at risk for **Plummer-Vinson syndrome.** This syndrome is characterized by atrophic glossitis, esophageal webs, and anemia.

What are the common causes of microcytic, hypochromic anemia?

Microcytic anemia results from either decreased hemoglobin production or faulty hemoglobin function. Common causes include iron deficiency, thalassemia, sideroblastic anemia, and lead poisoning.

CASE 26

A mother brings her 4-month-old infant to the pediatrician because the child has had watery diarrhea almost daily for the past month. Previously a good eater, the baby is now refusing to feed and is irritable most of the time. While holding the baby, the mother also calls attention to a mass in his belly that has not resolved in several days.

What is the most common tumor in infants?

Neuroblastoma is a malignancy of the sympathetic nervous system that arises during embryonic development. In the embryo, **neuroblasts** (pluripotent sympathetic stem cells) invaginate and migrate along the neuraxis to the adrenal medulla, the sympathetic ganglia, and various other sites. Figure 8-20 shows a large neuroblastoma occupying the right flank in an older child. The site of disease presentation depends on the area of neuroblast migration.

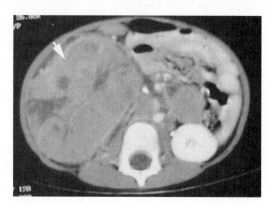

FIGURE 8-20. Abdominal neuroblastoma arising from the right retro-peritoneum (arrow). (Reproduced, with permission, from Brunicardi FC, et al. *Schwartz's Principles of Surgery,* 8th ed. New York: McGraw-Hill, 2005.)

What are the types of small, round, blue-cell tumors?

- Neuroblastoma is a common tumor of the adrenal medulla in children. It is characterized by homovanillic acid (dopamine breakdown product) present in urine. It is associated with the *N-myc* oncogene.
- Wilms tumor is the most common childhood renal malignancy and presents with flank mass and hematuria. It is associated with deletion of *WT1* on chromosome 11.
- Acute leukemia is caused by unregulated growth of leukocytes in the bone marrow.
- Mesothelioma is associated with smoking and asbestos exposure.
- Rhabdomyosarcoma is a tumor of skeletal muscle.
- Medulloblastoma is a highly malignant cerebellar tumor. It often compresses the 4th ventricle to cause hydrocephalus.
- Retinoblastoma is associated with 13q mutation of *Rb* gene.

What prognostic factors are important in this condition?

Tumor stage and the patient's age at diagnosis are the two most important prognostic factors. Patients with localized disease, regardless of age, have a favorable prognosis (5-year survival rate: 80%–90%). Overall, younger age at diagnosis carries a more favorable prognosis.

What are the likely biopsy findings in this condition?

Histologically, neuroblastoma presents as dense nests of small, round, blue tumor cells with hyperchromatic nuclei. **Homer-Wright pseudorosettes** are seen in 10%–15% of cases. These pseudorosettes are composed of neuroblasts surrounding neuritic processes and are pathognomonic for neuroblastoma.

What are the appropriate treatments for this condition?

For patients with localized disease, surgical excision is curative. For more advanced disease, treatment consists of surgical excision followed by chemotherapy. Chemotherapy for neuroblastoma consists of combination regimens, typically vincristine, cyclophosphamide, and doxorubicin. Other regimens include etoposide in combination with either cisplatin or carboplatin.

■ CASE 27

A 62-year-old African American man comes to his physician complaining of lower back pain of recent onset. His medical history is unremarkable except for two recent attacks of pneumonia that were successfully treated. Relevant laboratory values are as follows:

Sodium: 140 mEq/L   Potassium: 4.0 mEq/L
Phosphate: 3.6 mg/dL   Calcium: 14 mg/dL
Bicarbonate: 25 mEq/L   Blood urea nitrogen (BUN): 15 mg/dL
Chloride: 106 mEq/L   Creatinine: 2.0 mg/dL
Magnesium: 1.8 mg/dL

What is the most likely diagnosis?

Back pain, increased recent susceptibility to infection, and elevated serum calcium and creatinine levels strongly suggest multiple myeloma.

What is the pathophysiology of this condition?

Multiple myeloma is a clonal proliferation of B cells that have differentiated into plasma cells. These mature B cells cause lytic lesions in the bones, called **punched-out lesions.** These cells produce massive quantities of identical immunoglobulin molecules, usually IgG or IgA, that are either κ or λ light chain (κ more common than λ). Rarely, IgD or nonsecretory myeloma is diagnosed.

What renal complications are associated with this condition?

The large amount of **Bence Jones proteins** (free immunoglobulin light chains) found in the urine of patients with multiple myeloma causes azotemia. Other renal complications include inflammation with potential giant cell formation and metastatic calcification.

What other tests can be used to confirm the diagnosis?

A complete blood count should be ordered. Patients with multiple myeloma may be anemic as a result of tumor cells overcrowding myeloid precursor cells. Electrophoresis with immunofixation will demonstrate **M protein,** the term given to the massively produced immunoglobulin. Urinalysis of a 24-hour collection may reveal the presence of a Bence Jones protein. Bone marrow biopsy shows a two- to fourfold increase in plasma cells; biopsy results are essential for the diagnosis of multiple myeloma. Other immunoglobulins may be low, which can add to the risk of infection. Due to hyperglobulinemia, RBCs on peripheral blood smear will clump in a **rouleaux formation** (Figure 8-21).

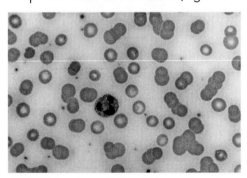

FIGURE 8-21. Rouleaux formation of multiple myeloma on peripheral blood smear. (Reproduced, with permission, from Lichtman MA, et al. *Lichtman's Atlas of Hematology.* New York: McGraw-Hill, 2007: Figure VII.C.61.)

What is MGUS?

Monoclonal gammopathy of undetermined significance (MGUS) is a precursor (premalignant) lesion if the M protein level is < 3 g/dL, there is < 10% plasma cells in the bone marrow, and there are no clinical manifestations of multiple myeloma present. The CRAB mnemonic can be used to remember the clinical characteristics that are *not* present in MGUS but *are* present in multiple myeloma: elevated Calcium, Renal failure, Anemia, and Bone lesions. Twenty-five percent to 30% of those with MGUS may go on to develop a lymphoproliferative disorder in their lifetime.

◾ CASE 28

A 30-year-old woman comes to her physician complaining of a headache that has affected her intermittently for the past 6 months. The frontally located headache occurs on most days and is typically dull but sometimes piercing. Over the same time period, the woman has also had profound weakness in her right arm to the point that she is sometimes unable to hold her 1-year-old daughter or to comb her hair. She also reports an intermittent sensation of "pins and needles" in her right hand.

What is the most likely diagnosis?

Oligodendroglioma. These relatively rare, slow-growing tumors are responsible for 2%–4% of primary brain tumors. They occur with equal incidence in women and men. They originate from glial cells, which myelinate central nervous system axons.

Where do the tumors of this condition typically occur?

Oligodendrogliomas almost always (92% of cases) occur supratentorially and are most often found in the frontal lobes. Lesions are typically peripheral. Most oligodendrogliomas arise in the cortex and extend into the white matter of the cerebral hemispheres.

What symptoms are typically associated with this condition?

The clinical presentation of oligodendrogliomas is typically attributable to compression of adjacent structures by the tumor:

- Headache.
- Mental status changes.
- Paresis.
- Seizures.

Because they are slow-growing tumors, they may have a more insidious presentation, whereas the anaplastic forms present with more rapid neurologic decline.

What are the likely histology findings in this condition?

"Fried egg" cells are typically seen on histologic section. These cells have characteristic round nuclei with clear cytoplasm. The tumors often calcify (30% of cases), and calcifications may be apparent on histologic section.

What is the prognosis for patients with this condition?

About 50% of patients with oligodendrogliomas survive > 5 years, and the 10-year survival rate is 25%–34%. Mortality increases with features of increasing nuclear atypia, necrosis, and mitosis. Some oligodendrogliomas contain astrocytic components and are termed **mixed gliomas**. Patients with highly anaplastic oligodendrogliomas have a median survival of < 2 years.

■ CASE 29

A 49-year-old woman presents to her gynecologist because her menstrual periods have become irregular. The patient also reports she has hair growing on her face and has developed mild acne, which she has not had since she was a teenager. On physical examination, the patient's abdomen is somewhat distended and there is a palpable mass on the left adnexum.

What is the most likely diagnosis?

A palpable adnexal mass in conjunction with abdominal swelling suggests ovarian cancer, which is often accompanied by ascites. The patient's irregular periods may simply be normal menopause, but the triad of irregular periods, facial hair, and acne suggest androgen excess. The **Sertoli-Leydig ovarian tumor** is an androgen-producing neoplasm that presents with hirsutism in 50% of patients.

From what cell line does the tumor involved in this condition originate?

The Sertoli-Leydig cell tumor is of sex cord–stromal origin. Tumors from this origin are relatively rare and account for only 5% of ovarian neoplasms. They consist of mixtures of stromal fibroblasts, granulosa cells, theca cells, and cells that resemble testicular Sertoli cells and Leydig cells.

What do Sertoli and Leydig cells produce?

- Sertoli cells contain aromatase and convert testosterone to estrogen. In men, follicle-stimulating hormone stimulates Sertoli cells in spermatogenesis.
- Leydig cells, which are stimulated by luteinizing hormone, secrete testosterone.

What other tumors have the same origin?

Other stromal ovarian tumors include:

- **Fibromas,** solid tumors consisting of cells that resemble fibroblasts.
- **Thecoma** tumors, which contain fibroblasts plus lipid-containing cells.
- **Granulosa cell** tumors, which consist of estrogen-secreting granulosa cells and may present with abnormal vaginal bleeding or endometrial hyperplasia.

What are the likely histology findings in this condition?

The Sertoli-Leydig cell tumor is usually composed of large cells with eosinophilic cytoplasm arranged into tubules and surrounded by a fibrous stroma. Sertoli cells are found lining the tubules, and Leydig cells may be found in the stroma.

What is the lymphatic drainage of the ovaries?

Like that of the testicles, the ovaries' lymphatic drainage is to the lumbar and para-aortic lymph nodes. The ovarian lymph vessels travel with the venous drainage in the broad ligament.

What is the treatment and prognosis of this condition?

These tumors are almost always benign and have an excellent long-term prognosis; treatment with unilateral oophorectomy is highly successful.

CASE 30

A 54-year-old diabetic African-American man presents to his primary care physician after his wife noted scleral icterus and a recent unintentional 11.4-kg (25-lb) weight loss. The patient denies abdominal pain. Physical examination reveals a mass in the right upper quadrant of the abdomen. Relevant laboratory findings are as follows:

Alkaline phosphatase: 127 U/L
Direct bilirubin: 6 mg/dL
Calcium: 10.6 mg/dL

What is the most likely diagnosis?
Pancreatic cancer.

What is the classic presentation of this condition?
The classic presentation of pancreatic cancer is painless jaundice. Weight loss, abdominal pain, and pruritus are also common.

What is the pathophysiology of this condition?
Pancreatic tumors form mostly in the head and neck of the pancreas from the endocrine and exocrine portions of the pancreas. The majority of pancreatic cancers are exocrine in origin.

What risk factors are associated with this condition?

- African American race.
- Cigarette smoking.
- History of chronic pancreatitis.
- History of diabetes mellitus.
- Male gender.
- Diet high in fried meats.

What are the common sites of invasion for this condition?
Pancreatic cancer can invade the duodenum, the ampulla of Vater, and the common bile duct. Figure 8-22 shows a pancreatic adenocarcinoma, which appears as a large, heterogeneously enhancing mass at the head of the pancreas.

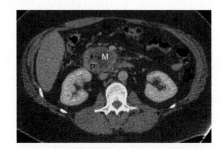

FIGURE 8-22. CT of pancreatic cancer. (Reproduced, with permission, from Chen MYM, et al. *Basic Radiology*, 2nd ed. New York: McGraw-Hill, 2011: Figure 11-70.)

What is the most common form/location of this condition?
More than 80% of pancreatic tumors are adenocarcinomas, and 60% are found in the head of the pancreas. Notably, with pancreatic adenocarcinoma, the tumor marker CA19-9 is often elevated.

What are the common sites of metastasis?
Metastasis often begins in the regional lymph nodes and spreads to the liver or, less often, to the lungs. Pancreatic cancer can also directly invade the duodenum, stomach, and colon.

With treatment, what is the prognosis of this condition?
Approximately 90% of patients die within 1 year of diagnosis; however, if resection of the cancer is possible and the cancer is caught in an early stage, 5-year survival increases to 30%. For a cancer in the head/neck of the pancreas, resection is performed with a Whipple procedure; for a cancer in the tail, resection is performed with a distal pancreatectomy. In a Whipple procedure, the stomach antrum, part of the duodenum, head of the pancreas, common bile duct, and gallbladder are removed. The remaining pancreas, common hepatic duct, and remaining stomach are all sewn into the jejunum.

■ CASE 31

During the course of an annual physical examination, a previously healthy 70-year-old man mentions recent weakness and rib pain. His appetite has been good, and he has not experienced fevers, nausea, vomiting, or changes in bowel habits. Physical examination reveals splenomegaly. Results of a complete blood count are as follows:

WBC count: 10,000/mm³
Hemoglobin: 22 g/dL
Hematocrit: 62%
Platelet count: 425,000/mm³

What is the most likely diagnosis?

Polycythemia vera, also known as **primary erythrocytosis.** This patient's elevated hemoglobin concentration is a sign of an increased RBC count. An increased RBC mass (> 32 mL/kg in women and > 36 mL/kg in men) is diagnostic of polycythemia vera absent of secondary causes. Polycythemia vera is one of the myeloproliferative syndromes, which also include essential thrombocytosis, CML, and myeloid metaplasia.

Levels of which hormone should be measured to establish the diagnosis?

Polycythemia vera may be primary or secondary in nature. **Erythropoietin** levels can help distinguish between the two.

- Erythropoietin levels will be decreased or normal in primary polycythemia (polycythemia vera).
- In secondary polycythemia, increased erythropoiesis results from increased erythropoietin stimulation (eg, erythropoietin-secreting tumor, hypoxemia, altitude, or erythropoietin receptor mutations).

Which two types of carcinoma are associated with this condition?

Renal cell carcinoma and **hepatocellular carcinoma.** In a healthy adult, the kidneys produce a majority of the body's erythropoietin, and the liver is a secondary source.

What is a myeloproliferative disorder?

It is a disorder in which there is clinical expansion of multipotent hematopoietic stem cells. Isolated cell lines may be affected; if megakaryocyte expansion occurs, an essential thrombocytosis is seen.

How can an uncorrected ventricular septal defect (VSD) lead to this condition?

In patients with uncorrected VSD, atrial septal defect, or patent ductus arteriosus, blood is shunted from the left side of the heart to the right side, which exposes the pulmonary vasculature to systemic blood pressures. Over time, the pulmonary vasculature adapts by increasing pulmonary resistance, and blood flow through the shunt is reversed to flow from right to left. This reversal of flow is known as **Eisenmenger syndrome.** Right-to-left shunts cause hypoxemia and cyanosis, a potent stimulus for erythropoietin secretion and a cause of secondary polycythemia.

What are the appropriate treatments for this condition?

Phlebotomy can reduce the risk of blood clots in patients with polycythemia to that of the normal population. In high-risk patients (the elderly or those with a history of clots), hydroxyurea may be useful for controlling the hematocrit.

■ CASE 32

A 3-year-old boy is brought to the pediatrician by his parents who noticed that his right eye has turned "white" (Figure 8-23). When they referred back to earlier photographs, the child's eyes were normally colored. The boy denies any pain or irritation in his eyes, and he does not complain of loss of vision. The parents deny any trauma to the area, and there is no family history of ocular disease. On physical examination, the boy's extraocular movements are intact and symmetrical, his pupillary light reflexes are normal, and he has intact central and peripheral vision in both eyes. However, when he is asked to fixate at a point in distance, the boy's right eye deviates toward his nose (esotropia). Funduscopic examination reveals a chalky, white-gray retinal mass in the right eye.

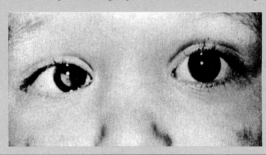

FIGURE 8-23. (Reproduced, with permission, from Riordan-Eva P, Whitcher JP. *Vaughan & Asbury's General Ophthalmology*, 16th ed. New York: McGraw-Hill, 2004: Figure 10-32.)

What is the most likely diagnosis?
Leukocoria found in a young child suggests **retinoblastoma.**

What conditions should be considered in the differential diagnosis?
Conditions that present similarly to leukocoria include the following:
- Congenital cataracts.
- Developmental abnormalities of the vitreous/retina.
- Inflammatory conditions.

What is the pathogenesis of this condition?
Retinoblastoma results from mutations of both alleles of the **Rb gene,** on chromosome 13q14, which codes for a tumor suppressor protein. The Rb protein binds and sequesters transcription factors of the E2F family to prevent the G1-to-S phase transition. Loss of Rb thus promotes deregulation of this transition and increased growth.

What is the "two-hit hypothesis"?
The **two-hit hypothesis** (Knudsen hypothesis) suggests that two separate mutations are required for tumorigenesis involving a suppressor gene. In heritable disease, patients inherit a mutated germline allele from a parent and acquire a second somatic mutation later in development. This often causes binocular and multifocal disease. In noninherited disease, two spontaneous mutations arise in a single retinal cell during development, causing uniocular, unifocal disease.

What secondary malignancies is this patient at risk of developing?
Osteogenic sarcoma, soft tissue sarcoma, and malignant melanoma commonly develop in patients with retinoblastoma. Metastatic spread occurs rapidly through direct infiltration or via the subarachnoid space, blood, and lymphatics.

What is the appropriate treatment for this condition?
The treatment of choice for retinoblastoma is enucleation of the affected eye; the goal is to remove a large portion of the optic nerve, as it is the most common path for metastasis to the brain. Other treatment options include external-beam radiation therapy, cryotherapy, and chemotherapy. With treatment, 5-year survival for retinoblastoma is > 90%.

◼ CASE 33

A 20-year-old African-American woman visits her physician complaining of episodes of extreme pain and discomfort in her legs and lower back. She has experienced these recurrent episodes, accompanied by extreme fatigue, since she was a child. On physical examination, she appears jaundiced and has a hematocrit of 23% and a hemoglobin level of 7 g/dL. She reports she has family members who experienced the same symptoms.

What is the most likely diagnosis?

Sickle cell anemia.

What is the typical presentation of this condition?

Sickle cell anemia develops at approximately 6 months of age when hemoglobin S (HbS) replaces hemoglobin F (HbF). Painful crises, which are believed to be a result of hypoxic tissue injury from microvascular occlusions, often occur.

What is the pathophysiology of this condition?

HbS is the result of a single missense mutation in the beta-globin gene of hemoglobin (negatively charged glutamate is replaced by neutrally charged valine and position 6). This makes hemoglobin susceptible to polymerization in conditions of low oxygen or dehydration (Figure 8-24), dramatically reducing the flexibility of the RBC membrane. Any organ can be affected by the vascular congestion, thrombosis, and infarction caused by sickling cells, so patients tend to have multiple health problems. The combination of sickle cell anemia and β-thalassemia is common and can also result in sickle crises.

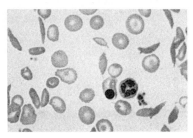

FIGURE 8-24. **Peripheral blood smear of sickle cell anemia.** (Reproduced, with permission, from Fauci AS, et al. *Harrison's Principles of Internal Medicine*, 17th ed. New York: McGraw-Hill, 2008: Figure 99-4.)

What complications are common in patients with this condition?

- Painful (vaso-occlusive) crisis.
- Aplastic crisis (cessation of erythropoiesis due to parvovirus B19 infection).
- Splenic sequestration crisis.
- Autosplenectomy, which increases susceptibility to encapsulated organisms, like *Pneumococcus*.
- Increased susceptibility to *Salmonella* osteomyelitis.
- Priapism.
- Stroke.
- Leg ulcers.
- Acute chest syndrome (fat emboli, infection, and vaso-occlusion).
- Dactylitis.

What are the typical radiologic findings in this condition?

The marrow expansion caused by the profound anemia can lead to resorption of bone and subsequent new bone formation on the external aspect of the skull. This leads to a "crew cut" appearance on skull radiographs.

What is the appropriate treatment for this condition?

Appropriate supportive care, including pain control and intravenous fluids, for acute sickle complications is the mainstay of therapy. Attention to the psychological impact of this disease, with social and psychiatric support, is essential to help patients deal with this disabling, painful disease. Additional medical therapy includes hydroxyurea, which increases HbF production, thereby reducing the number of cells with the potential to sickle. Exchange transfusion with normal RBCs may reduce the sickle RBC percentage and is used to treat the life-threatening complications of acute chest syndrome, stroke, and splenic sequestration.

■ CASE 34

A 55-year-old woman presents to her physician complaining of a 2- to 3-month history of cough. The cough was initially nonproductive but has become progressively more productive of sputum and occasionally blood. She has a 50-pack-year history of cigarette smoking. Physical examination reveals marked wheezing, and an x-ray of the chest demonstrates hilar enlargement and a perihilar mass on the right side. The mass is biopsied, and the histologic specimen is shown in Figure 8-25A and B.

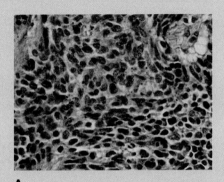
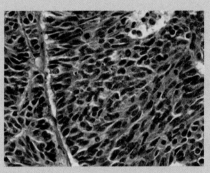

A   B

FIGURE 8-25. (Reproduced, with permission, from Kantarjian HM, et al. *MD Anderson Manual of Medical Oncology,* New York: McGraw-Hill, 2006: Figure 11-1.)

What is the most likely diagnosis?

Small cell lung carcinoma (SCLC). SCLC often presents as a hilar or mediastinal mass.

What risk factors are associated with this condition?

Smoking is the major risk factor for the development of most lung cancers. Large cell lung cancer and bronchoalveolar carcinoma, however, are not thought to be related to smoking.

Exposure to other substances, including asbestos, polycyclic aromatic hydrocarbons, and ionizing radiation also increases the risk for SCLC.

What are the most common sites of metastasis for this condition?

Small cell lung cancers metastasize to virtually every organ in the body, usually early in the onset of disease. Brain metastases are common, with resulting neurologic deficits. Bone metastases result in bone pain or fractures and can cause spinal cord compression. Liver, supraclavicular lymph nodes, and adrenal metastases are also common.

What are the appropriate treatments for this condition?

Most patients with SCLC have unresectable disease at the time of presentation. In the rare patient with small peripheral lesions and no metastases, surgical resection may be an option. Treatment for SCLC involves chemotherapy, typically etoposide plus cisplatin, with or without radiotherapy. In patients who do not receive chemotherapy or radiation, mean survival is 6–17 months, while survival for treated patients can average > 24 months.

What other syndrome is this patient at greatly increased risk for developing?

She is at risk for developing Lambert-Eaton myasthenic syndrome (a paraneoplastic syndrome). This condition, which is similar to myasthenia gravis, is caused by autoantibodies against the P/Q-type calcium channels in the presynaptic neuromuscular junction. It causes weakness of the proximal musculature, especially of the lower limbs. Cranial nerves are commonly affected, which often manifests as ptosis of the eyelids and diplopia.

CASE 35

Upon presentation to his family physician, an 8-month-old boy is noted to have jaundice and dyspnea. Physical examination reveals tachycardia and splenomegaly. The mother recalls a long family history of "blood disease." A Coombs test is negative. Relevant laboratory findings are as follows:

Hemoglobin: 8.5 g/dL
Hematocrit: 29%
MCV: 85 fL
Mean corpuscular hemoglobin concentration (MCHC): 400 g/L

What is the most likely diagnosis?

Hereditary spherocytosis, an autosomal dominant form of hemolytic anemia.

What protein defect causes this condition?

RBC membrane defects are the result of mutations in **spectrin** or **ankyrin** (erythrocyte skeletal proteins). This results in a decreased membrane/volume ratio, which makes the cells more fragile. Therefore, a positive result on **osmotic fragility testing** is typically pathognomonic for the disease. Cells are trapped in the spleen, where they are destroyed.

What are the typical peripheral blood smear findings in this condition?

Small RBCs without central pallor (**spherocytes**) (Figure 8-26) are seen on a peripheral blood smear.

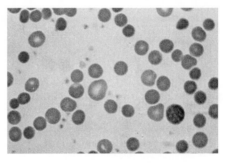

FIGURE 8-26. **Histology of spherocytosis.** (Reproduced, with permission, from Kasper DL, et al. *Harrison's Principles of Internal Medicine,* 16th ed. New York: McGraw-Hill, 2005: 609.)

What blood tests and findings can help establish the diagnosis?

- An osmotic fragility test may confirm the presence of fragile sphere-shaped RBCs.
- The MCHC is increased because of a reduction in membrane surface area in the setting of a constant hemoglobin concentration.
- MCV remains normal because the overall volume remains stable.
- High reticulocyte counts (5%–10%).
- Indirect bilirubin levels are elevated.

What test could be used to differentiate this condition from autoimmune etiologies?

A direct Coombs test is used to distinguish hereditary spherocytosis from warm antibody hemolysis: Hereditary spherocytosis is Coombs negative, whereas warm antibody hemolysis is Coombs positive. A positive result on a direct Coombs test indicates the presence of antibodies on RBCs. A positive result on an indirect Coombs test indicates the presence of antibodies in the serum.

What are the appropriate treatments for this condition?

Splenectomy is curative and should be considered in patients with severe disease. Surgery also helps prevent gallstone formation. Folate supplementation can be useful.

■ CASE 36

A 27-year-old man is brought to the emergency department by ambulance after a motor vehicle accident. He was a restrained passenger in a two-car collision. He is complaining of left upper quadrant pain. On physical examination he appears restless and agitated, and he is noted to be tachycardic and tachypneic.

What organ is most likely injured in this case?

The spleen. It is an important organ in immune function and hematopoiesis. The primary function of the spleen is clearance of abnormal RBCs, microorganisms, and particulate matter from the bloodstream. Additionally, it is involved in hematopoiesis (extramedullary hematopoiesis) and synthesis of IgG, properdin, and tuftsin.

What is the normal size of this organ?

A normal spleen weighs 150 g and is nonpalpable. Spleens that are prominent below the costal margin typically weigh 750–1000 g. Figure 8-27A is a CT scan of a man with splenic injury due to blunt trauma. This scan, obtained soon after contrast administration, shows multiple large lacerations of the spleen, hematoma, and perihepatic free fluid. Figure 8-27B, obtained after the contrast had cleared, more clearly shows a large laceration on the posterior surface of the spleen extending anteriorly to the hilum.

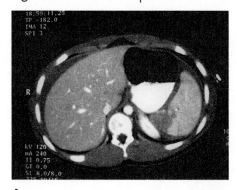 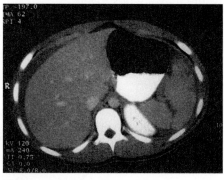

A   B

FIGURE 8-27. (A) CT of spleen early after contrast administration in a patient with blunt trauma to the spleen. (B) CT of spleen after contrast clears more clearly shows splenic laceration. (Reproduced, with permission, from Stone CK, Humphries RL. *Current Emergency Diagnosis & Treatment*, 5th ed. New York: McGraw-Hill, 2004: 471.)

Where is the injured organ located?

The spleen is located under the rib cage in the left upper quadrant of the abdomen, below the diaphragm. Therefore, during palpation, descent of an enlarged spleen is felt on inspiration.

Where is the most common site of referred pain in this injury?

Left shoulder and trapezius ridge tenderness (C3–C5 dermatomes, same as the roots of the phrenic nerve) may also be present as a result of subdiaphragmatic phrenic nerve irritation. Referred pain is due to subdiaphragmatic pooling of blood.

Why is a blunt injury to this organ so concerning?

The spleen is a highly vascular organ that filters up to 15% of the total blood volume per minute. The spleen can hold an average of 40–50 mL of RBCs in reserve and can pool significantly more blood.

What is the major concern for a patient postsplenectomy?

The major concern is sepsis from encapsulated bacterial organisms. *Streptococcus pneumoniae, Neisseria meningitidis,* and *Haemophilus influenzae* vaccinations are essential since encapsulated organisms are usually cleared by the spleen. Vaccinations are usually given several weeks before splenectomy, if possible, or 2 weeks after in an emergent case. Antibiotic prophylaxis for dental procedures and empiric treatment for fever are also vital given the immunocompromised state of the asplenic patient.

■ CASE 37

A 36-year-old sexually active man goes to his doctor after noticing that his left testicle has been swollen for the past few weeks. The patient has noticed a dull, achy sensation in this testicle but no acute pain. On physical examination, the left testicle is larger than the right, and a nontender, round, firm, rubbery mass is palpated. Transillumination with a penlight reveals an opaque mass. Laboratory tests reveal a normal chemistry panel, normal complete blood count, elevated LDH level, normal serum human chorionic gonadotropin (hCG) level, and normal α-fetoprotein (AFP) level.

What is the most likely diagnosis?

Testicular tumor, as suggested by the presence of a painless, nontransilluminating testicular mass. In a young man, the most likely diagnosis is a **seminoma**, which has a peak incidence of age 35 years and accounts for approximately 35% of testicular tumors. This diagnosis is further supported by the elevated LDH level, normal hCG level (elevated in 20% of seminomas), and normal AFP level.

What is the differential diagnosis of a scrotal mass?

Conditions to consider in the differential of a scrotal mass include the following:

- Orchitis.
- Epididymitis.
- Hydrocele.
- Spermatocele.
- Varicocele.
- Hernia.
- Cancer (nonseminomatous and nongerminal).

Epididymitis and orchitis are accompanied by a painful testicle and an elevated WBC count, differentiating them from seminoma. Elevated AFP levels suggest a nonseminomatous germ cell cancer. Fluid collections, like a hydrocele, transilluminate. A hernia may be reducible or irreducible; if it is irreducible, the patient will likely be in significant pain from the presence of incarcerated bowel.

What is the analogous condition in women?

The analogous ovarian tumor is the **dysgerminoma**, the most common germ cell tumor in women. It is usually malignant and is more common in younger patients. Like seminomas, it can produce LDH. It can also produce alkaline phosphatase.

What is the lymphatic drainage of this tumor?

Understanding the lymphatic drainage of the testicles is important in considering metastases. Because the testicles descend from the abdomen during development, the lymph vessels ascend to the lumbar and para-aortic lymph nodes. This contrasts with the lymph drainage of the scrotum, which is an outpouching of skin. The lymph vessels of the scrotum drain to the superficial inguinal nodes.

What other conditions are characterized by an elevated hCG level?

Only 10%–20% of seminomas present with elevated hCG levels. Tumors in women that are likely to present with an elevated hCG level include hydatidiform moles, choriocarcinomas, and gestational trophoblastic tumors.

■ CASE 38

A 45-year-old woman presents to the emergency department with the sudden onset of confusion, severe headaches, and blurred vision. These symptoms have been progressive over the past week. On physical examination, she is febrile and disoriented with diffuse petechial hemorrhages throughout her body. Relevant laboratory results are as follows:

Serum BUN: 42 mg/dL
Serum creatinine: 4.0 mg/dL
Hemoglobin: 9.6 g/dL
Hematocrit: 29%
MCV: 90 fL
WBC count: 7800/mm³ with a normal differential
Platelet count: 36,000/mm³
Peripheral blood smear shows schistocytes and reticulocytes

What is the most likely diagnosis?

Thrombotic thrombocytopenic purpura/hemolytic-uremic syndrome (TTP/HUS).

What are the five cardinal symptoms of this condition?

• Transient neurological problems.
• Fever.
• Thrombocytopenia.
• Microangiopathic hemolytic anemia.
• Acute renal insufficiency.

What is the pathogenesis of these symptoms?

TTP/HUS involves the widespread development of hyaline thrombi composed of platelet aggregates in the microcirculation. This consumption of platelets leads to thrombocytopenia and microangiopathic hemolytic anemia, which can cause widespread organ dysfunction.

What would this patient's coagulation studies show?

Coagulation studies will be within **normal** limits. This is predominantly a thrombocytopenic disease with no coagulation cascade abnormalities.

Which inherited risk factor predisposes patients to this condition?

A deficiency of the **von Willebrand metalloproteinase** (ADAMTS-13) is an inherited factor that causes very large von Willebrand factor multimers to accumulate in the plasma and promote clot formation.

What is the appropriate management for this condition?

Plasma exchange reverses the platelet consumption that is responsible for the thrombus formation. Severe cases may also require adjunctive **immunosuppressive treatment** with prednisone. Platelet transfusion is contraindicated because it may lead to new or worsening thrombosis and subsequent neurologic symptoms. Prompt initiation of treatment is essential to avoid irreversible renal failure and possibly death.

What is a common cause of this condition in children?

Typically, TTP/HUS is preceded by severe bloody diarrhea due most often to enterohemorrhagic *Escherichia coli* O157:H7 infection. This is thought to be due to systemic absorption of a Shiga-like toxin that binds to and damages endothelial cells, inciting platelet activation and thrombosis.

■CASE 39

A 2-year-old boy is brought to his family physician by his parents who are concerned about the multiple bruises on the boy's shins and hands. They report that the child seems to get large bruises with minimal injury and bleeds profusely when his teeth are brushed. They also report that a month ago he fell and hit his head on a coffee table, and they could not stop the bleeding for hours. On questioning, they reveal that the child has a grandmother with a bleeding disorder. The physician is concerned about child abuse but orders laboratory tests. Relevant findings are as follows:

Bleeding time: 14 minutes
PT: 12 seconds
PTT: 41 seconds

What is the most likely diagnosis?

Von Willebrand disease (vWD) is the most common inherited bleeding disorder. It is the result of a quantitative (type 1 or 3) or qualitative (type 2) defect in **von Willebrand factor** (vWF). vWF is a large protein made by endothelial cells and megakaryocytes. It is a carrier for factor VIII and is a cofactor for platelet adhesion. There are now more specific tests that measure vWF antigen levels and activity (ristocetin cofactor assay) directly.

What clinical findings are commonly associated with this condition?

vWD disturbs both primary and secondary hemostasis. Its role in adhesion of platelets to exposed subendothelium leads to **increased bleeding time** and an overall clinical picture of platelet dysfunction (mucous membrane bleeding, petechiae, and purpura) with vWF defects. The role of vWF as a carrier protein for factor VIII means that severe vWF deficiency leads to a clinical picture similar to a coagulation factor deficit ("pseudo-hemophilia"): "deep bleeds" such as hemarthroses (bleeding into joints), easy bruising, and macrohemorrhages. Patients often have a positive family history.

What do the PT and PTT values reflect?

The PT reflects changes in factor II, V, VII, IX, or X. The PTT reflects changes in any of the coagulation factors except factors VII and XIII, and it can be elevated in vWD.

How would the PT and PTT values differ with the administration of warfarin versus heparin?

Heparin affects the intrinsic pathway, causing increased PTT. **Warfarin** affects the extrinsic pathway, increasing PTT and PT. PT should always be monitored with patients taking warfarin (mnemonic: **WEPT** = **W**arfarin affects the **E**xtrinsic pathway, increasing **PT**.

Which coagulation factors require vitamin K for synthesis?

Factors II, VII, IX, and X and proteins C and S require vitamin K for synthesis. Warfarin interferes with vitamin K, leading to a clinical picture that is similar to vitamin K deficiency. The liver is important in the synthesis and metabolism of vitamin K and the coagulation factors (except VIII). Therefore, liver disease can also produce a similar clinical picture.

What are the appropriate treatments for this condition?

Treatment for mild bleeding in type 1 disease involves the use of desmopressin, which causes release of vWF from endothelial stores. Severe disease may be treated with factor VIII concentrates that contain high vWF antigen. Cryoprecipitate is no longer used as viruses cannot be inactivated (high infection risk).

Musculoskeletal

9

Musculoskeletal

■ CASE 1

A 62-year-old woman presents to her physician with a 2-day history of right-sided chest pain. She describes a sharp, nagging pressure medial to her right breast. Her vital signs are stable. Physical examination reveals point tenderness over the chest wall, and the pain is exacerbated by movement of her trunk and deep inspiration. There is no swelling or erythema. No other tender points are found. Echocardiogram, electrocardiogram, and chest radiograph are all normal.

What is the pathophysiology of this condition?

Costochondritis, inflammation of the costochondral or costosternal joints, causes localized pain and tenderness. Often, more than one of the seven costochondral joints is affected, especially between the second and fifth costosternal junctions. Repetitive minor trauma or repetitive activities are the likely causes, but bacterial and fungal infections (not likely here given the lack of swelling, erythema) and thoracic surgery may also be implicated.

What is the innervation of the intercostal space?

The intercostal nerves (thoracic spinal and ventral rami) supply general sensory innervation to the skin of the thoracic and anterior abdominal walls. The dermatomes follow a girdle-like distribution. The sensory nerves also supply the parietal pleura and parietal peritoneum. The intercostal nerves also have motor innervation through the ventral rami of T1–T12. Intercostal nerve 1 participates in the brachial plexus; nerves 2–6 innervate the thorax; and nerves 7–12 innervate the anterior abdominal wall.

What other conditions should be considered in the differential diagnosis?

Although the localized areas of tenderness suggest a musculoskeletal cause, serious conditions such as myocardial infarction and pericarditis (which has an abnormal echocardiogram, pain changes with position, and frictional rub on auscultation) need to be ruled out. Other considerations include pleuritic pain, which could be a manifestation of pneumonia, pulmonary embolism, pneumothorax, or pleuritis. Pleuritis can be seen in inflammatory conditions such as systemic lupus erythematosus (abnormal serology), fibromyalgia (tender points), and gastroesophageal reflux disorder.

What is the blood supply of the intercostal space?

At each space, there is a posterior artery and anterior set of arteries (Figure 9-1). The bottom nine posterior arteries originate from the descending thoracic aorta, whereas the anterior artery originates from the internal thoracic. The posterior intercostal vein, artery, and nerve run together as a neurovascular bundle along the lower border of each rib. Therefore, during thoracentesis the needle must be inserted just above the lower rib in the intercostal space to avoid injury to the vessels and nerve.

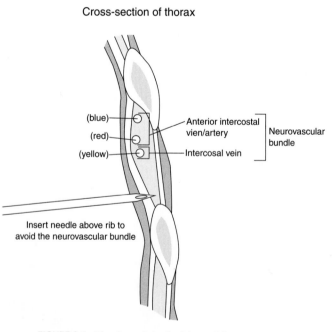

Cross-section of thorax

(blue) — Anterior intercostal vien/artery

(red) — Neurovascular bundle

(yellow) — Intercosal vein

Insert needle above rib to avoid the neurovascular bundle

FIGURE 9-1. **Blood supply to the intercostal space.**

CASE 2

A 63-year-old farmer has noticed an area of discoloration on her cheek that seems to have grown dramatically over the past 2 years. On physical examination, there is a well-demarcated 1.5-cm rough, scaly, erythematous patch. Biopsy of the lesion reveals hyperkeratosis, atypical keratinocytes, and basal cells that invade through the basement membrane.

What is the most likely diagnosis?

The patient's biopsy shows atypical keratinocytes that have invaded the basement membrane; therefore, malignancy is present. Although basal cell carcinoma (BCC) is the most common type of skin cancer, the description of the lesion suggests squamous cell carcinoma (SCC).

Cutaneous SCC is the second most common tumor of the skin. It arises from the malignant proliferation of epidermal keratinocytes. The condition typically presents as a firm, well-demarcated lesion that is scaling, crusting, or ulcerated. Histologic examination is necessary for a diagnosis.

What precursor lesion can lead to this condition?

Actinic keratosis (AK), a dysplastic lesion of the epidermis, can lead to SCC. These lesions occur only on sun-exposed skin and consist of hyperkeratotic papules that have a coarse, sandpaper feel; some may present as a "cutaneous horn."

What risk factors are associated with this condition?

The most important risk factor for SCC is **sunlight exposure** in which ultraviolet (UV) rays cause DNA damage. Other exogenous factors include ionizing radiation, immunosuppression, chronic inflammation (from burns, scars, or ulcers), and arsenic exposure.

What inherited disorders predispose patients to this condition?

Xeroderma pigmentosum is a rare autosomal recessive disorder that displays a defect in DNA excision repair, which impairs the ability to repair UV-induced DNA damage. **Albinism** is also associated with SCC because of the generalized pigment loss due to dysfunction and deficiency of melanocytes.

What is the prognosis for patients with this condition?

Even though cutaneous SCC can be locally invasive, it rarely metastasizes (1%–5% of cases). Therefore, more than 90% of patients can be cured with local excision.

■ CASE 3

A 17-year-old boy is brought to the emergency department by ambulance after a gunshot wound to the left flank. On survey, one entry site is noted with no exit wound; x-rays of the chest and abdomen show that the bullet dislodged in the left flank. During assessment, the patient goes into hypovolemic shock with a steadily decreasing blood pressure, last measured at 60/35. He is rushed to the operating room for exploratory laparotomy. Relevant laboratory findings are as follows:

Hematocrit: 22%
White blood cell (WBC) count: 17,000/mm³
Blood pressure: 60/35 mm Hg

What retroperitoneal structures of the abdomen could the bullet have hit?
A useful mnemonic for abdominal retroperitoneal viscera is **SAD PUCKER**:

- Suprarenal gland (adrenal gland)
- Aorta / IVC
- Duodenum (second and third segments)
- Pancreas
- Ureters
- Colon (ascending and descending)
- Kidneys
- Esophagus
- Rectum

What layers of the lateral and anterior abdominal wall would the bullet have to penetrate to reach the peritoneum?
The **lateral** abdominal wall layers are:

Skin → Camper fascia → Scarpa fascia → deep fascia → external oblique muscle → internal oblique muscle → transversus abdominis muscle → fascia → extraperitoneal fat → peritoneum

The **anterior** abdominal wall layers superior to the arcuate line (the horizontal line inferior to the umbilicus demarcating the lower limit of the posterior layer of the rectus sheath and the point at which the inferior epigastric vessels perforate the rectus abdominis) are:

Skin → Camper fascia → Scarpa fascia → deep fascia → external oblique*→ anterior internal oblique* → rectus abdominis → posterior internal oblique* → abdominis* → transversalis fascia → extraparietal fat → parietal peritoneum

(*Aponeurosis of these muscles form the rectus sheath.)

What is the blood supply to the kidney?
Renal artery → segmental artery → lobar artery → arcuate artery → afferent arteriole → glomerulus → efferent arteriole → vasa recta → segmental vein → renal vein

What is the blood supply to the spleen?
The main blood supply is from the splenic artery, which is a branch of the celiac trunk (the other two branches are the L gastric and common hepatic arteries). The L gastro-omental and short gastric are branches off the splenic artery.

What organs supply the splenic vein?
The splenic vein starts at the hilus of the spleen and receives blood from the stomach, pancreas, and inferior mesenteric vein. The splenic vein joins with the superior mesenteric vein to form the hepatic portal vein.

What are the histologic layers of the skin?
Listed superficially to deep: stratum corneum, lucidum (only in palms and soles), granulosum, spinosum, basale.

CASE 4

A 12-year-old Caucasian boy complains of 6 weeks of pain and swelling over his right midthigh, particularly at night. He denies any trauma or recent illness. Physical examination reveals a firmly attached soft tissue mass of the right leg with overlying tenderness and warmth. Erythema is absent. X-ray of the leg shows a large, poorly demarcated lytic lesion with periosteal reaction in the right femoral diaphysis with extension to the soft tissue (Figure 9-2). A biopsy of the mass reveals sheets of primitive round cells with small uniform nuclei, scant cytoplasm, and positive PAS staining.

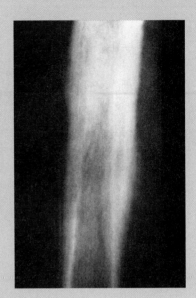

FIGURE 9-2. (Reproduced, with permission, from Skinner HB. *Current Diagnosis & Treatment in Orthopedics,* 4th ed. New York: McGraw-Hill, 2006: 336.)

What is the most likely diagnosis?

The young age at clinical presentation along with the tenderness, warmth, and swelling around the mass without systemic signs of infection suggests Ewing sarcoma (Figure 9-2). This diagnosis is supported by the location of the lesion and the histologic appearance (small, round, blue neuroectodermal cells), which are characteristic of this neoplasm.

What conditions should be considered in the differential diagnosis?

- Infectious causes to consider include acute osteomyelitis.
- Benign lesions, such as eosinophilic granuloma and giant cell tumor of bone, should also be considered.
- Other common solid tumors of childhood, such as osteosarcoma, primary lymphoma, spindle cell sarcoma, acute leukemia, and metastasis from a neuroblastoma, must also be ruled out.

What are the other small cell tumors?

Other small cell tumors include neuroblastoma, Wilms tumor, medulloblastoma, and rhabdomyosarcoma.

What is the most likely chromosomal aberration leading to this condition?

In total, 85% of Ewing sarcoma cases demonstrate a t(11;22) translocation. This translocation leads to an overexpression of the *EWSR1* gene (encodes RNA binding proteins) on chromosome 22, which is translocated next to the *FLI1* gene on chromosome 11 (encodes transcription factors).

What is the appropriate treatment for this condition?

Ewing sarcoma is known to be a systemic disease due to the high relapse rate (80%–90%) of patients who undergo only local therapy. Therefore, most patients likely have subclinical microscopic metastatic disease at the time of diagnosis, which is treated with chemotherapy.

What percentage of patients have metastatic disease at the time of diagnosis?

Only 25% of patients have overt metastases at the time of diagnosis.

■ CASE 5

A 72-year-old woman with a history of osteoporosis presents to her primary care physician after falling 2 days earlier on a slippery sidewalk, landing on her left side. Since the fall, she has been unable to walk because of severe pain in her left hip. The pain is worse when she tries to move it. When asked to walk for assessment of her gait, she refuses, saying that it is too painful. Physical examination reveals normal vitals, extreme pain with both external and internal rotation of the hip, and tenderness over the anterolateral portion of the left hip.

What is the most likely diagnosis?

The most common causes of lateral hip paining elderly patients include osteoarthritis, bursitis, metastases, and femoral fracture. In this patient, the sudden onset of pain after the fall and inability to walk strongly suggest a **fracture of the neck of the femur** (Figure 9-3). Femoral neck fractures can be incomplete or complete with no, partial, or total displacement.

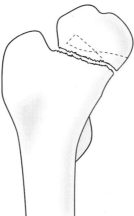

FIGURE 9-3. **Fracture at the neck of the femur.**

What is a potential complication of this condition?

Fracture of the neck of the femur may disrupt blood supply to the head of the femur. The major arterial supply to the head of the femur is the medial and lateral circumflex femoral arteries (branches of the deep femoral artery) and the artery of the ligament of the head of the femur (branch of the obturator artery). The circumflex arteries may be disrupted by a fracture of the femoral neck, leaving only the artery of the ligament (a branch of the obturator) as a supply. Disruption of the blood supply may cause **avascular necrosis** of the femoral head.

What bones form the hip joint?

The hip joint consists of the head of the femur articulating with the acetabulum. The acetabulum is formed by the ilium, ischium, and pubis. The fibrocartilaginous rim, the acetabular labrum, attaches to the acetabular margin and deepens the acetabular cup.

Six weeks later, repeat x-ray shows a callus. What does the callus indicate about the patient's stage of healing?

Bone healing is often divided into three stages:

- **Inflammatory phase:** A hematoma forms at the site of fracture to help deliver the building blocks of new bone formation. Reabsorption occurs at the edges of bone, which is why fractures are more likely to be seen on x-ray several days after the injury.
- **Reparative phase:** New blood vessels that supply nutrients to the cartilage begin to form at the fracture site, followed by callus formation. The osteoprogenitor cells that form the callus derive from the inner surface of the periosteum, not from the marrow or the epiphyseal plate. The patient is in this stage of healing.
- **Remodeling phase:** The endochondral callus becomes ossified and bone undergoes structural remodelling (a process that is much slower in elders than in children).

■ CASE 6

A 2-week-old term boy is brought to his pediatrician because his parents have noticed he has a large, full right scrotum. The left scrotum and testicle are normal. On physical examination, the right scrotum appears to be filled with a volume of fluid that is reduced by applying pressure. A small reducible bulging mass is also seen in the inguinal area on the right.

What is the most likely diagnosis?

In a newborn, a painless collection of fluid in the scrotum is almost certainly a hydrocele. It should resolve on its own by 1 year. The fact that the fluid in the scrotum is reducible indicates that the hydrocele was caused by a communication with the intraperitoneal fluid via a **hernia.**

What would the differential diagnosis be if the patient were a child instead of a neonate?

In a child with a painless scrotal mass, tumor and varicocele (a collection of dilated and tortuous veins of the pampiniform plexus, occurring mostly on the left side) must be considered. On palpation, a tumor is firm (as opposed to fluid-filled). Also, a hydrocele is transilluminated under light, whereas a tumor and a varicocele are not.

What structures define the Hesselbach triangle?

The Hesselbach triangle is formed by the lateral border of the rectus abdominis muscle, the inguinal ligament, and the inferior epigastric vessels.

What distinguishes the two major types of this condition?

Direct hernias protrude through a weakness in the floor of the inguinal canal within the Hesselbach triangle (directly through the triangle) medial to the inferior epigastric vessels to enter the external ring into the scrotal sac. **Indirect hernias** enter the inguinal canal lateral to the Hesselbach triangle (lateral to the inferior epigastric vessels) indirectly through the internal inguinal ring (located in the fascia transversalis), then via the inguinal canal to the external inguinal ring located above and lateral to the pubic tubercle, and finally into the scrotal sac (Figure 9-4).

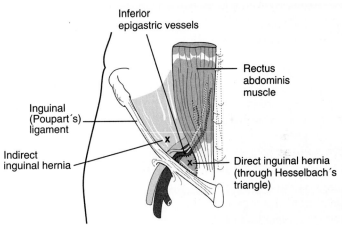

FIGURE 9-4. **Direct and indirect inguinal hernia.** (Reproduced, with permission, from Le T, et al. *First Aid for the USMLE Step 1: 2012.* New York: McGraw-Hill, 2012: 345.)

Which type of this condition is more common in infants and children?

Indirect inguinal hernias are more common in children, as they result from a congenital failure of the processus vaginalis to close.

What are the contents of the normal spermatic cord?

The spermatic cord in the inguinal canal contains the testicular artery and veins, lymphatic vessels, and the vas deferens. The sheath of the cord is formed by the internal spermatic fascia, the cremasteric muscle, and the external spermatic fascia. The ilioinguinal nerve is in the sheath and exits at the external ring; it is vulnerable to injury in surgical repairs of hernias. The genital branch of the genitofemoral nerve supplies the cremaster muscle. The processus vaginalis is an extension of peritoneum that normally obliterates spontaneously between the upper pole of the testes and the internal inguinal ring. In some cases, however, it remains patent, increasing the risk of hydrocele and indirect hernia.

CASE 7

A 19-year-old woman athlete comes to the emergency department with her coach after injuring her left knee during sports practice. She says she heard a "pop" when she made a quick turn and then developed a sharp pain on the lateral side of her knee and her leg "collapsed."

What are the two main intracapsular ligaments in the knee?

The **anterior cruciate ligament** extends from the anterior intercondylar area of the tibial plateau and traverses superior and lateral to the medial surface of the lateral femoral condyle. The **posterior cruciate ligament** extends from the posterior intercondylar area of the tibial plateau and traverses superior and medial to the lateral surface of the medial condyle of the femur (Figure 9-5).

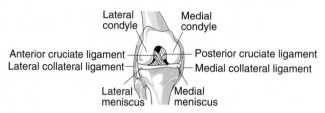

FIGURE 9-5. **Anatomy of the knee.** (Reproduced, with permission, from Le T, et al. *First Aid for the USMLE Step 1: 2008.* New York: McGraw-Hill, 2008: 343.)

What is the blood supply to the knee?

Blood supply to the knee consists of genicular branches of the following blood vessels:

- Anterior recurrent tibial artery.
- Anterior tibial artery.
- Descending branch of the lateral circumflex artery.
- Femoral artery.
- Patellar plexus.
- Popliteal artery.
- Posterior tibial artery.

What is the role of the meniscus?

The half-moon-shaped **meniscus** is cartilage that is found between the femur and tibia. The meniscus absorbs the impact load of the joint and is involved in stability. The meniscus is mostly avascular and is divided into the anterior horn, body, and posterior horn. A medial and lateral meniscus is connected by the transverse ligament.

How do the collateral and cruciate ligaments differ in function?

The cruciate ligaments remain tight in flexion and extension and relax at 30 degrees of flexion. The collateral ligaments are tight in extension and relaxed in flexion. Also, the cruciate ligaments prevent anterior and posterior displacement of the tibia. The collateral ligaments prevent abduction/adduction of the knee.

Which ligament of the knee is most often injured?

The medial collateral ligament is weaker than the anterior or the posterior cruciate ligaments, so medial collateral ligament injuries are more common. Anterior cruciate ligaments tears are much more common than posterior cruciate ligaments tears.

What is the terrible or unhappy triad?

This is a common contact-sport injury to the knee that occurs when lateral trauma is applied to the knee joint while the foot is fixed to the ground. Subsequently, the medial collateral ligament, lateral meniscus, and anterior cruciate ligament are damaged.

CASE 8

A 47-year-old man presents to his primary care physician concerned about a suspicious lesion on his shoulder that has increased in size over the past 2 years. He reports no other associated signs or symptoms. Physical examination reveals an 11-cm asymmetric, irregularly colored lesion with notched borders and no keratin plugs. It is slightly tender to palpation. Several other nevi are noted to be scattered over his chest and back.

What is the differential diagnosis and what is the most likely diagnosis?

Benign causes of an irregularly colored lesion include hemangioma, seborrheic keratosis, compound or junctional nevus, and pigmented dermatofibroma. But given the characteristics of this lesion, the most likely diagnosis is a **malignant melanoma**. The **ABCD** rules help distinguish melanoma from other lesions (Figure 9-6):

- **Asymmetry:** Malignant lesions are usually asymmetric.
- **Border irregularity:** Most melanomas lack smooth, round, uniform boundaries.
- **Color variegation:** Malignant lesions usually have variations in pigmentation and occasionally lose pigmentation.
- **Diameter:** A diameter > 6 mm greatly increases the chances of malignancy, and most lesions are > 10 mm.

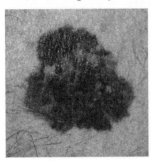

FIGURE 9-6. Malignant melanoma that demonstrates the ABCD criteria. (Reproduced, with permission, from Wolff K, et al. *Fitzpatrick's Dermatology in General Medicine,* 7th ed. New York: McGraw-Hill, 2008: 1138.)

Which cells are responsible for this lesion and what is their embryonic origin?

Melanomas originate from melanocytes, which are derived from neural crest tissue and reside in the epidermis or, less frequently, in the dermis.

What is the etiology of this lesion?

Malignant melanomas are more likely to appear on areas that receive **sun exposure.** Other risk factors include atypical/dysplastic nevi and family history,

What is the most important prognostic factor for this condition?

The most concerning factor is vertical invasion, as deeper lesions have a worse prognosis. Detection of melanoma at early stages is crucial and prognosis is excellent if treated early. However, after the tumor has penetrated the basement membrane and entered the subcutaneous fat, 5-year survival is only 49%. The S-100 protein can help determine prognosis; elevated S-100 serum levels correlate with a worse prognosis.

How and where does melanoma tend to spread?

Initial lesions usually spread superficially and horizontally across the skin and then enter a vertical growth phase into the deeper layers of the skin. Melanomas may then spread either lymphatically or hematogenously; earliest detectable metastases occur in regional lymph nodes. Classic sites of hematogenous spread include brain, lung, liver, and bone; however, melanomas are notorious for metastasizing to odd locations.

What is the appropriate treatment for this condition?

Surgical excision with optional regional node dissection for more advanced disease remains the first-line treatment.

■ CASE 9

A 3-year-old boy is brought to the pediatrician by his parents because he has been falling frequently and struggling to get up from a sitting or lying position, whereas he had previously done so with ease. His developmental history is notable for delayed motor skills; he began to walk at 18 months. The boy has a waddling gait and when sitting uses his arms to push himself into the upright position (Figure 9-7). Physical examination shows marked muscle weakness of the extremities, particularly of the proximal muscle groups, and hypertrophy of his calf muscles. The patient's maternal uncle, who died at 16 years of age, suffered from similar symptoms when he was younger.

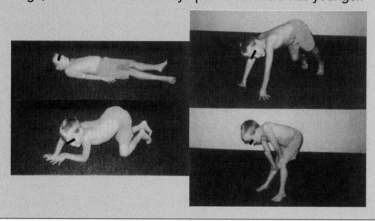

FIGURE 9-7. (Reproduced, with permission, from Kasper DL, et al. *Harrison's Principles of Internal Medicine,* 16th ed. New York: McGraw-Hill, 2005: 2526.)

What is the likely diagnosis and what is the pathogenesis of the disorder?

Duchenne muscular dystrophy (DMD) is an X-linked recessive (Xp21) disorder marked by a deficiency of functional **dystrophin,** a 23,000-kB protein that helps stabilize muscle fibers. Approximately one-third of cases are sporadic and due to spontaneous mutations (noninherited) that arise from a misalignment of chromosomes during a recombination event.

What is the prognosis for patients with this condition?

Patients with DMD are usually unable to walk by the end of the first decade and are confined to a wheelchair by 12 years of age. Most patients die by the end of the second decade; respiratory failure is the leading cause of death. Dilated cardiomyopathy and/or conduction abnormalities are common and can be fatal.

What tests are used to diagnose this condition?

If DMD is clinically suspected, serum creatine kinase levels are markedly elevated, and electromyography shows myopathic changes, genetic testing or a muscle biopsy can confirm the diagnosis. Muscle biopsy shows atrophic muscle fibers of various sizes in disarray, degeneration, and necrosis of individual muscle fibers with fibrous replacement.

The patient's parents have a second son who is 6 months of age. What is the chance that he, too, will develop this condition?

The chances are 50% (assuming that the first case was not sporadic). Because the mother is a carrier of this disorder, each son has a 50% chance of inheriting the X chromosome with the mutated allele from her.

Which band in a sarcomere stays constant in length during muscle contraction?

The A band, which corresponds to the length of the thick myosin filaments.

How would the presentation of a patient with Becker muscular dystrophy (BMD) differ from that of this patient?

The most obvious difference is the age of onset of symptoms and degree of clinical involvement. BMD patients typically remain ambulatory until at least 15 years of age and commonly into adulthood. Mental retardation and contractures are more common in BMD.

CASE 10

A 65-year-old man presents to his primary care physician complaining of a 10-year history of increasing morning stiffness and dull pain in his lower back and left hip. The pain is typically exacerbated by activity and relieved by rest. Physical examination reveals limited range of motion in the affected joints and tenderness on palpation without warmth or erythema. X-ray of the pelvis and lower spine shows joint space narrowing, subchondral sclerosis, and osteophyte formation (Figure 9-8).

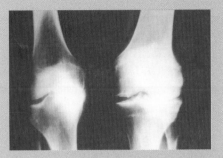

FIGURE 9-8. (Reproduced, with permission, from South-Paul JE, et al. *Current Diagnosis & Treatment in Family Medicine*, 2nd ed. New York: McGraw-Hill, 2008: 235.)

What is the likely diagnosis?

The asymmetric, gradually progressive joint pain and stiffness in this case point to **osteoarthritis** (x-ray findings confirm). Physical examination findings in osteoarthritis include tenderness to palpation without signs of inflammation, joint effusions, crepitus, and bony enlargement of affected joints.

What are the radiographic features of osteoarthritis?

Radiographic findings in osteoarthritis can be summarized by the mnemonic **LOSS**: **L**oss of joint space, **O**steophytes, and **S**ubchondral **S**clerosis.

What conditions should be considered in the differential?

- In an elderly patient with joint disease, the other conditions to consider are rheumatoid arthritis (RA), gout, pseudogout, and infectious monoarticular disease.
- In RA, joint stiffness (causing morning stiffness usually lasting > 30 minutes) increases with rest and improves with activity. Affected joints are soft, warm, and tender. Neither of these factors is the case in this patient.
- Infectious monoarticular disease is unlikely in this case given the lack of warmth or erythema.
- Gout is unlikely because the initial attack of acute gout is usually in the foot (first metatarsophalangeal joint) or knee and the pain is acute, not dull.
- Pseudogout can also be ruled out as it would likely present acutely in the hips and/or wrists with different radiographic findings, such as classification of cartilaginous structures.

What is the characteristic distribution of this condition?

Osteoarthritis most often affects large weight-bearing joints including the knees, hip, and spine, as well as the distal interphalangeal joint. In contrast, RA commonly affects the proximal interphalangeal and metacarpophalangeal joints. Osteoarthritis only rarely affects the elbows, wrists, and ankles.

What is the pathophysiology of this condition?

Osteoarthritis is characterized by degenerative noninflammatory changes in articular cartilage secondary to chondrocyte dysfunction. These changes may be caused by a complex interaction between metabolic, biochemical, and biomechanical factors with secondary components of inflammation. The result is progressive mechanical damage to the joint and bone eburnation, particularly in weight-bearing joints. This degeneration also causes reactive bone formation subchondrally and at the margins of affected joints.

What would arthrocentesis (tapping of the joint) likely show?

Arthrocentesis is mostly normal with perhaps mild pleocytosis, and modestly elevated protein.

What is the appropriate treatment for this condition?

Acetaminophen and nonsteroidal anti-inflammatory drugs remain the mainstays for analgesia. In a patient with a history of gastroduodenal disease, a gastroprotective agent could also be given. Occasionally, intra-articular glucocorticoids are used when symptoms persist in a few joints. Surgery may be required for refractory cases (joint replacement or fusion).

What risk factors are associated with this condition?

Risk factors for osteoarthritis include increased age, obesity, female gender, lack of osteoporosis, physically demanding occupations, previous injury, or genetic disorder such as Wilson disease and hemochromatosis.

■ CASE 11

A young Caucasian couple seeks genetic counseling before conceiving their first child. The man is concerned because he has had bilateral tumors removed from his acoustic nerves. His mother suffered from similar tumors, but his father did not. The woman reports two previous surgeries for the removal of spinal cord tumors; her father and sister had similar tumors. The woman's physical examination is significant for axillary freckles and approximately 15 light brown patches of skin averaging 3 cm in diameter.

What genetic syndromes do this man and woman have?

The woman has neurofibromatosis type 1 (NF1, or von Recklinghausen neurofibromatosis), and the man has neurofibromatosis type 2 (NF2). NF1 is characterized by café-au-lait spots, meningiomas, **neurofibromas** (subcutaneous nodules), and axillary freckling. NF2 presents with bilateral acoustic neuromas (vestibular schwannomas).

What is the probability that the couple will have an asymptomatic child?

NF1 and NF2 are both autosomal dominant genes. On the basis of their family histories, the man and woman must be heterozygous for NF2 and NF1, respectively. Thus, each mutant gene has a 50% chance of being inherited by the child. NF1 is on chromosome 17, and NF2 is on chromosome 22; therefore, the inheritance of each mutant gene occurs independently of the other. The probability of two independent events occurring at once is the product of the probability of each event: 50% × 50% = **25%**.

Which cell line is implicated in the formation of the woman's lesions?

Neural crest cells are involved. Most clinical signs of NF1 are related to abnormal descendants of neural crest cells.

What is the mechanism of tumor formation for the woman?

The *NF1* gene is a tumor suppressor gene belonging to a family of guanosine triphosphatase–activating proteins. Multiple loss-of-function mutations in this gene lead to tumor growth.

What is the path of the eighth cranial nerve (CN VIII) from the periphery to its site of entry into the central nervous system?

From the cochlea and vestibular canals in the petrous bone, CN VIII enters the cranial vault through the internal acoustic meatus to enter the brain stem at the junction of the pons and the medulla.

What other clinical features could a patient with the woman's condition have?

NF1 patients may have iris hamartomas (Lisch nodules), optic gliomas, distinctive bony lesions such as sphenoid dysplasia, and thinning of a long bone cortex with or without pseudarthrosis.

■ CASE 12

An 8-year-old girl is brought to the pediatrician for evaluation of recurrent skeletal fractures. Although she avoids contact sports, she has sustained three fractures of her femur, tibia, and elbow following seemingly minor trauma. The pediatrician notes the girl is short for her age and has mild scoliosis and blue sclerae. The girl's mother has blue sclerae as well.

What is the differential diagnosis for recurrent fractures in children?

- Accidental injury.
- Birth trauma.
- Bone fragility (including osteogenesis imperfecta and rickets).
- Child abuse (which accounts for the vast majority of cases).

What is the most likely diagnosis?

The most likely diagnosis is osteogenesis imperfecta (OI), which is an inherited disorder involving defects in type I collagen, usually due to mutations in the *COL1A1* or *COL1A2* gene. It is also known as **brittle bone disease,** and its most common form has autosomal dominant inheritance.

What pathologic findings are associated with this condition?

OI is associated with cardiac insufficiency, mitral valve prolapse, hearing loss, basilar skull deformities (causing nerve compression and other neurological sequelae) and kyphoscoliosis. Death due to multiple fractures or pulmonary failure is common in utero or soon after birth in severe forms, which are recessively inherited.

What are the four major types and locations of collagen?

- **Type I** collagen is found in bone, skin, tendon.
- **Type II** collagen is found in cartilage.
- **Type III** collagen is found in reticular tissue, arterial walls, and uterus.
- **Type IV** collagen is found in the basement membrane.

What steps are involved in collagen synthesis?

Procollagen strands containing a repeating Gly-Pro-X sequence are synthesized in the ribosome, hydrolyzed by prolyl hydrolase, and glycosylated in the rough endoplasmic reticulum and Golgi complex. Three procollagen strands associate in a triple helix and are secreted into the extracellular space, where the propeptides are cleaved, allowing for polymerization with other collagen molecules to form collagen fibrils.

What enzymes in collagen synthesis depend on ascorbic acid?

Proline hydroxylase (which hydroxylates prolyl and lysyl residues) cross-links collagen and depends on ascorbic acid. Vitamin C deficiency can lead to **scurvy,** which causes ulceration of the gums, bruising, anemia, poor wound healing, and hemorrhage due to deficient collagen synthesis.

■ CASE 13

A 62-year-old woman presents to her clinician with joint pain and morning stiffness for the past few years. The joint pain is present in both hands and feet bilaterally and has caused significant deformity and weakness. On physical examination, these joints are tender to palpation, warm, and swollen with no erythema. Her metacarpal joints display ulnar deviation bilaterally and subcutaneous nodules can be palpated at the elbow.

What is the most likely diagnosis?

Rheumatoid arthritis (RA). Clinical features of RA include the following:

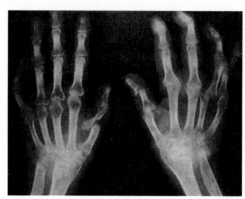

FIGURE 9-9. **Radiographic changes in rheumatoid arthritis.** Severe destruction of radiocarpal articulation with subluxation and ulnar deviation at the wrist; loss of ulnar styloid bilaterally; dislocation of the proximal interphalangeal joint of the left thumb and dislocation of the right fourth and fifth finger metacarpophalangeal joints and left metacarpophalangeal joint; diffuse joint space narrowing of many interphalangeal joints. (Reproduced, with permission, from Brunicardi FC, et al. *Schwartz's Principles of Surgery*, 8th ed. New York: McGraw-Hill, 2005: 1679.)

- Morning stiffness for more than 1 hour that is present for more than 6 weeks.
- Arthritis in three joints or more for more than 6 weeks.
- Arthritis of hand joints for more than 6 weeks.
- Symmetric joint swelling and involvement.
- Rheumatoid subcutaneous nodules.
- Positive serum rheumatoid factor and/or anti-cyclic citrullinated protein antibodies (anti-CCP).
- Abnormal C-reactive protein (CRP) and/or erythrocyte sedimentation rate (ESR).
- Typical radiographic changes (shown in Figure 9-9).

What is the pathophysiology of this condition?

RA is a chronic **systemic autoimmune inflammatory disorder** that destroys articular cartilage. While the etiology is unclear, the autoimmune reaction is mediated by CD4+ T cells, macrophages, and cytokines (tumor necrosis factor and interleukin-1), which promote the inflammatory response. Together these elements form a **pannus** that gradually erodes and disfigures joints.

What test can help diagnose this condition?

Although no specific laboratory test is diagnostic of RA, most patients have a **positive serum rheumatoid factor (RF; not perfectly sensitive nor specific)** and anti-CCP (similar sensitivity and better specificity than RF).

What joints are typically affected in this condition?

Symptoms usually develop symmetrically in the small joints of the hands and feet (metacarpophalangeal, proximal interphalangeal, metatarsophalangeal joints), as well as wrist, elbows, knees, and ankles. The cervical spine may also be involved.

What are the characteristic joint deformities in this condition?

Ulnar deviation/drift, swan-neck, and Boutonniere deformities of the fingers and the "bow-string" sign (prominence of the tendons in the extensor compartment of the hand) are all characteristic of RA. Occasionally patients present with synovial cysts from increased intra-articular pressure and eventual tendon rupture.

What are the primary pharmacologic therapies for this condition?

- Analgesics including acetaminophen.
- Nonsteroidal anti-inflammatory drugs.
- Glucocorticoids.
- Disease-modifying antirheumatic drugs such as methotrexate, hydroxychloroquine, or sulfasalazine.
- Anti-cytokine therapies such as etanercept, infliximab, and adalimumab.
- Other biologic agents such as abatacept and rituximab.

What are some nonarticular manifestations of this condition?

- Musculoskeletal manifestations include osteopenia, osteoporosis, muscle weakness, vasculitis, and skin symptoms such as rheumatoid nodules.
- Pulmonary manifestations include pleuritis, pleural effusion, and interstitial fibrosis.
- Cardiac manifestations include coronary artery disease and heart failure.
- Other manifestations include scleritis, anemia, and Felty syndrome (RA with splenomegaly and neutropenia).

■ CASE 14

A 65-year-old woman presents to the emergency department with sharp pain in her lower back after lifting some heavy objects while moving into a new home. The pain radiates to the anterior abdomen and is exacerbated by sitting and moving. On physical examination, she appears kyphotic with a "dowager hump." A plain film radiograph reveals multiple vertebral compression fractures.

What underlying condition contributed to these fractures?

Osteoporosis. This disease is characterized by reduced bone mass with microarchitectural disruption, porosity, and skeletal fragility. Osteoporosis is difficult to diagnose, as a fracture is often the first clinical manifestation.

What two factors contribute most to this condition?

The majority of postmenopausal women with osteoporosis have bone loss related to **age** and/or **estrogen deficiency.**
Estrogen naturally suppresses cytokines (such as interleukin-1 and -6) and receptor activator of nuclear κ-B ligand (RANKL,) which both increase osteoclast activity. RANKL interacts with RANK to promote development and function of osteoclasts. Denosumab is the first osteoporosis treatment that acts by blocking RANK-RANKL binding.

What secondary factors increase the risk of this condition?

- Physical inactivity.
- Calcium and vitamin D deficiency.
- Prolonged glucocorticoid therapy.
- Hyperparathyroidism.
- Hyperthyroidism.

What sites of fracture are most common in this condition?

Vertebral compression fractures are the most common clinical manifestation of osteoporosis. Most fractures are asymptomatic and usually an incidental finding on x-ray of the chest or abdomen. However, they may manifest as spinal deformity and shortened stature. **Hip** and **distal radius (Colles) fractures** are also common.

What tests and/or imaging tools can be used to test bone density?

Dual-energy x-ray absorptiometry **(DEXA) scans** are used to compare bone density to an age-matched reference population. Density more than two standard deviations below the expected range confirms the diagnosis.

What are the appropriate treatments for this condition?

- The mainstay of treatment and prevention of osteoporosis is **bisphosphonates** such as alendronate and risedronate. This is in addition to continuation of both calcium and vitamin D supplementation. These agents act by decreasing osteoclastic bone resorption. One of the side effects of bisphosphonates is esophagitis; thus, patients are instructed to take it with water and while standing or sitting upright (and remain so for at least 30 minutes).
- Raloxifene, a **selective estrogen receptor modulator** is also used in refractory cases.
- Intermittent administration of recombinant parathyroid hormone has also shown to be effective.

■ CASE 15

A 16-year-old boy is brought to the emergency department via ambulance after a motor vehicle accident. Physical examination reveals obvious trauma to the chest, and the patient is tachypneic and hypotensive. X-ray of the chest shows a hemothorax, and a chest tube is placed on the right.

What conditions should be considered in a patient with trauma to the chest?

Direct injury can cause pulmonary or myocardial contusion, rib or sternal fractures, diaphragmatic injury, vessel laceration, and aortic damage, which is often fatal. Conditions associated with chest trauma include pneumothorax, flail chest, hemothorax, and cardiac tamponade.

What important nerves are at risk in stab wounds to the thorax?

- Cardiac plexus.
- Recurrent laryngeal nerve.
- Phrenic nerve.
- Pulmonary plexus (contiguous with the cardiac plexus).
- Vagus nerve

What are the major arteries and veins of the thorax?

Arterial Supply	Venous Supply
Aortic arch	Azygos
Brachiocephalic trunk	Brachiocephalic
Common carotid	Internal thoracic
Internal thoracic	Jugular
Internal thoracic	
Left bronchial	
Subclavian	

Which side of the chest uses the thoracic duct for lymphatic drainage?

The lymphatic duct is used for lymphatic drainage for the entire lower body, left arm, left side of the head and neck, and the left side of the thorax. The right arm, right side of the head and neck, and right side of the thorax, however, use the right lymphatic duct. The thoracic duct drains into the venous system at the junction of the left jugular and subclavian veins.

What is the difference between the left and right mainstem bronchi?

The mainstem bronchus passes inferolaterally from the bifurcation of the trachea at the sternal angle to the hilum. The **right main bronchus** is shorter and wider and runs more vertically, allowing for passage of aspirates more easily than the left bronchus. The **left main bronchus** is longer and travels anterior to the esophagus between the thoracic aorta and the left pulmonary artery.

What are the clinical features in a patient with pneumothorax post trauma?

Fractured ribs from trauma or trauma itself can lead to a pneumothorax. Patients will often be tachypneic, hypoxic, and/or have decreased/absent breath sounds on the side of the pneumothorax. Imaging can confirm a pneumothorax. A chest tube is usually used to manage a pneumothorax from trauma. If there is a pneumohemothorax, separate chest tubes should be used to remove the blood and the air.

■ CASE 16

A 63-year-old woman complains that since falling on her outstretched hands 3 weeks ago, she can no longer use her right arm to remove books from the overhead shelves in her office. Further questioning reveals that she also has pain in her right shoulder at night that occasionally wakes her up and that she now avoids sleeping on her right side. Physical examination reveals tenderness to palpation below the right acromion. The patient also has pain at 60 degrees as she abducts her right arm and is unable to abduct with resistance. When she is asked to hold her right arm abducted at 45 degrees and laterally rotate her forearm against resistance, she is unable to do so.

Among the conditions that can cause shoulder pain in elderly patients, what is the most likely diagnosis in this case?

The most likely diagnosis in this case is a rotator cuff tear, which presents with both pain and weakness and is consistent with the physical examination findings. The subacromial bursa may also be involved, in which case pain is also felt at the insertion of the deltoid muscle in the middle of the upper arm.

Other common causes of shoulder pain include rotator cuff tendinitis, adhesive capsulitis (frozen shoulder), and subscapular bursitis.

- Rotator cuff tendinitis in unlikely in this case because it presents with pain but not weakness.
- Adhesive capsulitis is unlikely because it is characterized by an absolute loss of range of motion.
- Subscapular bursitis would localize pain to the upper back and have an audible popping sound with shrugging.

In a lidocaine injection test (in which the subacromial space is injected with lidocaine), rotator cuff tears show decreased pain but persistent weakness; rotator cuff tendinitis has normal strength; and frozen shoulder shows persistent loss of range of motion.

What events commonly precipitate this condition?

Rotator cuff tears are rare in patients younger than 40 years of age but common in patients older than 50 years of age with shoulder pain. However, sports injuries with rotator cuff tears are seen in young athletes. Other common causes of rotator cuff tears include the following:

- Direct blow to the affected shoulder.
- Falling onto an outstretched hand (as this patient did).
- History of recurrent rotator cuff tendinitis.
- Lifting a heavy object.
- Shoulder dislocation.

What other tendons are likely involved in this condition and what is their distal attachment?

The rotator cuff is made up of the tendons of the "SITS" muscles: Supraspinatus (the most commonly affected tendon with rotator cuff tears), Infraspinatus, and Teres minor insert on the greater tuberosity, and the Subscapularis inserts on the lesser tuberosity (Figure 9-10).

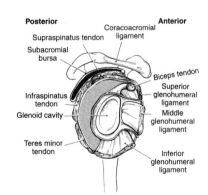

FIGURE 9-10. **Lateral view of shoulder illustrating coracoacromial arch with rotator cuff and subacromial bursa.** (Reproduced, with permission, from Tintinalli JE, et al. *Tintinalli's Emergency Medicine: A Comprehensive Study Guide*, 6th ed. New York: McGraw-Hill, 2004: 1780.)

What are the innervations and actions of these muscles?

- Supraspinatus: Suprascapular nerve (C4–C6); abduction of the arm for the initial 20 degrees (the deltoid abducts the arm beyond the initial 20 degrees).
- Infraspinatus: Suprascapular nerve (C4–C6); external rotation of the arm.
- Teres minor: Axillary nerve (C5–C6); aids in external rotation of the arm.
- Subscapularis: Upper and lower subscapular nerves (C5–C7); help with median rotation and adduction of the arm.

■ CASE 17

A 24-year-old woman presents to the clinic complaining of fatigue, muscle and joint aches, and intermittent fevers of over 2 months' duration. On physical examination, she displays a rash over her cheeks and nose as well as a friction rub on cardiac auscultation. Laboratory tests show the following:

Hemoglobin: 10.8 g/dL
Hematocrit: 32.8%
Platelet count: 145,000/mm^3
WBC count: 4350/mm^3
Urinalysis: 3+ proteinuria

What is the most likely diagnosis?

Systemic lupus erythematosus (SLE). SLE is a multisystem autoimmune connective tissue disease with a variable clinical presentation that most commonly affects young women in their 20s and 30s. Most manifestations of SLE are secondary to immune complex deposition.

What explains the friction rub on auscultation?

SLE patients can develop pericarditis leading to friction rub.

What laboratory tests can be used to confirm the diagnosis?

Antibody testing including antinuclear antibodies (ANA), antiphospholipid antibodies, antibodies to double-stranded DNA (dsDNA), and anti-Smith (Sm) antibodies are used to diagnose SLE. Positive anti-dsDNA and anti-Sm test results are the most specific for SLE. A positive ANA test is sensitive but not specific. High-yield fact: antiphospholipid antibodies also bind the cardiolipin antigen used in syphilis testing; therefore, lupus patients have a false-positive syphilis test.

What would a positive antihistone antibody suggest?

It would suggest **drug-induced lupus**, but the reason for this correlation is unknown. Common medications that can cause drug-induced lupus include hydralazine, procainamide, minocycline, penicillamine, and isoniazid.

What are the 11 classification criteria for this diagnosis?

For SLE, remember the mnemonic **SOAP BRAIN MD**: Serositis, Oral ulcers, Arthritis, Photosensitivity, Blood changes (SLE patients often have leukopenia, a mild anemia, and clinically insignificant thrombocytopenia), Renal involvement (proteinuria or casts), ANA, Immunologic changes, Neurologic signs (seizures, frank psychosis), Malar rash, and Discoid rash.

For the diagnosis of SLE, a patient must display a minimum of four out of 11 characteristics.

What are the typical renal findings in this condition?

Most SLE patients have an abnormal urinalysis. There are six classes of renal disease in SLE, which are usually differentiated with a renal biopsy. Immune complex (anti-DNA-DNA)–mediated glomerular diseases are most common. SLE nephropathy most commonly displays a nephrotic syndrome pattern with a histologic subtype of diffuse lupus nephritis (class IV). The pathologic finding on histology that is almost pathognomonic for SLE is **"wire loop"** lesions (tubuloreticular structures in the glomerular endothelial cells, which may also be seen in HIV nephropathy). Other findings include subepithelial or subendothelial deposits with inflammation.

■ CASE 18

A 54-year-old woman presents to the clinic with fatigue, difficulty swallowing, a nonproductive cough, stiffness in the joints of her hands, and tightness in her fingers. Additionally, she explains that her fingers occasionally become pale and painful when she forgets to wear gloves on cold days. On physical examination, her skin is taut and thickened over her hands and face. Her hands appear clawlike and have decreased motion at all of the small joints symmetrically.

What is the most likely diagnosis and what are the two forms of this condition?

Systemic sclerosis (scleroderma), an autoimmune connective tissue disorder (Figure 9-11). Scleroderma exists in two forms, **limited and diffuse**, both of which occur in the setting of Raynaud phenomenon (exaggerated vasoconstriction in response to cold or stress leading to sharply demarcated color changes of the fingertips). This patient displays the limited form in which the skin of the fingers, forearms, and face are often affected with distinctive thickening.

Diffuse systemic sclerosis eventually involves visceral organs as well as the gastrointestinal tract (particularly the esophagus), heart (myocardial fibrosis), muscles, lungs (interstitial lung disease is seen in the majority of patients, causing dyspnea on exertion and cough), and kidneys. This results in dysphagia, respiratory difficulty, arrhythmias, and mild proteinuria. The most concerning manifestation of this disease is malignant hypertension leading to renal failure.

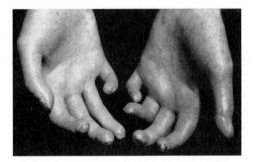

FIGURE 9-11. **Flexion deformities of the fingers and sclerodactyly.** The skin over the fingers and hands is taut and indurated. There is shortening and bony resorption of distal phalanges of the second and third fingers. Ulcers may develop over the distal phalanges and dorsal surfaces of the metacarpophalangeal and proximal interphalangeal joints. (Reproduced, with permission, from Kasper DL, et al. *Harrison's Principles of Internal Medicine*, 16th ed. New York: McGraw-Hill, 2005: 1984.)

What serologic marker is used to test for this condition?

Anti-DNA topoisomerase I **(Anti-Scl-70)** antibody is highly specific for systemic sclerosis. Anticentromere antibodies are more characteristic of limited scleroderma (CREST syndrome).

What is the pathogenesis of this condition?

The etiology of this condition is unknown; however, symptoms begin with vascular damage and are due to excessive synthesis of extracellular matrix, increased deposition of collagen in normal tissue, fibrosis, immune activation, and vascular damage.

What is CREST syndrome?

CREST is an acronym for the five findings in individuals with limited systemic sclerosis: **C**alcinosis, **R**aynaud phenomenon, **E**sophageal dysmotility, **S**clerodactyly, and **T**elangiectasia.

What is the appropriate treatment for this condition?

Most therapies are supportive; skin-softening agents and gloves are used to help skin sclerosis and Raynaud phenomenon. Bosentan and prostacyclin analogs might also be useful in pulmonary hypertension. Cytotoxics have a role in treating inflammatory lung disease.

■ CASE 19

After a difficult labor, a baby is delivered breech, with her arms above her head. Physical examination reveals that the newborn's right hand is slightly contracted, with the fingers curled toward the palm. The infant seems unable to extend the fingers on the right hand.

What is the most likely diagnosis?

Klumpke palsy results from birth injury to the lower trunk of the brachial plexus (C8 and T1 nerve roots). It is a proximal brachial plexus neuropathy.

What motor deficits are likely to result from this condition?

The C8 and T1 nerve roots contribute to the ulnar and median nerves. The muscles affected are the medial part of the flexor digitorum profundus and the flexor carpi ulnaris (the only extrinsic muscles of the forearm supplied by the ulnar nerve), and all intrinsic muscles of the hand, including those innervated by the ulnar nerve (interosseous muscles, the second and third lumbrical muscles, and the adductor pollicis brevis muscles), and those innervated by the median nerve (thenar muscles and the first two lumbrical muscles). Over time, wasting of the thenar and hypothenar eminences occurs. Marked wasting between the metacarpals on both palmar and dorsal surfaces of the hand results from paralysis of the lumbricals and interossei.

What sensory deficits are involved in this condition?

The lower trunk from C8 and T1 contributes to the medial cutaneous nerves of the arm, forearm, and the ulnar and median nerves. Thus, in this patient, loss of sensation will occur on the medial side of the arm; the forearm; the dorsal and palmar surface of the fifth finger and half of the fourth finger; the palmar surface of the first, second, and third fingers and lateral half of the fourth finger extending onto the nail beds on the dorsal surface as far as the distal interphalangeal joints; and the palmar surface of the hand.

What other injuries can cause this condition?

- **Thoracic outlet syndrome:** This is a congenital defect in which a cervical rib or a scalenus minimus muscle compresses the lower trunk at C8 and T1.
- **Trauma:** Injuries to the inferior brachial plexus are much less common than injuries to the superior brachial plexus; traumatic injury can occur when a person grabs something to break a fall, or a baby's upper limb is pulled too hard during delivery.
- **Tumor infiltration:** Tumor infiltration from the apex of the lung (**Pancoast tumor**) can be associated with compression of the stellate ganglion, resulting in **Horner syndrome.**

What is another nerve lesion that can cause claw hand?

An ulnar nerve injury will also present with claw hand. However, with ulnar nerve injury, only the little finger and the ring finger are clawed because the median nerve is spared (resulting in normal thenar muscles). Also, the sensory deficit involves only the ulnar nerve distribution: the palm and dorsal surfaces of the medial part of the hand and the dorsal and palmar surfaces of the fifth finger and half of the fourth finger.

▌CASE 20

A 40-year-old man presents to the clinic complaining of pain in his left big toe. The pain began suddenly this morning and woke him from sleep. He denies trauma to the area; however, the night before, he and his fiancée had a dinner of liver pâté, cheese, and wine. Physical examination reveals a warm, erythematous, and exquisitely tender left metatarsophalangeal joint. Arthrocentesis of the affected toe is performed. Laboratory studies are significant for a serum uric acid level of 9 mg/dL.

What is the differential diagnosis for acute joint pain?

The causes of acute joint pain can be categorized as follows:

- Infection: Septic arthritis can present with joint warmth, swelling, and pain. Patients may also complain of fever and a history of trauma.
- Autoimmune disease: Joint inflammation secondary to rheumatoid arthritis may lead to erythema, swelling, pain, and stiffness of one or many joints.
- Osteoarthritis: Joint pain increases with use. In this case, however, the patient's relatively young age and the presence of redness and joint swelling are not consistent with osteoarthritis.
- Crystal arthropathy: Deposition of crystals in joint spaces leads to pain and inflammation.

What is the most likely diagnosis?

Gout, secondary to hyperuricemia. Gout characteristically causes monoarticular arthritis, often of the first metatarsophalangeal joint (**podagra**).

What are common causes of this condition?

Uric acid overproduction, which can be due to:

- Excessive cell turnover (such as lymphoproliferative disease, hemolytic anemia, cytotoxic drugs, or severe muscle exertion).
- Excessive dietary alcohol or purine intake.
- Inherited enzyme defects such as Lesch-Nyhan syndrome (hypoxanthine guanine phosphoribosyltransferase deficiency.
- Phosphoribosylpyrophosphate (**PRPP**) synthetase overactivity.

Uric acid underexcretion, which can be due to:

- Dehydration.
- Impaired renal function.
- Lactic acidosis.
- Use of certain drugs (diuretics, salicylates, cyclosporine A).

What are the most likely findings of arthrocentesis?

Needle-shaped **negatively birefringent crystals** are diagnostic for gout. By contrast, findings of pseudogout include basophilic rhomboid crystals of calcium pyrophosphate composition.

What are the appropriate treatments for this condition?

For acute attacks:

- Nonsteroidal anti-inflammatory drugs (NSAIDs) to reduce inflammation.
- Colchicine, which depolymerizes microtubules, thus impairing leukocyte chemotaxis.

For prevention of future attacks:

- Probenecid to inhibit renal reabsorption of uric acid.
- Allopurinol to inhibit conversion of xanthine to uric acid by xanthine oxidase.
- Diet control, including reduced intake of purine-rich foods (eg, meat, beans, and spinach) and alcohol.

10

Neurology

■ CASE 1

A 73-year-old well-educated woman is brought to the physician by her daughter, who has become concerned about her mother's behavior. The mother volunteers at the local library shelving books, but for the past few months she has had trouble remembering where the books go. In addition, she often forgets to turn the stove off after cooking her family's long-time favorite dishes.

What is the most likely diagnosis?

This history is consistent with Alzheimer disease, which is characterized by loss of short-term memory and general preservation of long-term memory.

How are the causes of dementia classified?

Dementia is classified into reversible and irreversible causes. Reversible causes include major depression, hypothyroidism, and chronic subdural hematoma. Other irreversible causes are vascular dementia, normal-pressure hydrocephalus, and dementia with Lewy bodies.

What risk factors are associated with this condition?

Advancing age and a family history of Alzheimer disease are two well-known risk factors. Additionally, because the amyloid precursor protein (APP) is located on chromosome 21, patients with Down syndrome (trisomy 21) have increased APP levels; these patients often develop Alzheimer disease at 30–40 years of age. Presenilin 1 is located on chromosome 14 and is noteworthy for its association with early-onset Alzheimer disease. Abnormalities in this gene result in increased β-amyloid accumulation.

What are the likely gross pathology findings in this condition?

Neurofibrillary **tangles** and amyloid **plaques** (Figure 10-1) are commonly seen on autopsy. A high degree of cerebral atrophy in the frontal, temporal, and parietal regions is also present.

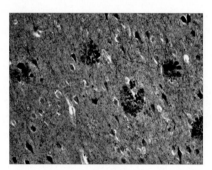

FIGURE 10-1. **Alzheimer disease.** Neurofibrillary tangles in Alzheimer disease. (Reproduced, with permission, from USMLERx.com.)

What biochemical mechanism is likely involved in the pathogenesis of this condition?

A preferential loss of acetylcholine and choline acetyltransferase in the cerebral cortex may play a role in the development of clinical disease.

What is the most appropriate treatment for this condition?

The acetylcholinesterase inhibitor class of medications, including tacrine, donepezil, rivastigmine, and galantamine, have been shown to slow the progress of memory loss. Memantine, an N-methyl-D-aspartate receptor antagonist, may protect from Alzheimer disease by blocking the excitotoxic effects of glutamate, independently of the effects of acetylcholinesterase inhibitors.

What is the prognosis for the patient's daughter?

Onset of the familial form of Alzheimer disease, which affects approximately 10% of patients with the disease, is usually 30–60 years of age. Because this patient was older than 70 years of age at onset, she likely does not have the familial form, and the daughter is unlikely to have an increased risk on the basis of family history alone.

■ CASE 2

A 35-year-old construction worker is taken to the emergency department (ED) after an accident in which a piece of metal became lodged in his back. The patient has excruciating pain at the site of his injury and is unable to move his right leg. In the ED, neurologic examination reveals paralysis of the right leg, ipsilateral hyperactive patellar reflex, and a positive Babinski sign. The patient can move his left leg without difficulty and has a normal patellar reflex and no Babinski sign. However, sensory testing reveals loss of temperature and pinprick sensation on the left leg up to the navel and loss of vibration sensation on the right leg up to the navel.

What is the most likely diagnosis?

Brown-Séquard syndrome due to a hemicord lesion. Brown-Séquard syndrome is characterized by ipsilateral spastic (upper motor neuron type) paralysis (1 in Figure 10-2), ipsilateral loss of vibration and position sensation (2 in Figure 10-2), and contralateral loss of pain and temperature sensation (3 in Figure 10-2).

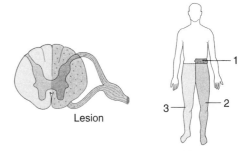

FIGURE 10-2. **Brown-Séquard syndrome.** (Reproduced, with permission, from Le T, Bhushan V, Tolles J. *First Aid for the USMLE Step 1: 2011.* New York: McGraw-Hill, 2011: 412.)

At what level is the lesion located?

The loss of sensation up to the navel suggests that the lesion is near T10, because the dermatome that includes the navel is supplied by T10.

Damage to which tracts is causing the ipsilateral deficits in this case?

The motor deficits are due to damage to the **lateral corticospinal tract** (Figure 10-3), which carries motor neurons from the cortex that have decussated in the pyramids. The loss of vibration and position sense is due to damage to the **dorsal columns**, which carry information from sensory nerves that enter through the dorsal root, ascend to the caudal medulla (where the primary neuron synapses), and then cross to ascend to the contralateral sensory cortex. These deficits are ipsilateral because the tracts cross the midline high in the spinal cord.

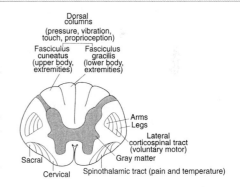

FIGURE 10-3. **Spinal cord and associated tracts.** (Reproduced, with permission, from Le T, Bhushan V, Tolles J. *First Aid for the USMLE Step 1: 2011.* New York: McGraw-Hill, 2011: 409.)

Damage to which tracts is causing the contralateral deficits in this case?

The loss of pain and temperature sensation is due to damage to the **spinothalamic tract** (Figure 10-3). The sensory neurons that travel in the anterolateral tract enter the spinal cord through the dorsal root, synapse almost immediately, and cross the midline (within one or two levels) via the anterior commissure to ascend to the cortex.

If the lesion were above T1, how would the presentation differ?

A hemicord lesion above T1, in addition to the findings above, will present as **Horner syndrome**, which consists of ptosis, miosis, and anhidrosis (droopy eyelid, constricted pupil, and decreased sweating).

CASE 3

A 38-year-old man presents to his primary care physician with a complaint of progressive weakness in his hands and feet. The patient states that these symptoms have slowly progressed over the past few months. Initially, he was unable to manipulate small objects such as picking up a coin or buttoning his shirt. Now he complains of difficulty grasping a gallon of milk and notices the muscles in his hands twitching. He often trips while walking because he feels he cannot lift his toes up and lacks coordination. In addition, he says that the muscles in his leg occasionally cramp or spasm.

What is the most likely diagnosis?

Amyotrophic lateral sclerosis (ALS), or Lou Gehrig disease, is a neurodegenerative disorder that causes progressive muscle weakness. There are several ALS variants classified on the basis of their pattern of distribution. Progressive bulbar palsy affects the motor nuclei of cranial nerves, and pseudobulbar palsy describes any condition that causes bilateral corticobulbar disease. Progressive spinal muscular atrophy is a lower motor neuron deficit involving anterior horn cells of the spinal cord. Primary lateral sclerosis predominantly affects the upper motor neurons.

Where are the lesions located and how does this explain the hallmark findings?

The hallmark of this disorder is the presence of **both upper motor neuron (UMN) and lower motor neuron (LMN) lesions**. ALS affects **anterior horn motor neurons** in the spinal cord (LMN) and the lateral corticospinal tracts carrying UMNs from the cortex. Sensory and cognitive functions are generally preserved.

How is this condition distinguished from the ascending paralysis syndromes?

ALS has both UMN and LMN findings whereas Guillain Barré syndrome (or acute inflammatory demyelinating polyradiculoneuropathy) and chronic inflammatory demyelinating polyradiculoneuropathy are solely LMN diseases and present with characteristic decreased reflex response.

What distinguishes UMN signs from LMN signs?

UMN signs include hyperreflexivity, increased tone, positive Babinski sign, and muscle spasm. **LMN signs** include weakness, muscle atrophy, and muscle fasciculations.

What is the course of this disease?

ALS is currently an untreatable disease with progressive neurodegeneration and muscle weakness, resulting in death within 3–5 years of diagnosis. Riluzole can prolong survival by 2–3 months, likely by blocking glutamatergic transmission in the central nervous system (CNS). Supportive care, including dietary modification, respiratory assistance, and palliative care, is an important part of management. Neuromuscular respiratory failure is the primary cause of death.

CASE 4

A 16-year-old high school student goes to see the school nurse because of severe eye pain and a feeling that there is something "stuck" in his right eye. He does not wear contact lenses. He reports that he was recently working with machines in shop class without wearing protective goggles. Ophthalmologic examination reveals no visible foreign body in the eye; visual acuity is slightly decreased at 20/30; pupils are equal, round, and reactive to light bilaterally; corneal reflex is intact; and extraocular muscles are intact, although the student says his right eye hurts when he moves it.

What is the most likely diagnosis?

The student has a corneal abrasion, which typically presents with significant eye pain and a foreign body sensation. The patient will also have photophobia. This patient's history suggests the source for his eye injury: working with machinery without wearing protective eyewear. Other etiologies of acute unilateral vision impairment are optic neuritis, retinal detachment or tear, giant cell arteritis, and amaurosis fugax.

What is the pathway of the corneal blink reflex?

The excruciating pain experienced by this patient is due to the rich innervation of the cornea by the ophthalmic branch of cranial nerve (CN) V (V1). This nerve constitutes the afferent portion of the corneal blink reflex. After synapsing in the sensory nucleus of CN V, there is bilateral projection to the nucleus of CN VII. From there, motor neurons project to the orbicularis oculi muscles, causing a consensual blink response.

What space lies between the cornea and the lens?

The space between the cornea and the lens is the anterior compartment, which is subdivided by the iris into the anterior chamber and the posterior chamber (Figure 10-4). The entire anterior compartment is filled with aqueous humor, which is secreted by the ciliary body.

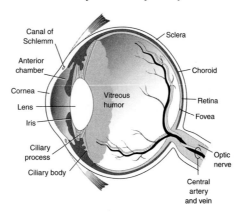

FIGURE 10-4. **The eye and retina.** (Reproduced, with permission, from Le T, Bhushan V, Tolles J. *First Aid for the USMLE Step 1: 2011.* New York: McGraw-Hill, 2011: 420.)

What space lies behind the lens?

Behind the lens is the posterior compartment (Figure 10-4), which is filled with vitreous humor, a gelatinous substance. At the anterior aspect of the posterior compartment, the lens is held in place by the suspensory ligament, which extends from the ciliary body of the choroid to the lens.

From what embryologic structures do the cornea, iris, ciliary body, lens, and retina develop?

The optic cup is an embryologic structure derived from neuroectoderm that gives rise to the retina, iris, and ciliary body. The lens is derived from surface ectoderm. The inner layers of the cornea are derived from mesenchyme, and the outer layer derives from the surface ectoderm.

■ CASE 5

A 70-year-old man with a history of rheumatoid arthritis comes to his physician complaining of weakness 1 day after a motor vehicle accident. Physical examination reveals intact sensation and strength in the lower extremities but weakness in the upper extremities bilaterally. The patient is able to move his arms parallel to the ground but is unable to lift his arms, forearms, or hands upward against gravity. Strength is rated 2/5. CT scan of the cervical spine rules out cervical spine fracture, and MRI demonstrates traumatic C6 disk herniation, buckling of the ligamentum flavum, and edema within the cervical cord in that area.

What is the most likely diagnosis?

Central cord syndrome. This syndrome is characterized by upper extremity weakness that exceeds lower extremity weakness and varying degrees of sensory loss below the level of the lesion.

What is the arterial supply to the cervical spinal cord?

The spinal cord is supplied by an anterior spinal artery (which is supplied by the vertebral arteries) that supplies the anterior two-thirds of the cord and by two posterior spinal arteries (which are supplied by the vertebral posterior inferior cerebellar arteries) that supply the dorsal columns and part of the posterior horns.

What is a vascular watershed zone?

A **watershed zone** is an area between two major arteries in which small branches of the arteries form anastomoses. Important watershed zones lie between the cerebral arteries (eg, middle and anterior cerebral arteries) and in the central spinal cord. These areas are susceptible to infarction during hypotension or hypoperfusion. In this case, edema and trauma impair blood flow to the cervical cord, and the predominant symptoms result from damage within the central cord watershed zone.

What is supplied by the long tracts in the areas labeled "Region A" in Figure 10-5?

Region A in Figure 10-5 indicates the most medial portions of the corticospinal tracts. These fibers supply the muscles of the upper extremity. Because they are medial structures, motor impairment of the upper extremities can occur after a smaller central cord lesion. The cross-hatched pattern in Figure 10-6 indicates the area of impairment that is associated with a central cord lesion.

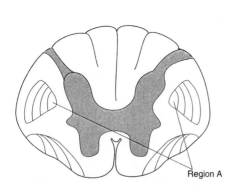

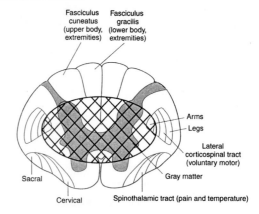

FIGURE 10-5. **Axial view of the spinal cord, showing the most medial portions of the corticospinal tracts (region A).** (Reproduced, with permission, from Le T, et al. *First Aid for the USMLE Step 1: 2008.* New York: McGraw-Hill, 2008: 371.)

FIGURE 10-6. **Axial view of the spinal cord, showing the area of impairment associated with a central cord lesion.** (Reproduced, with permission, from Le T, et al. *First Aid for the USMLE Step 1: 2008.* New York: McGraw-Hill, 2008: 371.)

What changes in the biceps, triceps, and brachioradialis reflexes are expected after damage to the anterior horn cells supplying the C6 nerve root?

The biceps reflex, which is regulated by fibers from C5 and C6, will be moderately diminished secondary to diminished lower motor neuron input. The triceps reflex is regulated primarily by C7 and should thus be unaffected by a C6 lesion. The brachioradialis reflex is primarily regulated by C6 and will thus be markedly diminished after a C6 lesion.

■ CASE 6

A 10-year-old boy is brought to the pediatrician by his parents for evaluation of short stature. The child is below the 10th percentile for height. Further evaluation reveals a bitemporal hemianopsia. MRI of the head reveals a suprasellar cystic, calcified mass (Figure 10-7).

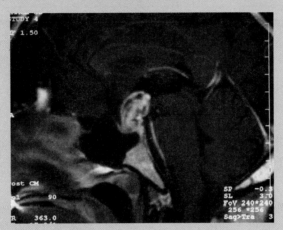

FIGURE 10-7. (Reproduced, with permission, from Riordan-Eva P, et al. *Vaughn & Asbury's General Ophthalmology*, 17th ed. New York: McGraw-Hill, 2008: 281.)

What is the most likely diagnosis?

The hallmark lesion for **craniopharyngioma** is a **suprasellar, cystic, calcified** mass. The differential diagnosis for a suprasellar mass includes optic gliomas, meningiomas, pituitary adenomas, and metastases.

What are other causes of short stature?

Other causes of short stature can arise from endocrine disorders including Cushing syndrome, growth hormone deficiency, hypothyroidism, and gastrointestinal disorders including malabsorption syndromes such as celiac disease, lactase deficiency, or inflammatory bowel disease.

From what tissue does the tumor in this condition derive?

Craniopharyngiomas are rare tumors derived from the Rathke pouch. The Rathke pouch is an invagination of **ectoderm** lining the primitive mouth that develops into the adenohypophysis.

What tests or imaging tools may be used to confirm the diagnosis?

CT scan or MRI of the head can visualize the cystic calcified suprasellar mass characteristic of craniopharyngioma. Plain radiographs of the skull can detect advanced cases. Testing of the pituitary axis and optic pathways can determine if the tumor has affected these structures.

What is the epidemiology of this condition?

Craniopharyngiomas exhibit a bimodal distribution, with one peak among children and the second among patients 55–65 years of age. It is the third most common intracranial tumor in children.

What are the clinical manifestations of this condition?

Craniopharyngiomas are slow-growing tumors with a highly variable clinical presentation. Symptoms occur because the tumor involves the pituitary gland or the optic chiasm. Patients may present with growth hormone deficiency, hypothyroidism, or central diabetes insipidus. Visual disturbances and headaches are common.

■ CASE 7

A 45-year-old woman presents to her physician with a 3-month history of anxiety, tremor, hyperreflexia, hair thinning, and an unintentional weight loss of 4.5 kg (10 lb). She is treated surgically. After surgery, her symptoms have resolved, but the patient now complains of hoarseness.

What is the cause of the patient's hoarseness?

This patient underwent surgery for hyperthyroidism. Damage to the recurrent laryngeal nerve may occur as the surgeon is ligating the inferior thyroid artery, which is adjacent to the nerve.

What cranial nerve is involved in this patient?

The recurrent laryngeal nerve is a branch of the vagus nerve (CN X).

This nerve provides motor innervation to which structures?

The recurrent laryngeal nerve innervates all intrinsic muscles of the larynx except for the cricothyroid, which is innervated by the external laryngeal nerve (also a branch of CN X).

What is the course of this nerve?

The left recurrent laryngeal nerve branches off the vagus nerve at the level of the aortic arch, wraps posteriorly around the aorta, and ascends superiorly to the larynx (Figure 10-8). The right recurrent laryngeal nerve branches off the vagus at the level of the right subclavian artery and vein and wraps around the artery to ascend posteriorly to the larynx. Because the left recurrent laryngeal nerve has a long course arising from the vagus in the superior mediastinum, it is prone to injury from abnormal structures, such as enlarged lymph nodes, aneurysm of the arch of the aorta, a retrosternal goiter, or a thymoma.

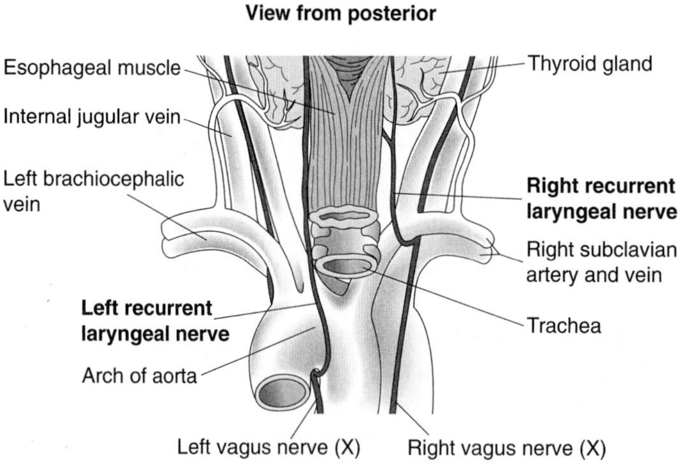

FIGURE 10-8. **Course of the recurrent laryngeal nerve.** (Reproduced, with permission, from Bhushan V, et al. *First Aid for the USMLE Step 1: 2005.* New York: McGraw-Hill, 2005: 83.)

What other structures can be damaged during this surgery?

Surgical technique focuses on preservation of the parathyroid glands, and hypoparathyroidism can occur after surgery. For this reason surgeons often remove the parathyroid gland and reimplant it elsewhere in the neck.

What are other scenarios in which this nerve may be injured?

Left atrial enlargement (eg, from mitral regurgitation) and tumor in the apex of the right upper lobe of the lung can impinge on and injure the recurrent laryngeal nerve. Injury of the left recurrent laryngeal nerve may also result in compression by abnormal structures in the superior mediastinum, as described above.

■ CASE 8

A 72-year-old woman falls while at home and lands face down. She is unable to get up and remains prone on the floor overnight until a neighbor notices her missing and calls 911. She is taken to the emergency department where she is noted to have several hematomas on her face and a large hematoma on her right upper thigh. On physical examination, the patient is unable to flex her right hip or extend her right lower leg. Patellar reflex cannot be elicited on the right. Leg adduction and abduction are intact bilaterally.

What is the most likely diagnosis?

Weakness of the quadriceps muscles and hip flexors (which are innervated by the femoral nerve) and lack of patellar reflex suggests femoral neuropathy (L2–L4). The cause of the neuropathy in this case is a hematoma (secondary to trauma) compressing the nerve. Because both the hip flexors (L2–L3) and the quadriceps muscles (L3–L4) are involved, the nerve is affected above the inguinal ligament. If the compression had affected the nerve distal to the inguinal ligament where the nerve branches into anterior and posterior divisions, a deficiency in either the hip flexors (anterior) or the quadriceps muscles (posterior), but not both, would be expected.

What sensory defects are expected in this patient?

The femoral nerve innervates the skin of the anterior and medial thigh; thus, light touch sensation is decreased in these areas. The lateral aspect of the thigh is innervated by the lateral femoral cutaneous nerve (L2–L3) and is spared in an isolated femoral neuropathy. The **saphenous nerve** is a cutaneous branch of the femoral nerve that arises from the femoral nerve in the femoral triangle. It innervates the skin of the anteromedial knee, leg, and foot to the medial side of the big toe. Because this lesion is above the femoral ligament, the saphenous nerve distribution is also involved.

What other structures are found with this nerve in the femoral triangle?

The femoral nerve is the largest branch of the lumbar plexus and, after forming in the abdomen, runs posterolaterally to the inguinal ligament. It crosses under the inguinal ligament lateral to the psoas muscle and enters the femoral triangle. In the **femoral triangle** (bounded by the sartorius muscle, inguinal ligament, and adductor longus), it runs lateral to the femoral artery, which is lateral to the femoral vein. The vessels are enclosed within the femoral sheath and the nerve is outside it.

Why is thigh adduction spared in this patient?

The major muscles responsible for thigh adduction are the adductor longus, adductor brevis, adductor magnus, and the gracilis, which are innervated by the obturator nerve (L2–L4). Because this is a peripheral neuropathy, not pathology of the nerve root, the obturator nerve is spared and so is thigh adduction.

What other clinical scenarios can be associated with this condition?

- Diabetic vasculitic damage.
- Direct penetrating trauma.
- Hip fracture.
- Iliac aneurysms.
- Incorrect placement of the femoral line.
- Prolonged hip flexion during gynecologic or urologic procedures.
- Tumor.

■ CASE 9

A 70-year-old man with a history of hypertension goes to his ophthalmologist for a routine eye examination. He has needed to wear eyeglasses while driving since he was 18 years of age. Ocular examination reveals increased intraocular pressure in both eyes. On a field test, there is significant loss of peripheral vision, and funduscopic examination reveals cupping.

What is the most likely diagnosis?

Open-angle glaucoma is the most common form of glaucoma in the United States (90%) and presents as progressive, painless visual loss. Closed-angle glaucoma is painful and can cause additional symptoms such as seeing halos around lights and red eye.

What is the pathophysiology of this condition?

Open-angle glaucoma is caused by elevated intraocular pressure resulting from obstruction of flow of aqueous humor through the normal outflow channels (Figure 10-9).

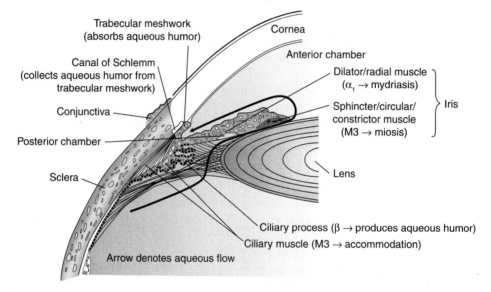

FIGURE 10-9. Aqueous humor pathways. (Reproduced, with permission, from Le T, Bhushan V, Tolles J. *First Aid for the USMLE Step 1: 2011.* New York: McGraw-Hill, 2011: 420.)

What are the appropriate treatments for this condition?

The direct cholinergic agonists pilocarpine and carbachol are used to treat open-angle glaucoma. These agents act by stimulating ciliary muscle contraction, thereby relieving tension in the suspensory ligament. Cholinomimetics also stimulate the sphincter pupillae of the iris, which widens the canal of Schlemm and constricts the pupil (miosis). Adverse effects include nausea, vomiting, diarrhea, salivation, sweating, vasodilation, and bronchoconstriction.

What effect does pilocarpine have on cardiac muscle?

Pilocarpine is an M3/M2 muscarinic receptor agonist. Cardiac cells have M2 receptors that, when activated, stimulate a G protein that inhibits adenyl cyclase and increases potassium conductance. Pilocarpine stimulation decreases the heart rate and the force of contraction (**negative inotrope**).

What additional classes of drugs are useful in treating this condition?

Other drug classes used to treat open-angle glaucoma include the following:

- Adrenergic agonists such as epinephrine.
- β-Blockers and acetazolamide (a carbonic anhydrase inhibitor), which decrease aqueous humor secretion.
- Prostaglandins, which increase the outflow of aqueous humor.

CASE 10

A 52-year-old man is brought to the emergency department after sustaining his first tonic-clonic seizure. The patient states he has had a bitemporal dull, constant headache for the last 2 weeks. MRI of the head is shown in Figure 10-10.

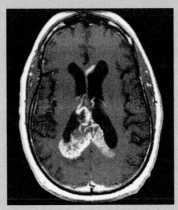

FIGURE 10-10. (Reproduced, with permission, from Kantarjian HM, et al. *MD Anderson Manual of Medical Oncology*. New York: McGraw-Hill, 2006: 796.)

What is the most likely diagnosis?

Glioblastoma multiforme (GBM), the most common primary brain tumor. GBM represents almost 20% of all primary intracranial tumors.

Where are these lesions typically located?

Glioblastomas are found supratentorially in the cerebral hemispheres and often cross hemispheres via the corpus callosum ("butterfly glioma") (Figure 10-10).

What are the histologic findings in this condition?

Glioblastomas are composed of highly malignant astrocytes that are visualized with a glial fibrillary acidic protein stain. Histology of glioblastomas shows pseudopalisading tumor cells surrounding focal areas of necrosis (Figure 10-11).

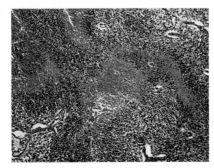

FIGURE 10-11. **Glioblastoma multiforme.** Histology shows necrosis with surrounding pseudopalisading of malignant tumor cells. (Reproduced, with permission, from Le T, Bhushan V, Tolles J. *First Aid for the USMLE Step 1: 2011*. New York: McGraw-Hill, 2011: Image 48B.)

What is the treatment for this condition?

Treatment is largely palliative and only moderately increases survival time. Treatment may include surgical resection, radiation, and chemotherapy.

What are other common adult brain tumors?

The most common cause of brain tumors in adults is metastases, and their presentation depends on location. Meningiomas derive from dura mater or arachnoid and are usually benign, but severity depends on location. Astrocytoma arises in brain parenchyma, has a better prognosis than GBM, and presents with seizures, headaches, and focal deficits.

What is the natural history of this condition?

Glioblastoma is an aggressive tumor; without treatment, most patients die within 3 months of diagnosis. With treatment, the median survival time is 1 year, and < 10% of patients survive 5 years.

▮ CASE 11

A 27-year-old man comes to his physician complaining of a tingling sensation in his toes and progressive weakness in both legs. On questioning, he says that he had bloody diarrhea, nausea, vomiting, and cramps 3 weeks ago that lasted for a few days. He has not traveled recently and has not eaten anything out of the ordinary. Physical examination reveals markedly decreased patellar and Achilles tendon reflexes bilaterally.

What is the most likely diagnosis?

Guillain-Barré syndrome (GBS), or acute inflammatory demyelinating polyradiculoneuropathy, is characterized by symmetric ascending muscle weakness or paralysis that begins in the lower extremities. Hyporeflexia or areflexia is invariable but may not be present early in the course of disease.

What physical findings are commonly associated with this condition?

Findings in GBS include ascending paresthesias, cranial nerve deficits leading to dysphagia, dysarthria, facial weakness, papilledema, autonomic dysfunction, and respiratory muscle paralysis in extreme cases. Figure 10-12 shows papilledema of the optic nerve head in GBS, along with the vascular congestion, elevation of the nerve head, and blurred disc margins often seen in papilledema, papillitis, and compressive lesions of the optic nerve.

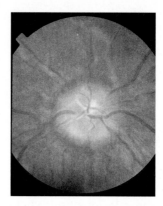

FIGURE 10-12. Papilledema of the optic nerve. (Reproduced, with permission, from Tintinalli JE, et al. *Tintinalli's Emergency Medicine: A Comprehensive Study Guide*, 6th ed. New York: McGraw-Hill, 2004: 1464.)

In what settings does this condition usually occur?

GBS often occurs 1–3 weeks after a gastrointestinal or upper respiratory tract infection, vaccination, or allergic reaction. Common associated infections include *Campylobacter jejuni* and herpesvirus. Although a preceding event is present in most patients, approximately one third of patients with GBS report no such events during the preceding 1–4 weeks.

What is the etiology of this condition?

GBS is thought to be an autoimmune reaction that develops in response to a previous infection or other medical condition. This process results in aberrant demyelination of peripheral nerves and ventral motor nerve roots. Cranial nerve roots can also be affected.

What laboratory finding is likely in this condition?

Cerebrospinal fluid (CSF) reveals a markedly elevated protein concentration with a normal cell count, commonly referred to as **albuminocytologic dissociation.** This contrasts the increased cell counts typical of CNS infection. Increased CSF protein can lead to papilledema.

What is the appropriate treatment for this condition?

The first element of GBS management is supportive care and treatment of the underlying condition with either IVIG antibody or plasmapheresis. Pulmonary function should be monitored with peak flow studies to assess for respiratory failure. Rehabilitation may be required to restore function.

If this patient's symptoms worsen over the next few months with no signs of improvement, what alternative diagnosis should be considered?

Chronic inflammatory demyelinating polyradiculopathy is a chronic, progressive, or chronic progressive counterpart of GBS that often presents with similar symptoms.

■ CASE 12

A 45-year-old man comes to the physician for a routine visit. On physical examination, his right eye appears abnormal (Figure 10-13). In addition, his right pupil is constricted but reacts normally to light and accommodation. The right side of the patient's face is dry and flushed. On questioning, he states the right side of his face has become abnormally dry.

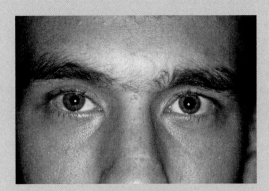

FIGURE 10-13. (Reproduced, with permission, from Tintinalli JE, et al. *Tintinalli's Emergency Medicine: A Comprehensive Study Guide*, 6th ed. New York: McGraw-Hill, 2004: 1463.)

What is the most likely diagnosis?

Horner syndrome.

What is the pathophysiology of this condition?

Horner syndrome results from a disruption in the sympathetic innervation of the face and subsequent uninhibited parasympathetic activity, which produces the classic symptoms: ipsilateral **P**tosis (slight drooping of the eyelid), **A**nhidrosis (absence of sweating), and **M**iosis (pupillary constriction) (mnemonic: **PAM**).

What nerve pathway is disrupted in this condition?

The first neuron of the sympathetic pathway begins in the hypothalamus and synapses in the intermediolateral column of the spinal cord near T1 (Figure 10-14). The second, preganglionic, neuron travels to the superior cervical ganglion. The third and final neuron of the pathway innervates the pupil, the sweat glands of the face, and the smooth muscle of the eyelid.

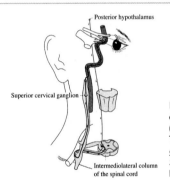

FIGURE 10-14. **Nerve pathways disrupted in Horner syndrome.** (Reproduced, with permission, from Tintinalli JE, et al. *Tintinalli's Emergency Medicine: A Comprehensive Study Guide*, 6th ed. New York: McGraw-Hill, 2004: 1463.)

If this patient presented with nystagmus to the right side and frequent falling, what acute condition should be considered?

Wallenberg syndrome results from a stroke in the lateral medullary region supplied by the posterior inferior cerebellar artery. It can present with ipsilateral Horner syndrome, nystagmus to the side of the lesion, ipsilateral limb ataxia, and vertigo. Another distinguishing feature is impaired pain and temperature sensation in the ipsilateral face and contralateral hemibody.

What are other common causes of this condition?

Any pathology that interrupts the described pathway can cause Horner syndrome. These include Pancoast tumor, neck trauma, carotid dissection, cervical cord lesions, and multiple sclerosis. Many cases of Horner syndrome are idiopathic.

What is Pancoast tumor?

Pancoast tumor is a carcinoma that usually occurs in the apex of the lung. It can cause Horner syndrome and ulnar nerve pain.

■ CASE 13

The parents of a term, 1-year-old girl are concerned because the child's head seems abnormally large. Their pediatrician notes that the child's head circumference has accelerated beyond her established growth curve in the past month. Axial CT of the head (Figure 10-15) demonstrates dilated atria of the lateral ventricles and a rounded third ventricle.

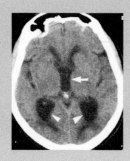

FIGURE 10-15. (Reproduced, with permission, from Brunicardi FC, et al. *Schwartz's Principles of Surgery*, 8th ed. New York: McGraw-Hill, 2005: 1650.)

What is the most likely diagnosis?

Hydrocephalus is defined as an excessive volume of cerebrospinal fluid (CSF) within the ventricles of the brain. Because CSF is trapped within the ventricular system, this case is an example of a **noncommunicating hydrocephalus**. A **communicating hydrocephalus** can occur in states of excess CSF production. CT scan of the head shows a dilated ventricular system (Figure 10-15) with dilated atria of the lateral ventricles (arrowheads) and rounded third ventricle (arrow).

Other causes of disproportionally large head size or growth include trauma, Canavan disease, and Hurler syndrome.

Where is CSF produced?

CSF is produced by the choroid plexus epithelium within the cerebral ventricles (Figure 10-16). The lateral ventricle communicates with the third ventricle via the foramen of Monro. The third ventricle communicates with the fourth ventricle via the aqueduct of Sylvius. The fourth ventricle communicates with the subarachnoid space via the foramen of Luschka (laterally) and the foramen of Magendie (medially).

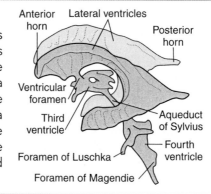

FIGURE 10-16. **Anatomy of the ventricular system.** (Reproduced, with permission, from Le T, Bhushan V, Tolles J. *First Aid for the USMLE Step 1: 2011.* New York: McGraw-Hill, 2011: 408.)

How is CSF reabsorbed?

Arachnoid villus cells, which are located in the superior sagittal sinus, return CSF to the bloodstream within vacuoles (through a process called **pinocytosis**).

What forms the blood-brain barrier?

Capillary and choroid endothelial cells form the **blood-brain barrier.** Tight junctions of capillary endothelium within the brain impede the passage of water and solutes. Within the choroid plexus, the choroid endothelium regulates the transport of water and solutes.

What is the pathophysiology of this condition?

Hydrocephalus results from a mismatch of CSF production and reabsorption in which the rate of production exceeds reabsorption. Causes of hydrocephalus include the following:

- Excess CSF production (eg, choroid plexus papilloma).
- Impaired CSF reabsorption (due to obstruction or disruption of arachnoid villi).
- Blockage of the flow of CSF.

What is the appropriate treatment for this condition?

Treatment is surgical and involves a ventriculoperitoneal shunt, which allows for reabsorption of fluid in the peritoneum.

■ CASE 14

A 39-year-old man is concerned about his health because his father died at 45 years of age after several years of dementia, uncontrollable twitching, and dance-like movements in his extremities. On further questioning, the patient reports that many members of his family have had similar symptoms. The patient's knowledge of his family history allows the physician to construct a detailed family tree (Figure 10-17; the asterisk represents the patient).

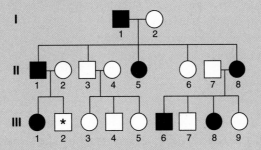

FIGURE 10-17. **Right homonymous hemianopia.**

What condition is the patient at risk for developing?

Huntington disease is characterized by dementia, choreoathetoid movements of the face and extremities, and early death. Huntington disease has an autosomal dominant inheritance. Other causes of early-onset dementia include early-onset Alzheimer disease, multiple sclerosis, HIV infection, or Creutzfeldt-Jakob disease (much rarer).

What is the genetic basis of this condition?

A mutation in chromosome 4 results in expansion of trinucleotide CAG repeats, which may decrease transcription of a striatal neurotrophic factor (brain-derived neurotrophic factor).

What neuronal pathology in patients with this condition makes CT imaging useful?

Patients with Huntington disease have marked atrophy of the striatum, including the caudate and putamen, representing degeneration and loss of γ-aminobutyric acid–ergic and cholinergic neurons.

What other conditions often present with similar movement abnormalities?

Sydenham chorea in rheumatic fever, tardive dyskinesia, and Wilson disease are among other diseases associated with choreoathetoid movements.

What is the prognosis for this patient?

Expansion of trinucleotide repeats over successive generations leads to earlier manifestations of disease in offspring; this is called **anticipation.** The patient's father died at age 45 years and likely developed Huntington disease many years earlier. If this patient had the genetic mutation, he might already be expected to show symptoms.

What other conditions are associated with trinucleotide repeats?

Fragile X syndrome, myotonic dystrophy, and spinocerebellar ataxia types I and II are also associated with trinucleotide repeats.

■ CASE 15

A 75-year-old woman visits an ophthalmologist because she has noticed a gradual decline in both her distance and near vision during the past 2 years. In particular, she has difficulty reading, focusing on objects in front of her, and adjusting her vision to the dark. She denies pain in her eye or any associated trauma. Funduscopic examination reveals deposits in the macula (Figure 10-18) and abnormal vision as assessed by the Amsler grid (Figure 10-19). Her peripheral vision and extraocular movements are intact.

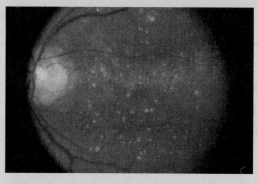

FIGURE 10-18. (Courtesy of Richard E. Wyszynski, MD, as published in Knoop KJ. Stack LB, Storrow AB. *Atlas of Emergency Medicine*, 2nd ed. New York: McGraw-Hill, 2002: 77.)

What is the abnormality in this patient's vision as assessed by the Amsler grid?

The **Amsler grid** assesses the degree of central vision loss (Figure 10-19A). In this assessment, patients cover one eye and, with the open eye, focus on the dot at the center of the grid. Patients with vision deficits in their macula see a distortion of the grid (Figure 10-19B).

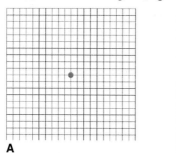 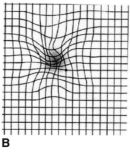

A   B

FIGURE 10-19. **Amsler grid.** (A) Normal grid. (B) Patient's view.

What is the most likely diagnosis?

Age-related macular degeneration (ARMD), in which central vision is blurred, is a significant cause of vision loss in the elderly. By contrast, glaucoma typically affects peripheral vision while sparing central vision. Central vision loss can also be caused by optic neuritis and cataracts.

What are the two variants of this condition?

There are dry and wet forms of macular degeneration. The **dry form** (85% of cases) typically progresses more slowly and occurs earlier in the disease process. The **wet form**, although rarer (% of cases), causes the majority of significant blindness in patients.

What are the histologic features of the retina in this condition?

Drusen are extracellular protein and lipid deposits in the retina, which appear on funduscopic examination as yellow or white spots in the eye (Figure 10-18). Irregularity and, in later stages, atrophy of the retinal pigmented epithelium also occur. In wet ARMD, new vessels from the choroid may grow into the subretinal space, causing **metamorphopsia** (a wavy distortion of vision), hemorrhage, and scarring.

What is the macula?

The **macula,** which is located temporal to the optic disc, is the area of the retina that is specialized for fine-detail vision. The center of the macula is the **fovea,** which has the highest density of cone photoreceptor cells in the retina and the smallest amount of convergence to bipolar cells. This provides for exquisite detail in visual perception.

■ CASE 16

A 67-year-old man with a history of hypertension and coronary artery disease presents to the ophthalmologist complaining that, for the past month, he has noticed decreased vision on his right side two or three times a week. Each episode lasts about 20 minutes and is accompanied by a severe retro-orbital headache. During the episodes, he is unable to read and bumps into objects on his right. Yesterday, he experienced the same visual loss, which has not resolved. Automated perimetry visual field testing reveals the pattern shown in Figure 10-20, with areas of visual loss in black.

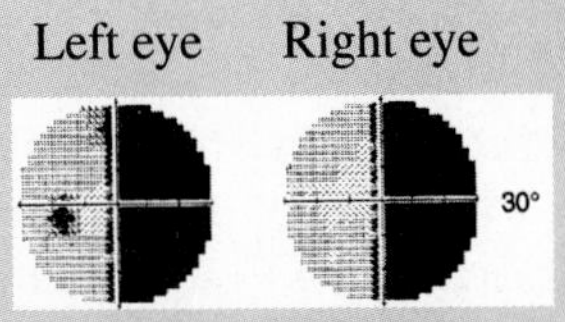

Left eye   Right eye

FIGURE 10-20. (Adapted, with permission, from Kasper DL, et al. *Harrison's Principles of Internal Medicine,* 16th ed. New York: McGraw-Hill, 2005: 165.)

What is this visual field defect?

The defect is a **right homonymous hemianopia** likely caused by a stroke. The patient's symptoms suggest that he has experienced a number of transient ischemic attacks (TIAs). The classical definition of a TIA is a vascular event that causes neurologic deficits that last < 24 hours. Clinically, it is defined as a neurologic deficit that lasts < 1 hour in the absence of abnormal imaging findings.

What is the pathway from photoreceptors in the retina to the visual cortex?

Photoreceptors (rods and cones) synapse on **bipolar cells** that synapse on **ganglion** cells in the retina, which form the **optic nerve**.

The optic nerve travels posteriorly and merges to form the **optic chiasm** where nasal (medial) retinal fibers from both eyes cross. The nasal hemiretina fibers are responsible for the temporal visual fields. Once past the chiasm it is known as the **optic tract**, which synapses on the lateral geniculate nucleus **(LGN)** of the thalamus.

Axons exiting the LGN fan out posteriorly through the white matter. The inferior radiations carry information from the **inferior retina** or **superior visual field**, travel through the temporal lobe, and are known as the Meyer loop. The superior radiations carry information from the superior retina or inferior visual field and travel through the parietal lobe.

The **optic radiations** synapse in the **visual cortex** of the occipital lobe near the calcarine fissure. The superior radiations synapse superior to the calcarine fissure and the inferior radiations inferior to the fissure (Figure 10-21).

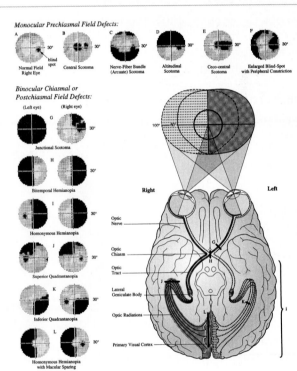

FIGURE 10-21. View of the visual fields and pathways. Lesion I illustrates the area affected in this patient with lesions possible in the left optic tract, the optic radiations, or the primary visual cortex. (Adapted, with permission, from Kasper DL, et al. *Harrison's Principles of Internal Medicine,* 16th ed. New York: McGraw-Hill, 2005: 165.)

Where along the optic pathway may a lesion be located to give this visual field defect?

A lesion in the left optic tract, posterior to the chiasm and anterior to the lateral geniculate nucleus, may be the cause, as may a large lesion affecting the upper and lower optic radiations or a lesion in the left visual cortex.

What visual field defect does a lesion in the right temporal lobe show?

The inferior optic radiations (Meyer loop) travel through the temporal lobe. A lesion to this area shows a left upper quadrantic anopia ("pie in the sky") as indicated by lesion J in Figure 10-21.

CASE 17

A 5-year-old boy is brought to the pediatrician by his mother for a follow-up appointment. Two months ago, the boy was seen for a chief complaint of morning headaches, vomiting, and decreased energy. A gastrointestinal illness was suspected. At this visit, the mother reports that her son's symptoms have worsened and that he now is falling and has a stumbling gait.

What is the likely diagnosis?

The history suggests **medulloblastoma**, a highly malignant tumor most often found in the cerebellum. The majority of patients are 4–8 years of age, and males are affected more than females. In children, 70% of intracranial tumors are infratentorial, whereas in adults 70% are supratentorial. Although medulloblastoma is the most common pediatric brain tumor, astrocytoma, brain stem glioma, and ependymomas are also common. Astrocytomas can occur anywhere in the hemispheres and the brain stem. In children, ependymomas typically occur in the fourth ventricle and are characterized by pseudorosettes, in which cells are arranged around vessels with ependymal processes directed toward the vessel wall.

How do cerebellar lesions present?

Lesions can occur in either the vermis or the hemispheres. Cerebellar lesions in the hemispheres cause ipsilateral limb ataxia and loss of muscle tone. Superior vermis lesions are characteristic of Wernicke encephalopathy and alcoholic cerebellar degeneration, presenting with the classic triad of gait or truncal ataxia, ophthalmoplegia, and confusion.

What imaging technique is used to visualize this condition?

On MRI of the head, medulloblastomas are heterogeneous enhancements located in the cerebellum, often extending into the fourth ventricle (Figure 10-22).

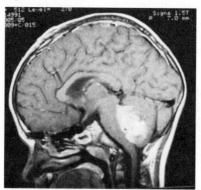

FIGURE 10-22. Sagittal MRI illustrates medulloblastoma involving the cerebellum and fourth ventricle. (Reproduced, with permission, from Ropper AH, et al. *Adams and Victor's Principles of Neurology*, 8th ed. New York: McGraw-Hill, 2005: 567.)

This condition may present with what other syndrome?

The association of inherited colonic syndromes with brain tumors is named Turcot syndrome. Patients with autosomal dominant familial adenomatous polyposis are at risk for medulloblastomas and gliomas. Patients with hereditary nonpolyposis colorectal cancer are at risk for gliomas only.

What is the morphology of this condition?

Medulloblastomas are rapidly growing, well-circumscribed friable tumors found exclusively in the cerebellum. Microscopically, **Horner-Wright rosettes**, described as circular patterns of tumor cells surrounding a center of neutrophils, can be seen.

What is the appropriate treatment for this condition?

Treatment consists of complete or near-complete surgical excision followed by radiation and chemotherapy. Current treatment protocols are designed to minimize damage to adjacent structures and prolong survival.

CASE 18

A 47-year-old woman is brought to the emergency department after a minor car accident. CT scan of the head without contrast reveals no intracranial hemorrhage. However, a spherical, 3-cm, bright enhancement abutting the falx cerebri is found incidentally. On physical examination, the patient has no neurologic deficits and denies headache, nausea, vomiting, or visual changes. MRI of the head is shown in Figure 10-23.

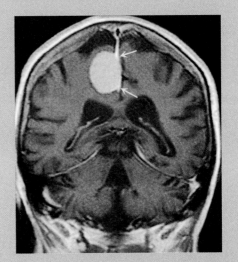

FIGURE 10-23. (Reproduced, with permission, from Kasper DL, et al. *Harrison's Principles of Internal Medicine*, 16th ed. New York: McGraw-Hill, 2005: 2456.)

What is the most likely diagnosis?

The location of the lesion on MRI scan is typical of a **meningioma.** Meningiomas are usually benign, slow-growing tumors arising from the arachnoid cells penetrating the dura. They are the second most common primary brain tumor.

Where are the lesions associated with this condition typically located?

Meningiomas are found along the dura, most often in the sylvian region, superior parasagittal region, and cerebellopontine angle. Other diseases that commonly involve the dura include lymphoma, metastatic carcinoma, and tuberculosis.

What are the histologic findings of this condition?

Meningiomas display psammoma bodies and elongated spindle cells arranged concentrically in a whorled pattern. Psammoma bodies are laminated, concentric calcified concretions formed by meningiomas (**head**), papillary adenocarcinomas of the thyroid (**neck**), malignant mesothelioma (**thorax**), and serous papillary cystadenocarcinoma of the ovary (**pelvis**).

What is the appropriate treatment for this condition?

For small, slow-growing, and asymptomatic tumors, careful observation is appropriate. Surgical resection is indicated for symptomatic tumors or quickly growing tumors. Complete resection is often curative; however, tumors can recur if incompletely resected.

What other symptoms are common in patients with this condition?

Because of their slow growth, many meningiomas are detected incidentally after neuroimaging for other reasons. However, large tumors may displace normal brain tissue and cause focal neurologic deficits such as visual disturbances, hearing loss, mental status changes, extremity weakness, obstructive hydrocephalus, and/or seizures.

CASE 19

A 10-year-old boy is brought to his pediatrician because of a painful ear. The pain began 1 week earlier with a runny nose and sinus pressure that progressed to ear pain and dizziness. Otoscopic examination reveals the findings in Figure 10-24. He has a low-grade fever of 37.8°C (100.0°F) but no other physical findings.

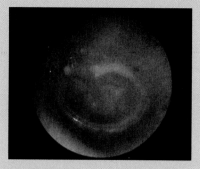

FIGURE 10-24. (Image courtesy of B. Welleschik.)

What is the most likely diagnosis?

Acute otitis media. The bulging, red tympanic membrane is a sign of middle ear infection. The clinical course suggests a viral upper respiratory infection leading to secondary involvement of the middle ear due to inflammation and congestion of the eustachian tube. The eustachian tube connects the middle ear to the nasopharynx.

From what embryologic structure is the tympanic membrane derived?

The tympanic membrane derives from the first pharyngeal membrane. The **pharyngeal membranes** constitute the tissue between the pharyngeal groove, or cleft, and the pharyngeal pouch. Only the first pharyngeal membrane is retained in the adult; the rest are obliterated during development.

What three bones are located in the middle ear?

The three bones located in the middle ear (auditory ossicles) are the malleus, incus, and stapes (Figure 10-25); together, they transmit sound from the tympanic membrane to the internal ear. The **malleus,** which articulates with the tympanic membrane, derives from the first branchial arch. The **incus,** which lies between the malleus and the stapes, derives from the first branchial arch. The **stapes,** which articulates with the oval window of the inner ear, derives from the second branchial arch.

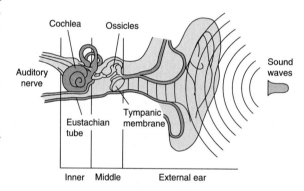

FIGURE 10-25. **Anatomy of the ear.** (Reproduced, with permission, from Lalwani AK. *Current Diagnosis & Treatment in Otolaryngology—Head & Neck Surgery,* 2nd ed. New York: McGraw-Hill, 2008: 578.)

What two muscles control the movement of the bones of the middle ear?

The tensor tympani inserts on the malleus and dampens the amplitude of the tympanic membrane oscillations, which prevents damage to the inner ear from loud sounds. Innervation is by the mandibular nerve (CN V3). The stapedius inserts onto the neck of the stapes and dampens movement of this ossicle. It is innervated by the facial nerve (CN VII). A lesion denervating the stapedius causes hypersensitivity to sound.

What organisms commonly cause pediatric ear infections?

In order of prevalence, common bacteria that cause middle ear infection are *Streptococcus pneumoniae, Haemophilus influenzae* (although rarely type B since the introduction of the conjugated vaccine), and *Moraxella catarrhalis.* Appropriate antibiotic coverage involves a β-lactamase such as amoxicillin. Less common organisms are group A streptococci, *Staphylococcus* aureus, *Pseudomonas,* and in newborns, gram-negative bacilli. Approximately 15%–20% of middle ear infections are due to viruses, including respiratory syncytial virus, rhinovirus, influenza viruses, and adenovirus.

■ CASE 20

A 54-year-old woman was successfully treated for small cell lung cancer 3 years ago. She received chemotherapy and radiation therapy and was declared disease-free via CT scan of the chest 1 year ago. She now comes to her primary care physician with a complaint of nausea, vomiting, and right-sided headaches of a few weeks' duration. A repeat CT scan of the head is shown in Figure 10-26.

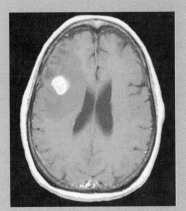

FIGURE 10-26. (Reproduced, with permission, from Kantarjian HM, et al. *MD Anderson Manual of Medical Oncology.* New York: McGraw-Hill, 2006: 797.)

What is the most likely diagnosis?

Metastatic brain tumor from her small cell lung cancer. Brain metastases are more prevalent than primary central nervous system tumors.

What is the differential diagnosis for this condition?

The differential diagnosis includes a primary brain tumor, metastatic tumor from a second primary brain tumor, infection, cerebral infarct, or radiation necrosis.

What types of cancer most often metastasize to the brain?

Lung, **B**reast, **S**kin (melanoma), **K**idney (renal cell carcinoma), and **G**astrointestinal (mnemonic: Lots of Bad Stuff Kills Glia) tumors can spread hematogenously to the brain.

Where are these lesions usually located in the brain?

Metastases are supratentorial, located at the **gray-white matter junction,** where the arterial vessels narrow sufficiently for tumor cells to lodge (Figure 10-26). They are also found at **watershed areas,** or vascular territories situated between two supplying arteries (eg, middle cerebral artery and anterior cerebral artery).

What are the common symptoms of this condition?

Symptoms include headaches, seizures, stroke, nausea, vomiting, cognitive dysfunction such as personality changes, and focal neurologic deficits such as aphasia or weakness.

What tests and/or imaging tools can help confirm the diagnosis?

MRI is the imaging modality of choice because of its superior sensitivity for soft tissue. Biopsy of the lesion is often indicated to confirm the diagnosis before a definitive treatment plan is chosen.

What paraneoplastic syndromes are associated with small cell lung carcinoma?

The most common paraneoplastic syndromes are the syndrome of inappropriate antidiuretic hormone secretion and the syndrome of ectopic adrenocorticotropic hormone; however, small cell lung cancer can also cause variable nonspecific neurologic symptoms.

■ CASE 21

An 18-year-old woman presents to her family physician for an evaluation of severe headaches. She describes her headaches as unilateral, beginning with a dull and steady ache and increasing in severity to a throbbing, debilitating pain after several hours. No aura is associated with the headaches, but they are exacerbated by motion and light. Consequently, the patient prefers to remain in a dark room when her headaches occur. She also states this is the second episode she has had; the first episode occurred approximately 4 weeks ago and dissipated within a few days.

What is the most likely diagnosis?
Migraine headache.

What signs and symptoms are commonly associated with this condition?
Migraines are unilateral in 60%–70% of cases; the remaining cases are typically bifrontal or, less frequently, bioccipital. The pain often begins with the gradual onset of a deep, steady ache that reaches a pulsatile, severe pain within several hours. Migraines are typically worsened by movement, loud noises, and bright lights. Although **auras** (temporary neurologic symptoms such as light flashes and zigzag lines or numbness and tingling in the arms and face) are commonly associated with migraine headaches, they are actually seen in only 20% of cases.

How is this condition differentiated from other, more serious pathologic conditions of the head?
The following warning signs indicate that a headache may be serious:
- Absence of similar episodes in the past.
- Association with vigorous exercise or trauma (suggesting carotid dissection).
- Change in mental status.
- Concurrent infection.
- Sudden onset within seconds to minutes (suggesting subarachnoid hemorrhage).

Physical findings pointing to potentially serious pathology include nuchal rigidity (meningitis), poor general appearance, or papilledema (elevated intracranial pressure).

How can this woman's headache be differentiated from pseudotumor cerebri, cluster headaches, or tension headaches?
Tension headaches are typically bilateral and are often described as a bandlike tightness or pressure (as if the patient were wearing a tight hat). They are typically not debilitating, and the pressure waxes and wanes over an unpredictable time course. Tension headaches are closely associated with stress.

Pseudotumor cerebri is commonly found in obese women and is a result of idiopathic intracranial hypertension. These headaches are commonly accompanied by nausea, vomiting, tinnitus, and vision changes. Pseudotumor cerebri is treated by therapeutic lumbar puncture, acetazolamide, or surgery in refractory cases.

Cluster headaches typically occur in males and are always unilateral. The pain often begins around the eye or temple, is sudden in onset (and could thus be mistaken for subarachnoid hemorrhage), and is described as deep and persistent. The pain often lasts for several hours and can be associated with tearing of the eyes and sweating.

What are the appropriate treatments for this condition?
- **Maintenance agents** include β-blockers, calcium channel blockers, tricyclics, and anticonvulsants.
- **Abortive agents** include nonsteroidal anti-inflammatory drugs, acetaminophen, triptans, and ergotamine agents.
- **Antiemetics** are often used for control of associated nausea and vomiting.

▌ CASE 22

A 12-year-old boy is brought by mother to the dermatologist for numerous skin lesions. Physical examination reveals 10 uniformly hyperpigmented macules, 15–25 mm in diameter, scattered over the patient's trunk and limbs. Freckling is present in both armpits, and dozens of soft, skin-colored, domed nodules have recently appeared on the patient's back. The dermatologist notes kyphosis and refers the patient to an ophthalmologist for further evaluation.

What is the most likely diagnosis?

Neurofibromatosis type 1 (NF1), or von Recklinghausen disease, is a common neurocutaneous disorder. NF1 has complete penetrance with variable expression. Diagnosis is made on clinical criteria. Although neurofibromatosis type 2 (NF2) can present with skin lesions, NF2 most commonly causes bilateral acoustic neuromas and eye lesions; approximately 50% of affected patients develop lesions in the spinal cord, cranial nerves, and meninges.

What are the genetics of this condition?

NF1 is an autosomal dominant disorder caused by mutation in the *NF1* gene found on chromosome **17**. Approximately 50% of NF1 cases are familial and the rest represent new mutations. *NF1* codes for the protein neurofibromin and is thought to be a tumor suppressor gene (mnemonic: "von Recklinghausen" has **17 letters** and is located on chromosome **17**).

What are the typical dermatologic findings of this condition?

The hallmark finding is six or more hyperpigmented macules called **café-au-lait** spots. In addition, **neurofibromas**, multiple soft fleshy tumors, usually develop during adolescence (Figure 10-27). **Freckling** is also present in the axilla and groin. Although NF2 often demonstrates neurofibromas, café-au-lait spots are rare in this condition.

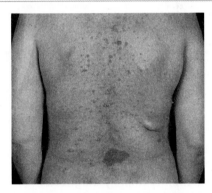

FIGURE 10-27. The multiple small skin-colored papules seen here are neurofibromas. The large hyperpigmented macule is a café-au-lait spot. (Reproduced, with permission, from Wolff K, et al. *Fitzpatrick's Color Atlas & Synopsis of Clinical Dermatology*, 5th ed. New York: McGraw-Hill, 2005: 465.)

What are the typical ophthalmologic findings in this condition?

Lisch nodules, which are raised, pigmented, hamartomas, are found on the iris (Figure 10-28).

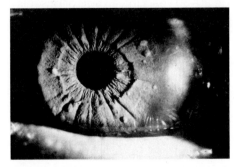

FIGURE 10-28. Multiple hamartomas (Lisch nodules) on the iris of this patient with neurofibromatosis type 1. (Reproduced, with permission, from Ropper AH, et al. *Adams and Victor's Principles of Neurology*, 8th ed. New York: McGraw-Hill, 2005: 870.)

Patients with this condition are predisposed to what tumors?

Optic gliomas may arise anywhere along the optic tract, particularly in the optic nerve or chiasm. Patients are also at increased risk for other central nervous system tumors such as astrocytomas and other gliomas. Peripheral neurofibromas can undergo malignant transformation into neurofibrosarcomas.

■ CASE 23

A 28-year-old previously healthy woman comes to the physician after suffering loss of vision in her right eye that resolved within a few hours. She also complains of weakness in her legs, urinary incontinence, and difficulty speaking. She has noticed a tremor in her right hand when writing and eating that has worsened over the past few weeks. Although she has had occasional tremors and troubled speech, her problems have never lasted this long and have never been accompanied by urinary incontinence or loss of vision. Upon questioning, she recalls that her mother had similar symptoms when she was young. Physical examination reveals left-sided facial droop, left tongue deviation, and lateral gaze weakness. An MRI is shown in Figure 10-29. Relevant laboratory findings are as follows:

White blood cell (WBC) count: 9100/mm³   Platelet count: 287,000/mm³
Hemoglobin: 13.3 g/dL   CSF IgG index: 0.89 (normal < 0.66)
Hematocrit: 37.1%

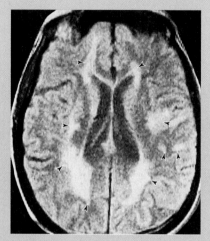

FIGURE 10-29. (Reproduced, with permission, from Waxman SG. *Clinical Neuroanatomy*, 25th ed. New York: McGraw-Hill, 2003: 307.)

What is the most likely diagnosis?
Multiple sclerosis (MS). The arrowheads in Figure 10-29 show the lesions of MS.

What risk factors are associated with this condition?
Risk factors for MS include the following:

• Age 20–50 years (mean age of onset is 30 years).
• Female gender (female/male ratio is 1.77:1.00).
• Having grown up in a temperate climate.
• Family history of MS.

What anatomic feature could explain the findings on physical examination?

A **medial brain stem lesion** involving cranial nerves VI, VII, and XII (Figure 10-30) leads to the constellation of facial droop, tongue deviation, and lateral gaze weakness. The intention tremor indicates cerebellar involvement.

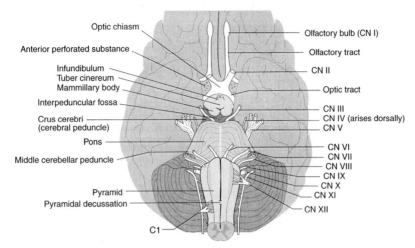

Optic chiasm
Anterior perforated substance
Infundibulum
Tuber cinereum
Mammillary body
Interpeduncular fossa
Crus cerebri (cerebral peduncle)
Pons
Middle cerebellar peduncle
Pyramid
Pyramidal decussation
C1

Olfactory bulb (CN I)
Olfactory tract
CN II
Optic tract
CN III
CN IV (arises dorsally)
CN V
CN VI
CN VII
CN VIII
CN IX
CN X
CN XI
CN XII

CNs that lie medially at brainstem: III, VI, XII. 3(×2) = 6(×2) = 12.

FIGURE 10-30. Brain stem anatomy. (Reproduced, with permission, from Le T, Bhushan V, Tolles J. *First Aid for the USMLE Step 1: 2011.* New York: McGraw-Hill, 2011: 415.)

What are the typical CSF findings in this condition?

Oligoclonal bands are seen in 85%–95% of cases. The presence of these immunoglobulins reflects the autoimmune nature of the disease. Oligoclonal bands are not specific to MS and can be elevated in Lyme disease, lupus, syphilis, Sjögren syndrome, and neurosarcoidosis. Similarly, the **IgG index** is elevated in > 90% of patients with definite MS. The total CSF WBC count is normal in most patients, but an elevated WBC count is nonspecific.

What is the likely finding on imaging of the brain?

Multiple **demyelinating plaques** are usually present in the brains of patients with MS, especially in the periventricular region, corpus callosum, and centrum semiovale.

What are the appropriate treatments for this condition?

Acute attacks are treated with high-dose corticosteroids; however, these drugs do not change the course of the disease. Interferon-β1b is the most common disease-modifying treatment. Supportive care including neurorehabilitation is important in preserving activities of daily living. Interferon-β binds a receptor and induces a transcriptional response that reduces T-cell proliferation and antigen presentation and alters cytokine levels.

■ CASE 24

A 25-year-old woman presents to her physician with difficulty chewing and swallowing food. She also complains of occasional double vision. She states her symptoms are often absent in the morning and appear to worsen as the day progresses.

What is the most likely diagnosis?

Myasthenia gravis. Differential includes Lambert-Eaton syndrome, which is a paraneoplastic syndrome associated with small cell lung cancer involving muscle weakness; however, strength improves if a contraction is maintained. In myasthenia gravis, symptoms worsen as activity progresses. Lambert-Eaton syndrome also typically spares the extraocular muscles.

What patient characteristics are typically associated with this diagnosis?

Myasthenia gravis is more commonly seen in women than in men, and most patients are older than 50 years of age when diagnosed.

What signs and symptoms are commonly associated with this condition?

Patients may present with a variety of findings, including ptosis, diplopia, dysarthria, difficulty chewing, and difficulty swallowing. Proximal muscle weakness is usually greater than distal muscle weakness. Weakness increases with use of the muscles.

What is the pathophysiology of this condition?

Patients develop antibodies against **acetylcholine** receptors. Because of a higher threshold of activation by acetylcholine, signal transmission across the neuromuscular junction is decreased. This process leads to muscle weakness. The Tensilon test assesses the response to edrophonium to distinguish myasthenia gravis from cholinergic crisis; because edrophonium is an anticholinesterase it will improve myasthenia gravis but worsen a cholinergic crisis.

What tumor is commonly associated with this condition?

Myasthenia gravis has been associated with an increased frequency of **thymomas**. It is thought that the thymus is the site of production of autoantibodies against acetylcholine receptors. Even in patients with no thymus neoplasm, **thymectomy** has been shown to improve symptoms in 85% of cases.

What is the appropriate treatment for this condition?

Anticholinesterase drugs are the mainstay of treatment. Pyridostigmine is the most common drug prescribed; however, neostigmine may still be used. Prophylactic thymectomy is indicated in patients younger than 60 years of age. Corticosteroids and azathioprine are used in refractory cases. Plasmapheresis and IVIG can provide temporary relief.

■ CASE 25

A 16-year-old boy presents to his pediatrician with a few months' history of progressive hearing loss in both ears. His deteriorating hearing has been accompanied by ringing in his ears (tinnitus). The pediatrician notices hyperpigmented macules on the patient's arms and legs. MRI of the head is shown in Figure 10-31.

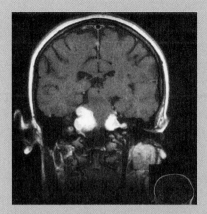

FIGURE 10-31. (Reproduced, with permission, from Riordan-Eva P, et al. *Vaughn & Asbury's General Ophthalmology*, 17th ed. New York: McGraw-Hill, 2008: 301.)

What is the most likely diagnosis?

Neurofibromatosis type 2 (NF2) is an autosomal dominant disorder whose hallmark is bilateral acoustic neuromas. Perforation of the eardrum, ototoxic medication, otosclerosis, or Ménière disease can also cause acquired hearing loss in children.

What is the pathogenesis of this condition?

Mutation of the gene *merlin* found on chromosome **22** (mnemonic: **type 2 = 22**). *Merlin* codes for a protein involved in cytoskeleton components responsible for contact inhibition of tumor progression.

What other signs and symptoms are common in patients with this condition?

Blurry or cloudy vision due to juvenile cataracts is also seen in NF2. Patients may also present with skin findings similar to those seen in neurofibromatosis type 1, such as café-au-lait spots.

What are the two forms of hearing loss?

- **Conductive hearing loss** involves the ear canal, tympanic membrane, middle ear, and ossicles.
- **Sensorineural hearing loss** involves the inner ear (cochlea), vestibulocochlear nerve, or central processing centers in the brain.

How do the Weber and Rinne tests distinguish between the two forms of hearing loss?

In the **Weber** test, a vibrating tuning fork is placed at the center of the patient's cranium. A patient with **unilateral conductive** hearing loss will have lateralization to the **affected ear** (ie, the tone will be louder in the affected ear). A patient with unilateral sensorineural hearing loss will have lateralization to the unaffected ear.

In the **Rinne** test, a vibrating tuning fork is placed on the mastoid process behind the ear (bone conduction; BC) and then next to the external auditory canal (air conduction; AC). Normally AC is greater than BC. A patient with **conductive** hearing loss will "hear" the vibration louder when the tuning fork is on the mastoid process than when it is near the external auditory canal (**BC > AC**). In a patient with sensorineural hearing loss the normal relationship (AC > BC) will be preserved. This patient has **bilateral** sensorineural hearing loss and tests normal in both examinations.

CASE 26

A 66-year-old man presents to his physician with a new-onset tremor in his right hand that worsens when he is sitting down watching television. He also experiences difficulty walking, and his friends complain that he has not been able to keep up with them on the golf course. His wife has noticed that he does not seem to get excited about anything.

What is the most likely diagnosis?

Parkinson disease typically presents with the following symptoms: Tremor that is worse at rest, Rigidity, Akinesia or bradykinesia, and Postural instability (mnemonic: **TRAP**).

What are the Parkinson plus syndromes?

The Parkinson plus syndromes and their associated symptoms are as follows:

- Dementia with Lewy bodies: Fluctuating cognition and visual hallucinations
- Multiple system atrophy: Autonomic instability
- Progressive supranuclear palsy: Early postural instability, loss of voluntary eye movements, and dysarthria
- Corticobasal degeneration: sensory loss, apraxia, aphasia, myoclonus, dementia

What neuropathologic findings are associated with this condition?

Parkinson disease is marked by significant neuronal loss in the **substantia nigra,** which decreases dopaminergic input into the basal ganglia. Characteristic findings include depigmentation of neurons in the substantia nigra and concentric eosinophilic cytoplasmic inclusions called **Lewy bodies** (Figure 10-32).

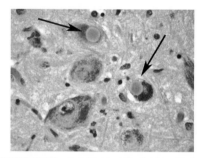

FIGURE 10-32. Lewy bodies in Parkinson disease. (Reproduced, with permission, from USMLERX.com.)

How does a loss of dopamine release from the substantia nigra decrease movement?

Dopamine produced by the substantia nigra activates the direct pathway and inactivates the direct pathway in the basal ganglia. In the direct pathway, dopamine activates the caudate nucleus; this inhibits the globus pallidus internus, which in turn inhibits the ventral lateral thalamus nucleus resulting in frontal motor stimulation. In the indirect pathway, dopamine inhibits the caudate, which inhibits the globus pallidus externus, which in turn inhibits the subthalamic nucleus resulting in stimulation of the globus pallidus internus (the opposite end result as the direct pathway) (Figure 10-33). In both, decreased dopamine results in inhibition of the frontal motor cortex and bradykinesia.

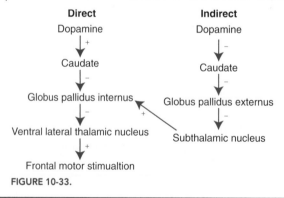

FIGURE 10-33.

What symptoms are likely to develop over time in this patient?

As the disease progresses, shuffling gait, masked facies, and dementia are likely to occur.

What are the appropriate treatments for this condition?

Carbidopa can be used with levodopa to treat Parkinson disease. Carbidopa, a peripheral dopa decarboxylase inhibitor, reduces peripheral conversion of levodopa. This augments its action in the central nervous system and reduces its action outside the central nervous system (where levodopa can cause arrhythmias and dyskinesias). Pramipexole and bromocriptine, which are direct dopaminergic agonists, can also be used to augment dopamine signaling. Catechol-*O*-methyltransferase increases the half-life of Sinemet. Anticholinergic drugs, amantadine, and monoamine oxidase-B inhibitors are also used in Parkinson disease.

What other etiologies might result in a similar presentation?

Typical antipsychotic agents have antidopaminergic activity. Thus, patients taking these medications for schizophrenia can exhibit Parkinson-like symptoms. 1-Methyl-4-phenyl-1,2,3,6-tetrahydropyridine and antiemetic agents can also induce Parkinson-like symptoms.

■ CASE 27

A 36-year-old woman presents to her primary care physician with a 6-month history of occasional milky discharge from her breasts, chronic headaches, and decreased libido. Her past medical history reveals long-standing amenorrhea and infertility. The patient denies any visual disturbances. Laboratory tests reveal a negative urine pregnancy test, a normal thyroid-stimulating hormone level, and a prolactin level of 88 µg/L (normal 5–20 µg/L).

What is the most likely diagnosis?

Hyperprolactinemia from a prolactin-secreting anterior pituitary adenoma. Classic symptoms in females are amenorrhea, infertility, and galactorrhea.

What class of drugs can cause this condition?

Hyperprolactinemia also occurs in patients on antipsychotic medication. Because dopamine inhibits prolactin production, the dopamine inhibitors cause hyperprolactinemia.

What is the differential diagnosis of a mass in the sella turcica?

The differential diagnosis includes pituitary adenoma, pituitary hyperplasia, craniopharyngioma, meningioma, germ cell tumor, chordoma, primary lymphoma, cyst, abscess, or arteriovenous fistula of the cavernous sinus.

What is the pathogenesis of elevated prolactin levels in this condition?

Dopamine secreted from the hypothalamus travels to the anterior pituitary where it inhibits prolactin secretion. A mass in the pituitary may compress the infundibulum, causing a "stalk effect," in which dopamine cannot reach its target. Thus, prolactin is continuously secreted. Physiologic hyperprolactinemia may occur during **pregnancy**. Pregnancy must always be ruled out in any female who presents with amenorrhea.

What other hormones are secreted from the anterior pituitary?

Adrenocorticotropic hormone, thyroid-stimulating hormone, growth hormone, luteinizing hormone, and follicle-stimulating hormone are also secreted. Although prolactinomas are the most common hyperfunctioning tumor, a pituitary adenoma may secrete any of the above hormones.

What is the appropriate treatment for this condition?

Reduction in tumor size, suppression of prolactin secretion, and return of menses are usually accomplished with a dopamine agonist such as **bromocriptine** or cabergoline. Both are ergot derivatives that act directly on dopamine receptors in the hypothalamus to decrease prolactin secretion. When medical management is no longer effective or the mass is very large, transsphenoidal surgery with resection of a large hyperfunctioning sellar mass is typically indicated.

What visual disturbance is classically seen with this condition?

Bitemporal hemianopia results when the growing pituitary tumor impinges on the optic chiasm (Figure 10-34).

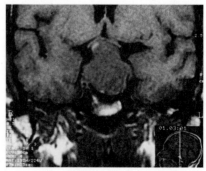

FIGURE 10-34. Pituitary adenoma. MRI showing a pituitary mass elevating the optic chiasm, causing bitemporal hemianopia. (Reproduced, with permission, from Riordan-Eva P, et al. *Vaughn & Asbury's General Ophthalmology*, 17th ed. New York: McGraw-Hill, 2008: 280.)

CASE 28

An emergency medical team is called to help a 60-year-old woman with small cell lung cancer who is unconscious at work. Her coworkers state that for about10 seconds before she lost consciousness, she pointed to her right hand as it began twitching rhythmically, then stiffened every muscle and fell down. After about 15 seconds, she became incontinent and her arms and legs began jerking rhythmically. She then was still, unresponsive, and unconscious for about 3 minutes. The medical team notes she is now breathing deeply but remains unresponsive.

What is the most likely diagnosis?

Seizure. Involvement of the left motor cortex is implicated because the seizure started with right-handed motor activity. In this patient a metastasis is the likely culprit. Seizures can also be caused by infection, ischemia, drug exposure or withdrawal, certain ion imbalances including hypoglycemia and hyponatremia, and trauma.

How is this condition classified?

This is a simple partial seizure with motor signs secondarily generalizing into a tonic-clonic seizure. During the first 10 seconds, the patient maintained consciousness, pointing to a **simple seizure** (complex seizures require a loss of consciousness). After the first 10 seconds, her simple partial seizure evolved into a generalized tonic-clonic seizure. The **tonic phase** is characterized by the immobile contraction of all muscles, and the **clonic phase** is characterized by the bilateral rhythmic jerking of the extremities.

Why is the patient breathing deeply after her incident?

The patient is likely responding to acidosis. A **respiratory acidosis** can develop from the loss of coordinated respirations during the seizure, and a **metabolic acidosis** can develop as muscles contract under anaerobic conditions and produce lactic acid.

What is the appropriate treatment for this condition?

Popular antiseizure medications include valproic acid, phenytoin, phenobarbital, primidone, and carbamazepine. Many antiseizure medications work by enhancing γ-aminobutyric acid (GABA) binding on chloride channels. GABA binding allows chloride ions to flow into neurons, thereby inhibiting neuronal firing. Barbiturates act on the same chloride channels and enhance GABA signaling by increasing the **duration** of chloride channel opening. Benzodiazepines act on the same channels and enhance GABA signaling, but they do so by increasing the **frequency** of chloride channel opening.

What are the most common adverse effects of treatment?

Adverse effects of seizure treatments are as follows:

- Valproate: Hepatotoxicity, neutropenia, thrombocytopenia, teratogenicity (neural tube defects in the fetus).
- Carbamazepine: Hepatotoxicity (check liver function), aplastic anemia, agranulocytosis.
- Phenytoin: Gingival hyperplasia, teratogenicity.
- Ethosuximide and lamotrigine: Stevens-Johnson syndrome (a bullous form of erythema multiforme that involves mucous membranes and large areas of the body).
- Carbamazepine and phenobarbital: Induction of cytochrome P450, resulting in drug interactions.

▌CASE 29

A 72-year-old woman is at home with her husband when he notices she sounds confused even though she had been speaking clearly just moments before. He brings her into the emergency department, where she is unable to follow commands. Her speech is fluent but does not make any sense. CT scan of the head is shown in Figure 10-35.

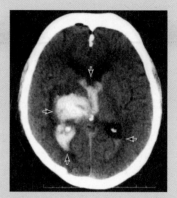

FIGURE 10-35. (Reproduced, with permission, from Aminoff MJ, et al. *Clinical Neurology*, 6th ed. New York: McGraw-Hill, 2005: 315.)

What is the most likely diagnosis?

Stroke. Figure 10-35 shows extensive hemorrhage in the thalamus (left arrow) and its extension into the third (top arrow), ipsilateral (bottom arrow), and lateral (right arrow) ventricles.

What risk factors are associated with this condition?

- Advanced age.
- Cardiovascular disease.
- Carotid disease.
- Diabetes mellitus.
- Dyslipidemia.
- Family or personal history of transient ischemic attack or stroke.
- Hypertension.
- Smoking.

What type of aphasia does the patient exhibit?

The combination of fluent but nonsensical speech and poor comprehension is characteristic of **Wernicke aphasia** (sensory aphasia). These patients also display poor repetition and naming ability. Other findings commonly associated with Wernicke aphasia include contralateral visual field cut (due to ischemia of optic radiation) and **anosognosia** (unawareness of one's deficit).

A lesion in what anatomic area causes these findings?

Wernicke aphasia is usually the result of ischemia in the superior temporal gyrus, which is supplied by the inferior division of the left middle cerebral artery.

What speech pattern results when this condition affects the inferior frontal gyrus?

The inferior frontal gyrus controls motor aspects of speech. A stroke in this area causes **Broca aphasia** (motor aphasia), which is characterized by nonfluent, agrammatic speech. Because of the proximity of the primary motor cortex for the face and arm, **dysarthria** (difficulty in articulating words) and right face and arm weakness are often associated with Broca aphasia. Comprehension is intact in these patients.

If the patient had nail-bed hemorrhages, nodules on her fingers and toes, and retinal hemorrhages, what diagnosis should be considered?

This constellation of symptoms suggests **infective endocarditis,** which is characterized by splinter hemorrhages, Osler nodes on the pads of the fingers and toes, and Roth spots on the retina. Infective endocarditis can lead to the release of thrombi from the valvular vegetations, resulting in embolic events.

■ CASE 30

A 35-year-old woman presents to the emergency department complaining of back pain. Six years ago, she was diagnosed with a 2.5-cm primary breast tumor with metastases to one axillary lymph node. At that time, she underwent a mastectomy and adjuvant chemotherapy. She had been feeling well until 3 months ago, when she began to develop back pain. The pain has become progressively worse, particularly when she lies down. She also notes some weakness in both legs but no leg pain. She denies fever, night sweats, weight loss, or headache. Physical examination reveals no cervical lymphadenopathy; 4/5 muscle strength in the lower extremities bilaterally; normal pain, vibration, and position sensation; 3+ patellar reflexes bilaterally; a positive Babinski reflex on the right; and normal anal sphincter tone.

What are common causes of back pain?

Common causes of back pain include the following:

- Musculoskeletal conditions (eg, muscle strain, osteoarthritis, compression fracture, or ankylosing spondylitis).
- Disk herniation.
- Metastases.
- Osteomyelitis.
- Referred pain from visceral disease (eg, gallstones or kidney stones, pancreatitis, or aortic aneurysm).

What is the most likely cause of this patient's back pain?

The patient's history of breast cancer raises concern for the development of metastases resulting in epidural **spinal cord compression.** Her leg weakness, hyperreflexia, and positive Babinski signs indicate upper motor neuron lesions, which are likely the cause of her weakness as well. Her pain at rest and lack of sciatica argue against disk herniation.

How do signs of upper motor neuron lesions contrast with those of lower motor neuron lesions?

As in this patient, upper motor neuron lesions are characterized by spastic paralysis, hyperreflexia, and a positive Babinski sign. By contrast, lower motor neuron lesions are associated with flaccid paralysis, muscle atrophy, muscle fasciculations and fibrillations, and hyporeflexia.

What are the most common metastases to bone?

The most common sources of bone metastases are cancers of the breast, prostate, lung, and kidney (renal cell carcinoma).

What are the appropriate treatments for this condition?

Treatment options include steroids such as dexamethasone, radiation therapy, and surgical decompression. Spinal cord compression is an oncologic emergency because neurologic dysfunction, if present, may become permanent if it is not immediately addressed.

■ CASE 31

A mother brings a 14-month-old girl to the neurologist for evaluation of new-onset seizures and right-sided hemiparesis. The infant has a purple-red superficial skin lesion distributed on the right forehead and upper eyelid. The infant has also failed to meet developmental milestones for her age.

What is the most likely diagnosis?

Sturge-Weber syndrome is a rare neurocutaneous congenital disorder with unknown etiology. The disorder manifests vascular malformations of the skin (**port-wine stain**; see Figure 10-36) and leptomeninges (leptomeningeal angiomatosis).

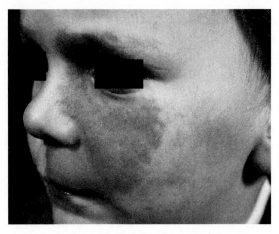

FIGURE 10-36. This young child has a port-wine stain in the distribution of the second branch of the trigeminal nerve. Patients with Sturge-Weber syndrome usually have port-wine stains on the forehead in the distribution of the **first** branch of the trigeminal nerve. (Reproduced, with permission, from Wolff K, et al. *Fitzpatrick's Color Atlas & Synopsis of Clinical Dermatology*, 5th ed. New York: McGraw-Hill, 2005: 187.)

What other tests or imaging tools can be used to confirm the diagnosis?

MRI is most useful for identifying a leptomeningeal angioma. Often, these tumors are ipsilateral to the port-wine stain. These lesions are responsible for the seizures, hemiparesis, and mental retardation in Sturge-Weber syndrome.

What ocular features may be present in this condition?

Many patients may also have **glaucoma. Heterochromia** of the iris (different-colored irises), visual field defects, and vascular malformations of the choroid may also be present.

What is the appropriate treatment for this condition?

Treatment is aimed at alleviating symptoms. Port-wine stains may be treated with laser therapy. Seizures can be managed with anticonvulsants. Patients with seizures refractory to pharmacotherapy may undergo surgical resection of the lesion, often involving a hemispherectomy of the affected side.

CASE 32

A 44-year-old woman with a history of hypertension presents to her physician with a severe headache. She says it is the most painful headache she has ever experienced. The headache began this morning while she was eating breakfast. Since then she has had two episodes of vomiting but denies abdominal pain or nausea. She denies any traumatic events. Cardiac examination reveals a midsystolic click with a late systolic murmur at the apex. CT scan of the head is shown in Figure 10-37.

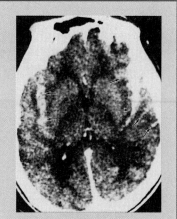

FIGURE 10-37. (Reproduced, with permission, from Waxman SG. *Clinical Neuroanatomy*, 25th ed. New York: McGraw-Hill, 2003: 186.)

What is the most likely diagnosis?

Subarachnoid hemorrhage (arrows in Figure 10-37). The classic presentation is a complaint of "the worst headache in my life" after a "thunderclap" sensation marking the onset of severe pain. Hypertension is the most common risk factor.

What are some common etiologies of this condition?

Most spontaneous subarachnoid hemorrhages occur as the result of the rupture of a **berry aneurysm** in the **circle of Willis.** Other causes are trauma or an arteriovenous malformation. The risk is increased by a history of hypertension. The most common location of a berry aneurysm is the anterior communicating artery, followed by the posterior communicating artery and then the middle cerebral artery.

Given this patient's symptoms, what is the pathophysiology of this condition?

The murmur on cardiac examination is characteristic of mitral valve prolapse, which is commonly seen in **Marfan syndrome.** Berry aneurysms have been associated with Marfan syndrome, Ehlers-Danlos syndrome, adult polycystic kidney disease, and coarctation of the aorta.

What are the typical findings from CT scan of the head and CSF analysis?

After a subarachnoid hemorrhage, CT scan of the head will show blood, in the subarachnoid space if the scan is performed within 24 hours of the bleed. The diagnostic finding in the CSF is xanthochromia, a yellow supernatant caused by bilirubin release from the breakdown of hemoglobin. There may also be gross blood in the fluid, but since this can also be due to a traumatic tap it is not considered a diagnostic finding unless there is a steady elevation in CSF red blood cell count over subsequent lumbar punctures.

Why was the patient vomiting?

Vomiting is a common sign of increased intracerebral pressure, which, in this patient, is secondary to the hemorrhage.

What is an important short-term sequela for patients with this condition?

Patients who have recently suffered a subarachnoid hemorrhage are prone to cerebral vasospasm, especially during the first week after the hemorrhage. Prophylaxis is typically achieved with nimodipine, a calcium channel blocker that improves outcomes in SAH.

▌CASE 33

A 73-year-old man falls while climbing the stairs to his apartment. He temporarily loses consciousness and awakens with a mild headache. His relatives do not notice any problems until 3 days later, when they begin to see a change in his mental status. Typically a pleasant man, he starts to yell at his family members for no reason. He does not recognize people he knows well. He is brought to the emergency department where a CT scan of the head is obtained (Figure 10-38).

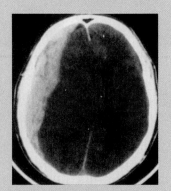

FIGURE 10-38. (Reproduced, with permission, from Aminoff MJ, et al. *Clinical Neurology*, 6th ed. New York: McGraw-Hill, 2005: 329.)

What is the most likely diagnosis?

The temporary loss of consciousness followed by gradual mental status change over the course of days or even weeks is the classic history of a **subdural hematoma**. The diagnosis is confirmed by CT scan, which shows a crescent-shaped area of hemorrhage that **crosses** cranial suture lines (Figure 10-38).

What is the source of bleeding in this type of injury?

Subdural hematomas result from head trauma that causes venous bleeding, most commonly from rupture of bridging veins within the dura, which then bleed into the space between the arachnoid and dura mater. The elderly and alcoholics are more prone to subdural hemorrhage due to cortical atrophy and subsequent increased tension on the bridging veins.

What explains the delayed onset of symptoms?

Venous bleeding results in a slowly expanding blood accumulation and gradual compression of the cerebrum. Symptoms result from the compression of cortical and subcortical structures and therefore are variably delayed depending on when specific intracranial areas are affected by the compression.

What is a CT scan likely to show if the patient experienced no loss of consciousness, followed shortly thereafter by mental status changes?

An immediate "lucid interval," or temporary conscious state, after a head trauma followed by rapid decline in function is more consistent with an **epidural hematoma**. Unlike subdural hematomas, epidural hematomas are due to arterial bleeding and thus cause a dramatic decline in mental status after an initial period of intact function. The CT scan of an epidural hematoma (Figure 10-39) shows a subosteal blood accumulation in the shape of a biconcave disk that **does not** cross suture lines.

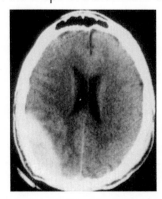

FIGURE 10-39. **Epidural hematoma.** (Reproduced, with permission, from Aminoff MJ, et al. *Clinical Neurology*, 6th ed. New York: McGraw-Hill, 2005: 329.)

What is the appropriate treatment for this condition?

Treatment for both acute subdural and epidural hematomas is decompression and evacuation of the blood via a craniotomy.

■ CASE 34

A 61-year-old man with a history of chronic diarrhea presents to the emergency department after fainting. He reports that he suddenly collapsed after getting up to go to the bathroom. He did not note any prodromal symptoms or vertigo. The patient has spent the past few days recovering from the flu, during which time he has had a poor appetite. He denies a history of seizures and has no known cardiac or valvular abnormalities. On admission, his blood pressure is 115/80 mm Hg supine and 90/70 mm Hg standing. His pulse is 88/min supine and 106/min standing. His respiratory rate is 20/min.

What are the most common causes of syncope?

The primary differential for syncope is divided into cardiogenic and noncardiogenic causes. Cardiogenic causes include arrhythmias, aortic stenosis, tamponade, and aortic dissection. Noncardiogenic causes include orthostatic hypotension and vasovagal, or neurogenic, syncope, which is a reflex drop in blood pressure caused by activation of the vagus nerve.

What is the most likely cause of syncope in this patient?

The most likely cause of syncope in this patient is orthostatic hypotension. Orthostatic hypotension is defined as a 20 mm Hg drop in systolic blood pressure or a 10 mm Hg drop in diastolic blood pressure from supine to standing position. When it is due to volume depletion, the postural hypotension is often accompanied by an increase in pulse rate > 20/min. Orthostatic hypotension in this patient is secondary to poor food and water intake and chronic diarrhea leading to volume depletion.

What signs of volume depletion are evident on physical examination?

Orthostatic hypotension, tachycardia, tachypnea, dry mucous membranes, and decreased skin turgor are signs of volume depletion evident on physical examination.

What common chronic disease can be associated with this condition?

Late-stage diabetes mellitus can be associated with orthostatic hypotension. This is due to autonomic neuropathy and is one of the microvascular complications of diabetes mellitus. The autonomic nervous system dysfunction causes a diminished compensatory response to decreased blood pressure.

How does the vascular system normally compensate for the decrease in venous return following an orthostatic change?

Mechanoreceptors in the heart react to the decrease in blood pressure and compensate by increasing sympathetic tone, decreasing vagal tone and causing release of antidiuretic hormone. This results in increased peripheral vascular resistance (increasing venous return) and an increase in cardiac output, thereby minimizing the drop in blood pressure.

■ CASE 35

A 57-year-old obese, right-handed man with a history of atrial fibrillation and mitral valve repair is brought to the emergency department by a coworker, who noticed a sudden onset of slurred speech and right-hand clumsiness. The coworker denied seeing any seizure-like activity or loss of consciousness. The patient can converse appropriately and denies any recent head trauma. Physical examination reveals an irregularly irregular heartbeat and a left carotid bruit. Neurologic examination reveals grossly intact cranial nerves with the exception of mildly decreased facial sensation on the right. He has 4/5 muscle strength and diminished sensation in the right arm. CT scan of the head is negative for bleeding or mass lesion. The patient's symptoms resolve spontaneously within 1 hour of onset.

What is the most likely diagnosis?

Transient ischemic attack (TIA). Classically, TIA has been defined as strokelike symptoms that resolve within 24 hours. However, increasingly sensitive imaging techniques have helped refine the definition of TIA; now it is defined as focal neurologic symptoms that last < 1 hour with no evidence of ischemic changes on radiologic studies.

What is the most likely cause of this patient's condition?

This TIA is most likely caused by an **embolic stroke**, as the patient has several risk factors for emboli:

- Carotid stenosis, usually from atherosclerosis, which can be a source of emboli.
- History of atrial fibrillation, which can predispose to embolus formation.
- Mitral valve repair, which can harbor vegetations that may embolize.

What findings on CT scan of the head suggest the presence of cerebral edema?

Signs of cerebral edema include loss of the gray matter–white matter junction; loss of prominence of sulci; and evidence of a mass effect, such as midline shift, decreased size of the lateral ventricle on the affected side, and uncal herniation.

What is the vascular distribution of the three major vessels supplying the cerebral cortex?

The anterior cerebral, middle cerebral, and posterior cerebral arteries are the three major vessels supplying the cortex. The anterior cerebral artery branches off the internal carotid artery and supplies the medial portion of motor cortex, the sensory cortex, and the majority of the frontal lobe. The middle cerebral artery also stems from the internal carotid artery and supplies the lateral portion of the motor cortex, temporal lobe, and the somatosensory cortex. The posterior cerebral artery stems from the basilar artery and supplies the visual cortex as well as the posterior parietal lobe (Figure 10-40).

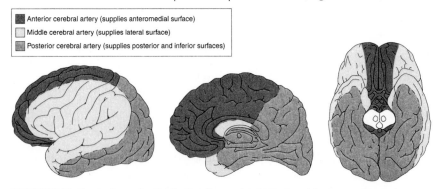

Anterior cerebral artery (supplies anteromedial surface)
Middle cerebral artery (supplies lateral surface)
Posterior cerebral artery (supplies posterior and inferior surfaces)

FIGURE 10-40. Cerebral vascular distribution. The arterial distribution of the three main vessels supplying the cortex. (Reproduced, with permission, from Le T, et al. *First Aid for the USMLE Step 1: 2010.* New York: McGraw-Hill, 2010: 400.)

What findings differentiate strokes due to occlusion of each of the three vessels?

Stroke symptoms correspond to the vascular distribution of each artery. A stroke of the anterior cerebral artery results in lower extremity deficits; a stroke of the middle cerebral artery results in face and upper extremity deficits; and a stroke of the posterior cerebral artery results primarily in visual deficits.

CASE 36

A 6-year-old boy with a history of mental retardation and seizures is brought by his mother to the pediatrician for an evaluation of skin lesions. The pediatrician notes firm, discrete, brown papules in the nasolabial folds and on the cheeks. Further examination reveals an elliptical, hypopigmented macule on the patient's abdomen and a pink-brown plaque with a cobblestone appearance on his lower back. Funduscopic examination reveals a flat, translucent lesion on the left retina.

What is the most likely diagnosis?

Tuberous sclerosis, an autosomal dominant syndrome manifested by numerous benign neoplasms of the brain, skin, heart, and kidney. Tuberous sclerosis demonstrates complete genetic penetrance but highly variable expressivity. Most cases arise from a sporadic mutation, but offspring of an affected individual will inherit the mutation in an autosomal dominant pattern.

What dermatologic and ophthalmic abnormalities are common in this condition?

- **Ash-leaf spots,** which are elliptical hypopigmented macules, may develop. In fair-skinned individuals, they can be visualized with a Wood's lamp (Figure 10-41).
- **Adenoma sebaceum,** which are small angiofibromas typically distributed in a malar fashion on the face, are also seen (Figure 10-42).
- **Shagreen patches,** which are firm, reddish, raised lesions with a leathery texture, are commonly found on the lumbar area of the back.
- **Retinal hamartomas,** which appear as gray or yellow lesions on funduscopic examination, may also be present.

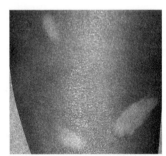

FIGURE 10-41. **Hypopigmented macules, or ash-leaf spots.** (Reproduced, with permission, from Wolff K, et al. *Fitzpatrick's Color Atlas & Synopsis of Clinical Pathology,* 5th ed. New York: McGraw-Hill, 2005: 461.)

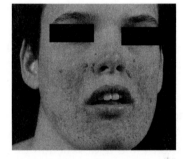

FIGURE 10-42. **Small angiofibromas in a malar pattern known as adenoma sebaceum.** (Reproduced, with permission, from Wolff K, et al. *Fitzpatrick's Color Atlas & Synopsis of Clinical Pathology,* 5th ed. New York: McGraw-Hill, 2005: 462.)

What are the cardiac and renal manifestations of the condition?

Patients classically present with **cardiac rhabdomyomas** that often regress spontaneously in the first few years of life. Renal manifestations include bilateral **angiomyolipomas** and cysts.

What brain lesions are typically seen in people with this condition?

Cortical tubers and subependymal nodules are common, and both are considered **hamartomas.** Subependymal nodules can undergo malignant transformation to subependymal giant cell **astrocytomas.** Consequences of cortical hamartomas are seizures and mental retardation.

What are the two other inheritable neurocutaneous disorders?

- **Neurofibromatosis I** is characterized by café-au-lait spots, neurofibromas on the skin, Lisch nodules, and optic gliomas. This condition is associated with astrocytomas and pheochromocytomas.
- **Von Hippel–Lindau syndrome** is characterized by hemangiomas of the skin and retina, hemangioblastomas in the central nervous system, and bilateral renal cell carcinoma. The inheritance pattern for all three conditions is **autosomal dominant.**

■ CASE 37

A 14-year-old boy is brought to his family physician complaining of weakness of his left hand and wrist for 2 days. He is a varsity tennis player and has been having difficulty playing and complains of a burning sensation in the fourth and fifth fingers of his left hand. He says he woke up 2 days ago with the change in sensation and strength after falling asleep with his left arm over the side of his bed. Physical examination reveals no evidence of fracture, but there is significant edema of his elbow and weakness of the medial digits of the left hand.

What is the most likely diagnosis?

Ulnar neuropathy due to nerve compression. Ulnar nerve injuries often present with acute onset of numbness/tingling in the fourth and fifth digits and weakness of wrist and fourth/fifth finger flexion. If severe, ulnar injury can present as a partial clawlike deformity known as the "Pope's blessing" (Figure 10-43).

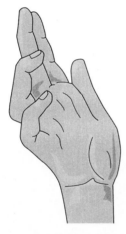

FIGURE 10-43. **Ulnar claw.** Extension of the fourth and fifth *metacarpophalangeal* joints with flexion of the interphalangeal joints. Distal ulnar nerve lesion. (Reproduced, with permission, from Le T, et al. *First Aid for the USMLE Step 1: 2011.* New York: McGraw-Hill, 2011: 375.)

What are the most common causes of this condition?

Injuries that cause ulnar neuropathy include direct trauma or prolonged pressure on the nerve. Symptoms occur when there is destruction of the myelin sheath or damage to axons sufficient to hinder nerve conduction. The most common site of ulnar nerve injury is at the elbow, because the nerve lies superficially in the groove between the medial epicondyle and the olecranon. A blow to the medial epicondyle often hits the nerve, causing tingling in the territory of the ulnar nerve and the so-called funny bone sensation.

What is the primary diagnosis to consider in the differential?

Medial epicondylitis, or "golfer's elbow," is an overuse injury affecting the muscle origins at the medial epicondyle, often due to repetitive swinging motions at the elbow joint. It causes medial elbow pain. It can result in irritation of the ulnar nerve.

What treatment is used to reduce the swelling at the elbow?

Anti-inflammatory agents such as corticosteroids and nonsteroidal anti-inflammatory drugs are used to treat ulnar neuropathy due to nerve compression and medial epicondylitis. Patients can also benefit from braces or casts that reduce movement at the elbow joint to decrease chronic inflammation.

■ CASE 38

A 72-year-old man with a history of coronary artery disease, diabetes, and hypertension is brought to the primary care physician by his wife. She reports a stepwise decline in her husband's function over the past year, beginning with lapses in memory, then subtle personality changes, and now difficulty talking. MRI scan of the head is shown in Figure 10-44.

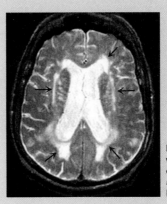

FIGURE 10-44. (Reproduced, with permission, from Kasper DL, et al. *Harrison's Principles of Internal Medicine*, 16th ed. New York: McGraw-Hill, 2005: 2401.)

What is the most likely diagnosis?

Multi-infarct dementia, also known as vascular dementia. Vascular dementia is the second most common cause of dementia after Alzheimer disease. It can be broadly categorized as either large vessel or small vessel in origin. Large-vessel disease results from recurrent infarctions or hemorrhage in the vessels that supply the cortical territories and is usually due to chronic atherosclerotic disease. It is characterized by a stepwise decline in cognitive, executive, and motor or language function. By contrast, small-vessel disease results from recurrent infarctions in subcortical and white matter regions of the brain and is usually due to poorly controlled hypertension. The stepwise decline in these patients can be subtle and may lack major defining events.

What are the risk factors for this condition?

History of stroke, advanced age, hypertension, vascular disease, diabetes, smoking, and dyslipidemia are all risk factors for vascular dementia. Treatment is aimed at any of these underlying causes. Antiplatelet therapy, especially aspirin and clopidogrel, may be used to prevent further cerebrovascular accidents.

What imaging tools can be used to confirm the diagnosis?

MRI is the best imaging choice to diagnose vascular dementia. The T2-weighted MRI shown in Figure 10-44 of a patient with diffuse white matter disease demonstrates numerous periventricular and corona radiata lesions.

What are the causes of dementia?

The etiologies of dementia can be broadly categorized as reversible or irreversible. The irreversible causes constitute the majority of cases; however, reversible causes should be sought out since treating them can significantly improve the patient's quality of life (Figure 10-45).

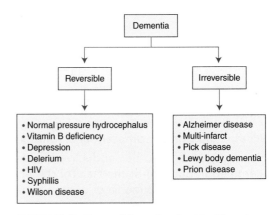

FIGURE 10-45. Causes of dementia categorized by potentially reversible and irreversible etiologies.

What characteristics differentiate delirium from dementia?

Delirium is characterized by an acute, rapid decrease in attention span with a waxing and waning level of consciousness. The patient may be difficult to arouse and classically has changes in mental status with visual hallucinations. The EEG in delirium shows nonspecific slowing. By contrast, dementia is more gradual in onset with **no changes in level of consciousness.** The EEG is usually normal in dementia.

■ CASE 39

A 45-year-old female visits her primary care physician because she noticed a sudden loss of hearing in her right ear. She says it started just a few days ago, but she does not recall any trauma or inciting event. She does not take any medications but says she was hospitalized 1 month ago for a serious urinary tract infection requiring some "powerful antibiotics." On further questioning, she also notes an increased sensation of ringing in her right ear. Otologic examination reveals a translucent, pink-gray tympanic membrane on the right. Weber testing lateralizes to the left ear. Rinne testing bilaterally reveals that air conduction is louder than bone conduction.

What is the most likely diagnosis?

This patient has sensorineural hearing loss. The recent hospital course suggests antibiotics, most commonly aminoglycosides, as the likely culprit. Sensorineural hearing loss is often associated with tinnitus. The otologic examination reveals a normal external ear canal and visualizes a normal tympanic membrane on the affected side. Weber testing lateralizes to the opposite ear, whereas Rinne testing in the affected ear is normal.

What is the mechanism underlying the findings on Weber and Rinne testing?

In sensorineural hearing loss, the cochlea or CN VIII is damaged. This means that sound signal does not transmit appropriately into the CNS; the result is hearing loss on the affected side. **Weber testing** is conducted by placing a vibrating tuning fork in the center of the patient's forehead and asking whether the volume is different between the two ears. In sensorineural hearing loss, Weber testing lateralizes to the opposite side because of normal sound signal to CNS transmission contralaterally (Figure 10-46A).

Rinne testing compares air conduction with mastoid bone conduction of sound. The vibrating tuning fork is placed just outside the external ear canal and then on the mastoid bone, and the patient is asked to identify which location produces a louder perception of sound (Figure 10-46B). There is no obstruction of air conduction in sensorineural hearing loss, so Rinne test results in a louder perception of sound through air conduction (as is the case in normal hearing function).

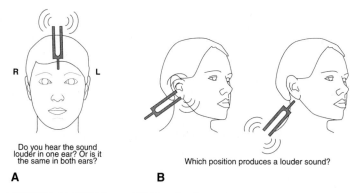

A Do you hear the sound louder in one ear? Or is it the same in both ears?

B Which position produces a louder sound?

FIGURE 10-46. (A) Weber and (B) Rinne hearing testing.

What is the primary differential diagnosis of this patient's hearing loss?

Hearing loss can also be conductive in nature. This occurs when there is an obstruction of the ear canal (cerumen impaction) or mechanical dysfunction of the middle ear apparatus (due to an inflammatory process such as otitis media or otitis externa) that helps transmit sound waves to the cochlea.

What would the Weber and Rinne tests find in conductive hearing loss?

In conductive hearing loss, the Weber test lateralizes to the affected ear. This is due to the reverberation and accentuation of sound caused by entrapment of sound waves behind the occlusion or site of dysfunction. The Rinne test results in greater bone conduction of sound in the affected ear because air conduction is obstructed.

CASE 40

A 14-year-old boy is sent to the emergency department by the nurse at his summer camp after he experienced a 1-minute seizure earlier that day. The boy has no previous history of seizure activity. In the ED, the boy complains of lethargy, vomiting, myalgia, severe headache, and neck stiffness. On further questioning, he reveals that he has had many of these symptoms for the past few days. A lumbar puncture is performed, and a Gram stain of the CSF is negative. The cells found in the boy's CSF are shown in Figure 10-47.

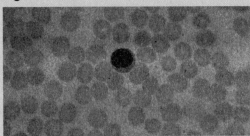

FIGURE 10-47. (Reproduced, with permission, from Berman I. *Color Atlas of Basic Histology*, 3rd ed. New York: McGraw-Hill, 2003: 107.)

What is the most likely diagnosis?

This presentation likely represents a viral meningitis.

What organisms are most likely to cause this condition?

The most common causative organism of viral meningitis is **echovirus**, which is part of the Enterovirus subgroup of the Picornaviridae family. Enterovirus outbreaks tend to occur during the summer and are often associated with summer camps. Other causative organisms include coxsackievirus (another enterovirus), adenovirus, HIV, cytomegalovirus, Epstein-Barr virus, and herpes simplex virus.

Detecting enteroviruses with polymerase chain reaction (PCR) assay requires modifying the standard PCR strategy. What type of enzyme is essential to this modification?

Reverse transcriptase is essential in this modified PCR. Because enteroviruses are RNA viruses, detection proceeds with reverse transcription PCR (RT-PCR). Normal transcription is the synthesis of RNA from DNA; this process is the **reverse**. Viral RNA is reverse transcribed into the complementary DNA (cDNA), and that cDNA can then be amplified using the standard PCR DNA amplification strategy.

What changes in this patient's CSF glucose and protein levels are most likely to be seen?

As with most cases of viral meningitis, CSF glucose concentration is typically normal (two-thirds of plasma glucose level) and CSF protein concentration is typically normal to slightly increased. CSF cell count reveals a lymphocytosis. This is in contrast to CSF findings in bacterial meningitis, in which protein is increased glucose is decreased and CSF cell count reveals a predominance of polymorphonuclear leukocytes (Table 3-1 in Chapter 3 for a comparison of CSF findings in bacterial, viral, and fungal meningitis).

Some viruses capable of causing this patient's symptoms are sensitive to acyclovir. What is the mechanism of action of this drug?

Acyclovir targets viral DNA polymerase. Herpesviruses are DNA viruses that are sensitive to acyclovir because they contain the viral thymidine kinase required to phosphorylate acyclovir. The phosphorylated acyclovir is a nucleic acid analog and will then be incorporated by viral DNA polymerase, disrupting replication. Picornaviruses, however, are RNA viruses that do not contain DNA polymerase, and therefore they are not sensitive to acyclovir.

What type of cell is shown in Figure 10-47?

The cell is a **lymphocyte**, which is characterized by its small size; most of the cell volume is occupied by the darkly stained and round nucleus. Lymphocytes play a key role in cellular immunity, particularly in combating infection. Lymphocytosis of the CSF is common in viral meningitis.

▮ CASE 41

A 26-year-old man is evaluated by a neurologist for recurrent headaches and changes in vision. A careful ophthalmologic examination reveals multiple groups of dilated blood vessels on both retinas, and an MRI of the brain demonstrates three hemangioblastomas of the cerebellum.

What is the most likely diagnosis?

Von Hippel–Lindau (VHL) disease is characterized by diffuse hemangioma formation, commonly in the retina and central nervous system, as well as by an increased incidence of renal cell carcinoma (RCC).

What is the pattern of inheritance for this condition?

VHL disease is inherited in an autosomal dominant fashion in 75% of cases. It is associated with deletion of the *VHL* gene, a tumor suppressor gene on the short arm of chromosome 3. Approximately 25% of cases occur sporadically. In the United States, the incidence of VHL disease is approximately 1:36,000.

What is the pathophysiology underlying the formation of hemangiomas in this condition?

One of the main functions of VHL protein is to regulate the activity of a transcription factor known as hypoxia-induced factor 1a (HIF1a). HIF1a activation induces the transcription of vascular endothelial growth factor (VEGF), which is responsible for the process of neovascularization. As its name suggests, HIF1a activation occurs under hypoxic conditions to facilitate the growth of new blood vessels in response to low oxygen levels. The VHL protein, as a tumor suppressor gene product, facilitates degradation of HIF1a in the presence of oxygen to restrict unnecessary neovascularization. However, the mutations in VHL disease cause HIF1a to be constitutively active. This causes the overproduction of VEGF and the formation hemangiomas.

What is the leading cause of death in patients with this condition?

RCC, predominantly the clear cell type, is the leading cause of death in patients with VHL; some case series report prevalence rates as high as 40%–75% at autopsy. In patients with VHL, RCC develops from malignant degeneration of renal cysts and is usually bilateral. The average age for development of RCC in patients with VHL is 44 years. Because of the high incidence of renal cysts and RCC in patients with VHL, periodic imaging of the kidneys is indicated in patients and at-risk relatives.

What other tumors or lesions are associated with this condition?

Patients with VHL disease are at risk for developing multiple cysts in the liver, epididymis, pancreas, and kidneys. Pheochromocytomas, rare pancreatic carcinomas, and endolymphatic sac tumors are also within the spectrum of VHL. Hemangioblastomas are typically in the cerebellum or medulla but may also occur in the spinal cord. In a significant number of patients, the hemangioblastomas release erythropoietin; these patients can present with polycythemia. Hemangiomas of the skin, mucous membranes, and retina are common.

■ CASE 42

A 55-year-old man is brought to the emergency department by a friend who has noticed that the patient has had memory lapses and difficulty with walking and balance. The patient has a 26-year history of excessive alcohol use. On further questioning, the patient is unable to provide a consistent history. When asked about his location, the patient states he is at home. Physical examination reveals nystagmus in the left eye and an ataxic gait.

What is the most likely diagnosis?

Excessive alcohol abuse is the primary culprit of **Wernicke-Korsakoff syndrome.** Wernicke encephalopathy presents as the triad of **nystagmus,** ataxia, and confusion. This may progress to Korsakoff syndrome, which consists of irreversible memory loss, confabulation, and personality changes.

What type of memory deficit is likely to be seen in this condition?

Patients with Wernicke-Korsakoff syndrome usually suffer from **anterograde amnesia,** which is characterized by an inability to form new memories but a general preservation of long-term memories. This is in contrast to **retrograde amnesia,** in which only long-term memories that precede the precipitating event are lost.

What is the pathophysiology of this condition?

This disease is seen in alcoholics with thiamine deficiency due to poor nutrition and absorption. Thiamine deficiency results in degeneration in a symmetric pattern in multiple cerebral areas, including the cerebellum, brain stem, and bilateral mammillary bodies (Figure 10-48; arrows show abnormal enhancement of the mammillary bodies).

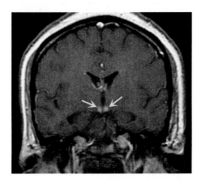

FIGURE 10-48. MRI of mammillary bodies in Wernicke encephalopathy. (Reproduced, with permission, from Kasper DL, et al. *Harrison's Principles of Internal Medicine*, 16th ed. New York: McGraw-Hill, 2005: 1636.)

For which essential biochemical pathways is thiamine required?

Thiamine (vitamin B_1) is needed in glycolysis as a cofactor for pyruvate dehydrogenase; in the tricarboxylic acid cycle as a cofactor for α-ketoglutarate dehydrogenase; in the hexose monophosphate shunt as a cofactor for transketolase; and in the breakdown of amino acids as a cofactor for branched-chain amino acid dehydrogenase.

What complication must be prevented when treating an alcoholic patient who is severely hypoglycemic and confabulating?

Glucose repletion in an alcoholic patient must always be accompanied by thiamine administration. Since thiamine is a cofactor in glycolysis, administration of glucose further depletes thiamine stores. This can lead to worsening of the Wernicke-Korsakoff syndrome.

What other disease can result from thiamine deficiency?

Beriberi is also caused by a deficiency of thiamine secondary to malnutrition. There are two forms of beriberi: dry and wet. Dry beriberi is characterized by peripheral neuropathy and symmetrical muscle wasting due to axonal loss. Wet beriberi is characterized by edema and high-output cardiac failure due to dilated cardiomyopathy.

11

Psychiatry

■ CASE 1

A mother brings her 8-year-old son to the pediatrician because she is concerned about his behavior. She states that her son is unable to finish activities at home and is easily distracted. He is unable to sit still long enough to complete his homework and is constantly "bouncing off the walls." The mother has received complaints from school about her son talking back to teachers and interacting poorly with peers. He may have to repeat the third grade.

What is the most likely diagnosis?

Attention deficit/hyperactivity disorder (ADHD). ADHD is estimated to affect up to 8% of U.S. school-age children. Males are more affected than females, and children in North America are diagnosed with ADHD more often than children in other countries.

What are the typical manifestations of this condition?

ADHD is characterized by hyperactivity, impulsivity, and inattention that lead to significant impairment. **Hyperactivity** manifests as fidgetiness and an inability to remain seated or play quietly. **Impulsivity** is displayed as the inability to wait for one's turn, talking when inappropriate, and constantly interrupting. **Inattention** is characterized by forgetfulness, poor concentration, an inability to finish tasks, and a lack of attention to detail. To meet the *Diagnostic and Statistical Manual of Mental Disorders* diagnostic criteria for ADHD, symptoms must be present before the age of 7 years, persist for at least 6 months, and be present in more than one setting (eg, at home and at school).

What are the known risk factors for this condition?

Pregnant women who smoke or use drugs are at increased risk for having children with ADHD. Genetics also plays an important role, as one in four children with ADHD has at least one relative with the condition.

What is the appropriate treatment for this condition?

Treatment includes behavioral interventions, pharmacological therapy, or both. Although it may seem counterintuitive, stimulants have shown great effect in treating patients with ADHD. Stimulants such as methylphenidate and dextroamphetamine act by increasing catecholamine release.

What is the natural course of this condition?

Many patients with ADHD find that they "outgrow" it during adolescence. For a subset of patients, however, the disorder continues into adulthood; these patients benefit from pharmacotherapy.

■ CASE 2

A mother brings her 3-year-old son to the physician because she believes he is not developing normally. She says he does not reach out for her with his arms, show joy, or follow her around like his siblings did. His language development is delayed, and he often mechanically repeats other people. He needs to have everything his way and has many rituals. She says he seems to be in a "world of his own." Testing shows normal hearing and a lower-than-average IQ.

What is the most likely diagnosis?

Autism.

What is the classic triad of findings in this condition?

The triad of impairments in autism is as follows:

- Impairments in social interaction: Decreased awareness of social stimuli, failure to respond to one's name when called, and inability to take turns with others.
- Severe language deficits: Delayed and abnormal speech, poor comprehension, and a tendency to echo questions.
- Repetitive and stereotyped patterns of behavior: examples include hand flapping, body rocking, and marked daily routines (eg, dressing rituals).

What is the epidemiology of this condition?

Autism is relatively rare, with a prevalence of approximately 2 per 1000 children. More common in boys (male-to-female ratio is approximately 4:1), autism presents in early childhood but is a lifelong condition. In addition, up to 70% of autistic children also meet the diagnostic criteria for mental retardation.

What is the etiology of this condition?

Autism is a heterogeneous disorder with a significant, although as yet uncharacterized, genetic component. There is no scientific evidence that vaccination causes autism.

What other conditions should be considered in the differential diagnosis?

Autism is the most severe of the pervasive developmental disorders, which also include Asperger syndrome, Rett disorder, and childhood disintegrative disorder.

- **Asperger syndrome** is a milder form of autism involving repetitive behavior and problems with social relationships. Unlike autistic children, children with Asperger have no cognitive or language delays. They often have stiff, monotonous speech, are clumsy, and express an unusually intense interest in a narrow subject area (eg, molecular structures or weather patterns).
- **Rett disorder** is a genetic syndrome seen in girls and characterized by regression in development at approximately 1 year of age.
- **Childhood disintegrative disorder** is a rare condition characterized by the onset of developmental delays at approximately 3 years of age.

What is the appropriate treatment for this condition?

Behavior therapy and educational interventions can help many autistic individuals reduce maladaptive behaviors and gain greater functional independence.

■ CASE 3

A 22-year-old woman presents to the clinic with an 8-day history of insomnia and increased energy. Her roommate is concerned because the patient has been talking rapidly and loudly. The patient has made several expensive purchases recently and is exhibiting uncharacteristically seductive behavior, dressing inappropriately for class, and drawing attention to herself. She denies substance abuse and urine toxicology screen is negative.

This patient displays symptoms of what category of psychiatric disorders?

This patient's symptoms are within the spectrum of mood disorders; specifically, she manifests symptoms of a manic episode of bipolar disorder. Other disorders in this class include major depressive disorder, dysthymic disorder, and bereavement.

What signs and symptoms are commonly associated with this disorder?

Bipolar disorder is characterized by periods of major **depression** alternating with **mania** or hypomania. Symptoms of mania may include the following:

- Increased goal-directed activity/psychomotor agitation.
- Decreased need for sleep.
- Elevated, expansive, or irritable mood.
- Pressured speech.
- Excessive involvement in pleasurable activities, including spending, gambling, substance use, or sex.

How is this disorder classified?

The *Diagnostic and Statistical Manual of Mental Disorders* requires that three or more of the above symptoms persist for at least 1 week to be classified as a **manic episode**. In addition, the symptoms must be severe enough to cause impairment in daily functioning. **Hypomanic episodes** display a milder variety of manic symptoms, do not cause gross functional impairment, and last only 4 days.

- **Bipolar I:** Distinct manic and depressive syndromes.
- **Bipolar II:** Distinct hypomanic and depressive syndromes.
- **Mixed:** Both manic and depressive symptoms concurrently over a period of time (often described as dysphoric mania or agitated depression).

What are the appropriate treatments for this disorder?

First-line drugs include mood stabilizers (lithium, valproate, or carbamazepine) and antipsychotic agents (olanzapine, haloperidol, or risperidone). Hospitalization may be necessary to ensure patient safety.

CASE 4

A 37-year-old pianist visits her physician because of difficulty sleeping in the past 3 weeks. She wakes up early in the morning, well before the usual time, and cannot get back to sleep. She says she does not enjoy playing the piano as much as she used to and finds it hard to concentrate when she tries to play. She notices a decrease in appetite and has lost 4.5 kg (10 lb) in the past month. On questioning, she reveals she had a similar episode about 1 year ago.

What is the most likely diagnosis?

Major depressive disorder.

What symptoms are commonly associated with this condition?

The diagnosis of major depressive disorder requires two or more episodes of five of the following symptoms, present for at least 2 weeks: **S**leep disturbances, decreased **I**nterest, **G**uilt, decreased **E**nergy, decreased **C**oncentration, change in **A**ppetite (usually decreased), **P**sychomotor retardation, and **S**uicidal ideations (mnemonic: SIG E CAPS) in addition to depressed mood. This patient cannot be diagnosed until additional symptoms are determined.

What other conditions can present with similar symptoms?

Bereavement can present with depressive symptoms within 1 year of the loss of a loved one, but symptoms are related to that loss. Grief is characterized by shock, denial, guilt, and somatic symptoms. Depressive symptoms can also suggest **dysthymia**, a milder form of depression with less intense symptoms that lasts at least 2 years. **Adjustment disorder with depressed mood** also presents as a milder form of depression, but symptoms are usually in response to a significant psychological stressor (eg, marital or financial problems) and usually last less than 6 months.

What is the epidemiology of this condition?

Women are diagnosed with major depression at approximately twice the rate of men. Studies show that living in urban areas, being of lower socioeconomic status, and being married (for women only) are independent risk factors for major depression.

What neurotransmitter disturbances are common in this condition?

Patients with major depressive disorder commonly have decreased levels of serotonin and norepinephrine. Dopamine may also be decreased in major depression.

What are the appropriate treatments for this condition?

Psychotherapy, antidepressants (including selective serotonin reuptake inhibitors, monoamine oxidase inhibitors, and tricyclic antidepressants), or both may be appropriate. Electroconvulsive therapy can be used for major depressive disorder that is refractory to other treatments.

■ CASE 5

A 51-year-old woman presents to her primary care physician because she is disturbingly anxious about everything. She is unable to identify a precipitating event or particular concern. She worries about her family, health, and finances. She has little respite and is frequently irritable, tired, and unable to concentrate. She has been a lifelong "worrier," but the symptoms have become so intense in the past 6 months that she thinks she may have to stop working.

What is the most likely diagnosis?
Generalized anxiety disorder (GAD).

What signs and symptoms are commonly associated with this condition?
The *Diagnostic and Statistical Manual of Mental Disorders* defines the major diagnostic criteria for GAD as excessive and uncontrollable anxiety occurring more days than not for at least 6 months. In addition, the anxiety is not the result of substance abuse and causes clinically significant impairment in social, occupational, or other areas of function. GAD may also be associated with the following symptoms:

- Difficulty concentrating.
- Fatigue.
- Insomnia.
- Irritability.
- Restlessness.

What other conditions should be considered in the differential diagnosis?
"Normal" worry and adjustment disorder should also be considered. Unlike individuals with normal anxiety, patients with GAD have evidence of social dysfunction secondary to the disorder. Adjustment disorder is characterized by emotional symptoms following an identifiable stressor (eg, divorce or loss of a job) and lasts < 6 months. By contrast, symptoms in GAD persist for > 6 months.

What are the appropriate treatments for this condition?
- Antidepressants (selective serotonin reuptake inhibitors).
- Buspirone (a serotonin receptor partial agonist).
- Benzodiazepines (fast-acting sedatives).
- Cognitive-behavioral therapy.

What is the danger of using benzodiazepines to treat this condition?
While benzodiazepines show beneficial effects in the short term, they are not recommended for long-term use, as they are associated with the development of tolerance, physical dependence, withdrawal, and addiction.

▮ CASE 6

A 29-year-old well-groomed man with no medical or psychiatric history consults a psychiatrist for evaluation. He notices that over the past 6 months he has been preoccupied with counting items, such as bricks in his driveway, raisins in his cereal, and tiles in the ceiling. He says he feels compelled to count to the number 30 particularly; for example, he does 30 push-ups in the morning, jogs for 30 minutes, and chews his food 30 times. He has not told anyone about his recent habit and does not believe it is interfering with his work. However, he is troubled by his own behavior and feels unable to stop. During the medical history, the patient reveals his 30th birthday is next week.

What is the most likely diagnosis?

The patient's obsessions (recurrent thoughts) and compulsions (recurrent acts) suggest obsessive-compulsive disorder (OCD). The *Diagnostic and Statistical Manual of Mental Disorders* defines the symptoms of OCD as follows:

- **Obsessions** are recurrent and persistent thoughts, impulses, or images that cause marked distress above and beyond real-life worries. The patient attempts to ignore or suppress them and recognizes that they are a product of the mind.
- **Compulsions** are repetitive behaviors (washing, ordering, checking) or mental acts (praying, counting) that a person is driven to perform in response to an obsession.

What is the epidemiology of this condition?

OCD occurs in approximately 3% of the general population. Males are much more frequently affected than females. The disorder often runs in families and may be associated with tic disorders (eg, Tourette syndrome).

What are the appropriate treatments for this condition?

Selective serotonin reuptake inhibitors and clomipramine are common pharmacologic treatments. Cognitive-behavioral therapy is also used with and without pharmacologic therapy.

What is cognitive-behavioral therapy?

Cognitive-behavioral therapy is a manualized, time-limited type of psychotherapy that seeks to modify a patient's emotions by identifying and adjusting maladaptive thought patterns and beliefs. In this patient, for example, turning 30 may represent the beginning of adulthood and the end to the impulsiveness of youth. The maladaptive thought may be, "If I count to 30, I am in control and an adult." The cognitive component of therapy will challenge this irrational thought. The behavioral component will allow him to combat the need to count or check.

What comorbidities are associated with this condition?

The prevalence of **major depressive disorder** among individuals with OCD is as high as 30%. Panic disorders and social phobia also commonly coexist with OCD.

■ CASE 7

A 48-year-old lawyer visits his physician for a routine physical examination. During the interview, he mentions difficulty at work. He has frequent arguments with his assistant because she cannot carry out tasks, and he constantly has to check on everything she does. He says his coworkers "don't do things the way I tell them to," and he feels he cannot delegate tasks because "they don't do things right." He also admits to frequent arguments with his wife, who does not put things where they are supposed to go. He cannot tolerate disorder. During the office visit, he takes copious notes.

What is the most likely diagnosis?

This patient exhibits traits consistent with obsessive-compulsive personality disorder (OCPD). Personality **traits** are patterns of relating to or thinking about the world that are exhibited in various social and personal contexts. A personality trait becomes a **personality disorder** when the traits are extreme and/or exclude other traits, causing personal distress, problems functioning, and an adverse impact on the social environment. A person is often not aware of maladaptive personality traits.

How are these conditions classified?

The *Diagnostic and Statistical Manual of Mental Disorders* divides personality disorders into three clusters:

- Individuals in **cluster A** are described as odd or eccentric ("weird") and may be diagnosed with paranoid, schizoid, or schizotypal personality disorder.
- Individuals in **cluster B** are described as dramatic, emotional, or erratic ("wild") and may be diagnosed with antisocial, borderline, histrionic, or narcissistic personality disorder.
- Individuals in **cluster C** are described as anxious or fearful ("worried") and may be diagnosed with avoidant personality disorder, dependent personality disorder, or OCPD. (This patient therefore falls into cluster C.)

How is this condition differentiated from obsessive-compulsive disorder?

Obsessive-compulsive disorder (OCD) is a disorder involving obsessions and compulsions, both of which are irresistible and unpleasant to the patient (**egodystonic**). In **OCPD**, patients have a rigid preoccupation with order and control. However, they view their beliefs and behaviors simply as part of who they are (**egosyntonic**).

What is the first-line treatment for this condition?

Both cognitive behavioral therapy and psychodynamic psychotherapy can be useful in patients with OCPD. Medications can be used to treat comorbid conditions like anxiety and depression.

■ CASE 8

A 20-year-old college student complains to her physician of sudden episodes of overwhelming anxiety. The episodes include palpitations, nausea, sweating, breathlessness, and an intense fear of dying. The episodes started about 8 months ago but are increasing in frequency. They begin suddenly at variable times during the day, and she must take deep breaths to calm herself down. The patient is confused and frustrated, and she goes to class only if she can sit in the back so she can leave if an attack occurs.

What is the most likely diagnosis?

Panic disorder.

How are panic attacks related to this condition?

Panic disorder requires repeated **panic attacks** (or episodes) with relevant behaviors or attitudes between attacks, such as worry about not being able to control the panic attacks. Patients tend to avoid situations where panic attacks occur and arrange their lives around fear of having an attack. This can lead to agoraphobia (ie, fear of having a panic attack in a place with no place to hide and no easy means of escape). A panic attack requires the presence of at least four of the following symptoms:

- Palpitations.
- Sweating.
- Trembling.
- Chest pain or discomfort.
- Fear of losing control.
- Fear of dying.
- Chills or hot flashes.

What other conditions must be ruled out before a diagnosis can be made?

Organic causes of symptoms (including tachycardia, hyperthyroidism, hyperparathyroidism, pheochromocytoma, hypoglycemia, seizure, and drug use) must be ruled out before panic disorder can be diagnosed.

What are the appropriate treatments for this condition?

Panic disorder is often treated with selective serotonin reuptake inhibitors (SSRIs), tricyclic antidepressants, and monoamine oxidase (MAO) inhibitors. These drugs influence levels of norepinephrine, serotonin, and γ-aminobutyric acid in the central nervous system. Benzodiazepines are also useful in the short term.

What syndrome can develop when SSRIs are used with MAO inhibitors?

Serotonin syndrome may result from the use of drugs that enhance serotonin signaling. MAO inhibitors and SSRIs enhance serotonin signaling through different mechanisms, so the risk of serotonin syndrome is higher when these drugs are taken together. Serotonin syndrome is more likely to occur with this combination of drugs because most MAO inhibitors irreversibly inhibit MAO. Symptoms of serotonin syndrome fit into three main categories:

- Autonomic dysfunction (eg, hyperthermia, tachycardia, unstable blood pressure, diarrhea, and sweating).
- Cognitive and behavioral changes (eg, agitation, confusion, and coma).
- Neuromuscular abnormalities (eg, hyperreflexia, shivering, myoclonus, and ataxia).

■ CASE 9

A 20-year-old man who returned from military service in Iraq a year ago visits his primary care physician complaining of a year's history of difficulty sleeping. He states that he gets only 4 hours of sleep per night. When he does fall asleep, he has recurring nightmares about a roadside bomb attack he suffered while driving a Humvee. The bomb killed his passenger and severely injured the patient. The patient states that he has difficulty driving because being in a car sometimes makes him "relive" the experience, and he avoids parking lots and busy freeways. He has no interest in returning to college and recently broke up with his girlfriend because she could not deal with his outbursts of anger and "numbness" to her feelings.

What is the most likely diagnosis?

Posttraumatic stress disorder (PTSD). PTSD is a complex and heterogeneous disorder characterized by reliving an extremely traumatic event with symptoms of increased arousal and avoidance. The disturbance must **last more than 1 month** and cause significant social and occupational distress.

What causes this condition?

PTSD is caused by any event that exposes an individual to real or threatened death or injury. The individual's response to the event must involve intense fear and horror. Examples include military combat, sexual or physical assault, accidents, and natural disasters.

How do patients with this condition relive the traumatic event?

Recurring distressing dreams or intrusive thoughts of the event are common. Patients may also describe flashbacks in which they feel as if the event is recurring. Flashbacks are often triggered by stimuli that are common to the traumatic event such as sights, smells, or sounds.

In what ways do patients cope with this condition?

PTSD patients often avoid thoughts, feelings, stimuli, and conversations that are associated with the trauma. Because of this, it is often difficult for patients to talk about their experience. They also display a restricted range of affect, often described as "numbness" or "detachment."

What symptoms may be present in this condition?

PTSD is characterized by hyperarousal that may manifest as insomnia, bouts of rage, hypervigilance, being easily startled, or having poor concentration.

What treatment options are available for this condition?

Selective serotonin reuptake inhibitors are usually the first line of treatment for PTSD. Tricyclic antidepressants and monoamine oxidase inhibitors can be used to decrease symptoms of hyperarousal. Effective psychotherapy includes cognitive behavior therapy, exposure therapy, and anxiety management.

■ CASE 10

A mother brings her 3-year-old daughter to the pediatrician. The mother reports that her daughter has gradually stopped speaking and is doing "weird" things with her hands. The mother states that although she was a normal baby and toddler, she has lost interest in her toys and looks at her family less. She does not speak at all and has screaming spells for hours during the day. Over time she has become unable to feed herself and constantly wrings her hands. Physical examination reveals decelerated head growth and stereotypic hand wringing.

What is the most likely diagnosis?

Rett disorder is a neurodevelopmental disorder characterized by initial normal development during the first 6–18 months of life followed by a **loss of speech** and loss of purposeful **hand movements.**

What are the genetics of this condition?

Rett disorder is an X-linked disorder affecting only females. Affected males die in utero. The disorder is caused by mutations in the *MECP2* gene, which encodes for a methyl-binding protein. This protein is most abundant in the brain and is thought to act as a gene suppressor during development.

What is the progression of this condition over time?

The course of this disorder is divided into stages:

- **Stage 1 (6–18 months):** Subtle delays in gross motor skills, less eye contact, and reduced interest in play.
- **Stage 2 (1–4 years):** Rapid loss of purposeful hand movements and loss of speech. Patients begin to display characteristic hand movements (wringing, tapping, clapping). Breathing abnormalities are common with periods of apnea and hyperventilation.
- **Stage 3 (2–10 years):** Ataxia, motor problems, and seizures.
- **Stage 4:** The final stage, marked by reduced mobility, curvature of the spine (scoliosis), and muscle rigidity.

What is the treatment and prognosis for patients with this condition?

Treatment for Rett disorder is aimed at alleviating symptoms with careful management of nutrition, pharmacotherapy for seizures, speech therapy for language dysfunction, and physical therapy for motor dysfunction. Patients can generally live for decades with successful management of symptoms.

CASE 11

The parents of a 22-year-old man bring him to the family physician because they have noticed a distinct change in their son's behavior over the past 4 months. The young man appears unkempt, does not have any friends at school, and has let his grades drop. He believes that a family neighbor has been sent to spy on him, and his parents hear him having conversations with imaginary partners. He denies any history of substance use and his urine toxicology is negative.

What is the most likely diagnosis?

The constellation of symptoms suggests schizophreniform disorder, which is the presence of psychotic symptoms for > 2 weeks but < 6 months. This contrasts a diagnosis of schizophrenia, which requires the presence of symptoms for at least 6 months. The majority of patients with schizophreniform disorder ultimately develop schizophrenia.

What symptoms are associated with this condition?

Patients with psychosis can present with positive and negative symptoms. **Positive symptoms** include formal thought disorder (disorganized speech and loosening of associations), delusions (often persecutory in nature), hallucinations (most commonly hearing voices), and ideas of reference (beliefs or perceptions that irrelevant, unrelated, or innocuous things are referring to a person directly or have a special significance for that person). **Negative symptoms** include flat affect, social withdrawal, and avolition (inability to initiate and maintain goal-directed activities).

What other conditions should be considered in the differential diagnosis?

- **Brief psychotic disorder:** The symptom criteria are the same as for schizophrenia, but the duration of symptoms is < 1 month. Prognosis is generally good.
- **Schizoaffective disorder:** The symptom criteria are the same as for schizophrenia, but the patient must also have at least one concurrent major mood episode (ie, major depressive disorder or mania).

What are the appropriate pharmacologic treatments for this condition?

- **Typical antipsychotics** (such as thioridazine, haloperidol, fluphenazine, and chlorpromazine) block dopamine-2 receptors. This class of drugs carries a higher rate of extrapyramidal side effects, including muscle rigidity, body posturing, akathisia (feeling of restlessness), and Parkinson-like tremors.
- **Atypical antipsychotics** (such as clozapine, olanzapine, and risperidone) block serotonin receptors and multiple subtypes of dopamine receptors.

CASE 12

A 28-year-old woman presents to her physician with abdominal pain that has persisted intermittently for a decade. The pain has been particularly intense for the past several weeks. She is unable to sleep at night and has "tried everything for the pain but it won't go away." She reports nausea and diarrhea. She also has longstanding complaints of chronic headaches, muscle spasms, and dyspareunia (painful sexual intercourse). Her chart shows multiple visits over the years for similar symptoms with only vague physical examination findings and no laboratory findings. She has had several investigative surgeries and procedures without results. She asks if she should have another surgery to find out what is wrong.

What is the most likely diagnosis?

Somatization disorder.

What are common symptoms of this condition?

To meet diagnostic criteria, patients must present with somatic complaints in at least four sites: two gastrointestinal, one neurologic, and one sexual.

How are other conditions in this category differentiated?

- **Body dysmorphic disorder:** Patients are excessively concerned with an imagined or slight physical defect, to the extent that social, occupational, and/or academic functioning is adversely affected.
- **Conversion disorder:** Patients present with a neurologic complaint (eg, numbness, blindness, or paralysis) that cannot be explained by any physiologic process. Patients may be completely unconcerned about their symptoms.
- **Hypochondriasis:** Patients persistently believe they have a particular disease, despite evidence to the contrary.
- **Pain disorder:** Patients complain of pain, but psychological factors contribute to the onset, severity, maintenance, and exacerbation of these complaints.

What other conditions must be distinguished from this condition?

In the above disorders, patients unconsciously mimic medical symptoms; in the following disorders, patients deliberately induce symptoms for personal gain:

- **Factitious disorder:** A condition in which patients consciously induce or mimic medical disorders (eg, by contaminating urine specimens or surreptitiously injecting insulin) in order to play the sick role (ie, to be taken care of to take advantage of the medical system).
- **Malingering:** A condition in which patients consciously feign medical disorders to provide secondary gain (eg, to get out of work or collect disability).

▊ CASE 13

A 38-year-old man having a severe asthma attack is brought to the emergency department and given IV steroids, which help to resolve his breathing. He is sent home on a steroid taper and seen in follow-up 2 days later when he reports insomnia and appears agitated. His speech is rapid and pressured, he has grandiose plans for the future, and he appears to have a euphoric affect. He is also tachycardic. When asked about his mood, he says he feels "sunny."

What is the most likely diagnosis?

Steroid-induced mania.

What drugs are most commonly associated with these symptoms?

Drug-induced mania can be secondary to ingestion of cocaine or amphetamines. Corticosteroids are a common iatrogenic cause of mood symptoms.

What signs and symptoms are commonly associated with this condition?

- Dilated pupils.
- ECG arrhythmia or ischemia.
- Hypertension.
- Mood elevation, general activation.
- Tachycardia.

What laboratory tests are useful in confirming the diagnosis?

Urine or serum toxicology screening can identify specific drugs the patient may have ingested. Medications should be reviewed for possible iatrogenic cause.

What are the appropriate treatments for this condition?

Steroids are appropriate but the dose should be reduced as much as clinically possible. If agitation or psychotic symptoms are present, haloperidol is useful, sometimes with lorazepam. Calcium channel blockers can be used for acute autonomic symptoms.

These symptoms could also be seen in which other psychiatric disorders?

These symptoms could also be evidence of delirium or a manic phase of bipolar disorder.

■ CASE 14

A 40-year-old woman is brought to the emergency department by her brother, who is worried about her "twitching of lips and tongue." The brother knows his sister was diagnosed with schizophrenia about a decade ago but has not seen her in years and is worried about these movements. The patient has achieved fairly good control of her psychotic symptoms with both oral and intramuscular depot antipsychotic agents. She recalls one prior visit shortly after she was diagnosed with schizophrenia to evaluate a neck spasm that was painful and "locked my neck to the left."

What is the most likely diagnosis?

Tardive dyskinesia. Extrapyramidal symptoms, such as stereotypic oral, buccal, or lingual movements and choreiform or athetoid movements, can occur after several months or years of therapy with antipsychotic agents. These symptoms are often irreversible.

What is the pathophysiology of this condition?

Although the exact mechanism is poorly understood, it is hypothesized that dopamine-2 receptor supersensitivity after long-term use of antidopaminergic drugs is the cause.

What risk factors are associated with this condition?

- Diabetes mellitus.
- History of movement disorders.
- Tobacco use.
- Typical antipsychotic agents (strong risk factor, especially at higher doses for longer periods).

What other movement abnormalities are associated with the use of antipsychotic agents?

- Acute dystonia is the earliest symptom to present (within hours) and is characterized by sustained muscle spasms of the face, neck (spasmodic torticollis), and eye (oculogyric crisis).
- Akathisia, characterized by extreme restlessness and an inability to sit still, is the most common extrapyramidal disorder.

What can be done to minimize the risk of these symptoms continuing?

Lowering the dose of typical antipsychotic agents can help resolve symptoms. However, this may produce a transient worsening of dyskinesia as receptors become desensitized. Switching patients to **atypical antipsychotic** agents is advised, as they are associated with fewer extrapyramidal symptoms. Clozapine is the least likely of all antipsychotic drugs to cause tardive dyskinesia and is also the only medication to treat it. However, its use is limited by the need for routine blood monitoring, a high degree of both benign and serious side effects, and its availability only as an oral preparation.

▌CASE 15

A mother brings her 6-year-old son to see the pediatrician because she is concerned about his facial movements. The mother states that her son has always "blinked too much," but recently he started jerking his head to the right and sticking out his tongue. She describes these as very quick movements that happen multiple times a day. She also reports that the child makes grunting noises. The boy says he does not know why he does these things but feels a sense of relief once he does them.

What is the most likely diagnosis?

This patient displays criteria for Tourette disorder, which is characterized by **multiple motor and vocal tics** present since childhood. A **tic** is a **sudden, stereotypical, repetitive movement or vocalization**. The tics in Tourette disorder occur many times a day for at least 1 year.

What is the epidemiology of this condition?

- Since the tics of Tourette disorder are believed to begin in childhood and remit with age, the prevalence is much higher among children than adults.
- Current data suggest that 1–10 children per 1000 have Tourette disorder, and it is believed to be three to four times more frequent in males than in females.
- Tourette disorder is frequently associated with other conditions, including obsessive-compulsive disorder and attention deficit/hyperactivity disorder.

What motor abnormalities are seen in this condition?

Motor tics can be simple or complex and can affect any part of the body. Often, patients will initially have simple tics such as blinking, shoulder shrugging, head jerking, or grimacing. Complex tics may involve jumping, squatting, turning, or obscene gestures (copropraxia).

What vocal abnormalities are seen in this condition?

The classic vocal tic is coprolalia, or involuntary vocalization of obscene words. Other vocal tics include echolalia (repetition of others), and sounds such as barking, coughing, sniffing, grunting, or snorting.

Are the tics of this condition involuntary?

Yes, the tics are involuntary, but for brief periods patients may be able to consciously suppress them. Patients often describe a sense of relief once the tic is performed.

What is the natural history of this condition?

Onset is usually during childhood and must occur before 18 years of age. The disorder may be lifelong, but many patients find that the severity of the tics decreases with age.

What is the appropriate treatment for this condition?

In many cases, education and reassurance may be sufficient. If the tics significantly interfere with the patient's social interactions, a dopamine antagonist (such as haloperidol) can be effective.

12

Renal

■ CASE 1

A 29-year-old woman who was involved in a motor vehicle accident is brought to the emergency department, where she is found to be hypotensive with severe internal bleeding. She is given several units of blood by transfusion and sent to the intensive care unit for monitoring. Within 36 hours, a slight decrease in urine output and an increase in blood urea nitrogen (BUN) are noted, and by 72 hours there is a dramatic drop in urine output. Laboratory studies at 72 hours are as follows:

Serum potassium: 5.1 mEq/L
BUN: 25 mg/dL
Serum creatinine: 2.5 mg/dL
Urinalysis: Mild hematuria, mild proteinuria, granular casts, and renal tubular epithelial cells in sediment
Fractional excretion of sodium (Fe_{Na}): 2.2%

What is the most likely diagnosis?

The patient most likely has acute tubular necrosis (ATN) secondary to renal ischemia as a consequence of shock due to the accident. ATN is the most common cause of acute kidney injury and is a result of direct injury to the renal tubular epithelia.

What are common causes of this condition?

Renal ischemia and nephrotoxins are the two general classes of causes of ATN. Hypotension and other prerenal diseases can cause renal ischemia. Common nephrotoxins include antibiotics (eg, aminoglycosides, amphotericin, foscarnet), radiocontrast, immunosuppressants (eg, cyclosporine, tacrolimus), chemotherapy agents (eg, cisplatin), and myoglobin (eg, in rhabdomyolysis).

What is the cause of the patient's azotemia?

ATN involves direct damage to renal tubular epithelial cells (the proximal tubule is particularly vulnerable to ischemic injury because of its high demand for adenosine triphosphate). In addition, the sloughing of intact tubular cells and necrotic cellular debris into the tubular lumen blocks the urinary luminal tract. This leads to a back leak of the filtrate and, consequently, a decrease in the glomerular filtration rate (GFR).

How do the laboratory findings help distinguish this condition from prerenal disease?

The microscopic findings on urinalysis and the BUN/creatinine values can help distinguish simple prerenal disease from ATN as follows:

- Muddy brown epithelial and granular cell casts in the urine are almost always pathognomonic for ATN.
- The BUN/creatinine ratio is approximately normal (10–20:1) in ATN but elevated (> 20:1) in prerenal disease.
- FeNa is usually < 1% in prerenal states, while the FeNa is usually > 1% in ATN.

Why is the BUN/creatinine ratio elevated in prerenal disease but not in intrinsic renal disease?

Urea is a water-soluble molecule that is passively reabsorbed in the proximal tubule (the area of the kidney most sensitive to hypoperfusion) where volume depletion increases reabsorption of sodium and water in parallel with an increase in BUN.

Creatinine is not reabsorbed in the proximal tubule; hence, when there is volume depletion, there is not a commensurate rise in serum creatinine. Creatinine is freely filtered, and then gets secreted in the tubules.

Thus, in cases of upper gastrointestinal bleeding or other causes of hypoperfusion, BUN is elevated but creatinine is normal.

What is the natural course of this condition?

Within 36 hours of injury, ATN undergoes an initiatory phase, during which time urine output decreases and BUN increases. Within 2–6 days, a maintenance phase begins, where urine output falls dramatically and there is a significant risk of death without treatment. Finally, the recovery phase typically occurs within 2–3 weeks.

How do the results of a fluid challenge test differ between this condition and prerenal disease?

A fluid challenge (the use of intravenous fluids to restore intravascular fluids) usually restores normal renal function in patients with simple prerenal disease (hypoperfused kidneys). However, in patients with ATN, renal dysfunction often persists despite fluid challenge. A fluid challenge is contraindicated in patients with volume overload (eg, heart failure).

How do the urinary sodium excretion and Fe_{Na} values differ between this condition and prerenal disease?

	U_{Na} (mEq/L)	Fe_{Na}
ATN	> 40	> 2%
Prerenal	< 20	< 1.0%

■ CASE 2

A 37-year-old man visits his physician because he has noticed blood in his urine over the past week. He denies increased frequency or dysuria. He admits intermittent aching back pain over the past few months, which he attributes to sitting at his desk for long periods of time each day at work. Ultrasound shows massively enlarged kidneys bilaterally. The surface of the right kidney is studded with several well-circumscribed cysts, and the left kidney demonstrates similar lesions. His blood pressure is 148/84 mm Hg.

What is the most likely diagnosis?

Autosomal dominant polycystic kidney disease (ADPKD). ADPKD has a prevalence of approximately 1:1,000 and is the leading genetic cause of chronic renal failure. It is diagnosed with imaging.

How is this condition inherited?

The disease is inherited in an autosomal dominant fashion. Approximately 85% of cases of ADPKD are due to a mutation in the *PKD1* gene on chromosome 16; the remainder of the cases are caused by mutations in *PKD2* on chromosome 4.

What is the presentation of this condition?

ADPKD may present at any age but is most frequently diagnosed in the third to fifth decades (although PKD type 2 inheritance has a later onset). Because ADPKD is dominantly inherited, patients may be aware of a family history of the disease. Patients can experience chronic flank pain due to calculi, urinary tract infection, or massively enlarged kidneys. Patients may also present with gross hematuria, and nocturia may be present if renal concentrating ability is impaired. Upon presentation, microscopic hematuria and proteinuria may be found, and hypertension at presentation is common.

What are the extrarenal manifestations of this condition?

Colonic diverticular disease is the most common extrarenal effect of ADPKD. Hepatic cysts (Figure 12-1) are present in 50%–70% of patients and are generally asymptomatic with little effect on liver function. There is also an association between ADPKD and berry aneurysms of the circle of Willis, which show familial clustering. Rupture of such aneurysms results in subarachnoid hemorrhage and increased mortality and morbidity. Mitral valve prolapse is found in 25% of patients with this disease. Most patients with APDKD die from cardiac causes. Cardiac hypertrophy and coronary disease are extremely common.

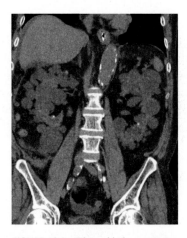

FIGURE 12-1. Bilateral kidney cysts in polycystic kidney disease. (Reproduced, with permission, from USMLERX.com.)

What is the prognosis for patients with this condition?

Progression to chronic renal failure is common, with 50% of patients developing **end-stage renal disease** by 60 years of age (ADPKD accounts for approximately 5% of patients who initiate dialysis annually). There is great variability in the progression of the disease even within families. Early age at diagnosis, male gender, recurrent infection, proteinuria, and hypertension are all associated with an early onset of renal failure. *PKD1* carriers tend to have a more severe course. At present, there is no proven treatment for ADPKD; management generally consists of controlling any associated hypertension and/or proteinuria to preserve the glomerular filtration rate, but renal replacement therapy is eventually indicated.

■ CASE 3

A 10-year-old boy is brought to his pediatrician for evaluation of bloody urine. A urine sample is positive for hemoglobin and RBC casts. The boy's maternal grandfather suffered from deafness and died of renal failure. The boy also has a 25-year-old male maternal cousin who uses a hearing aid and requires dialysis for end-stage renal disease. The family pedigree is shown in Figure 12-2; the boy is indicated by the arrow, his maternal grandfather by the number 1, and his maternal cousin by the number 2. Darkened symbols represent people with known renal disease.

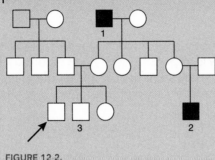

FIGURE 12-2.

What is the most likely diagnosis?

The most common causes of gross hematuria in a child are urinary tract infection and trauma. The most likely diagnosis in this case, however, is hereditary nephritis, or **Alport syndrome**, which consists of glomerular disease, sensorineural deafness, and ocular abnormalities, such as anterior lenticonus, a conical projection of the lens surface. These patients often progress to end-stage renal disease by the second decade of life.

This condition is due to a mutation in a gene that codes for which protein?

Alport syndrome is due to a defect in the gene that codes for the α5 subunit of **type IV collagen**. Type IV collagen is found primarily in the basal lamina. Tissue from patients with this mutation fails to stain for this protein.

Because of this mutation, the glomerulus loses the ability to selectively filter on the basis of what property?

The glomerulus loses the ability to filter on the basis of size. The glomerular basement membrane is primarily a size-selective (as well as charge-selective) filter; therefore, damage to the basement membrane leads to loss of size selectivity.

What is the probability that this patient's brother (person 3 in Figure 12-2) has the same disease?

The probability is 50%. The pedigree represents X-linked inheritance. Since the boy's mother is a carrier, each son has a 50% chance (one of two X chromosomes in the mother) of inheriting the mutation. There are also autosomal recessive and autosomal dominant variants of Alport syndrome.

What other screening tests, in addition to urinalysis, can be used to confirm the diagnosis?

Alport syndrome is associated with ocular abnormalities and deafness; therefore, an ophthalmological examination and a formal audiogram should be performed, as deficits may be subtle. Skin biopsies can also be useful in diagnosing Alport syndrome.

■ CASE 4

A 70-year-old woman presents to her physician complaining of a 3-day history of nausea and malaise. She states that she is essentially in good health, although she recently started taking omeprazole for her gastroesophageal reflux disease. The patient denies use of any other medications. Her physical examination reveals a temperature of 38°C (100.4°F), but it is otherwise unremarkable. Laboratory blood testing demonstrates eosinophilia and elevated serum creatinine. Urinalysis shows mild proteinuria. Urine microscopy is pending.

What is the most likely diagnosis?

There is a high clinical suspicion for drug-induced acute interstitial nephritis (AIN) because of the patient's recent initiation of a medication. Drug therapy is responsible for 71% of reported AIN cases, with infections (eg, *Legionella*, leptospirosis, cytomegalovirus, and streptococci) and autoimmune disorders (eg, systemic lupus erythematosus, Sjögren syndrome, sarcoidosis) responsible for the rest. AIN can develop between 1 week and 9 months of drug initiation.

What drugs are associated with this condition?

- Many medications have been associated with AIN, although methicillin remains the classic drug.
- Antibiotics are commonly associated with a high risk of causing AIN include penicillin, cephalosporins, rifampin, and sulfonamides.
- Nonsteroidal anti-inflammatory drugs (NSAIDs) are known to lead to AIN as well as to vasoconstriction of the afferent glomerular arterioles by inhibiting prostaglandin production.
- Proton pump inhibitors are increasingly reported as a cause of AIN.

What other symptoms are common in patients with this condition?

Other nonspecific complaints, such as weakness, fatigue, and anorexia, are common. Rash can sometimes accompany fever and eosinophilia to complete the classic triad of a drug-induced hypersensitivity reaction. However, only 10% of cases of drug-induced AIN manifest with all three signs.

What are the typical urinalysis findings?

Urinalysis often reveals pyuria and hematuria. WBC casts in the absence of a urinary infection is highly suggestive of AIN. Urine eosinophils increase the suspicion as well. Mild proteinuria may be found. Creatinine concentration can also be acutely elevated.

What kidney biopsy findings are common in this condition?

Kidney biopsy is the only way to confirm this condition. Renal tissue histopathology often shows interstitial edema with diffuse cellular infiltration of the interstitium by inflammatory cells including lymphocytes, monocytes, eosinophils, and granulocytes (Figure 12-3). Tubulitis may also be seen. The presence of granulomas may suggest an autoimmune cause, such as sarcoidosis.

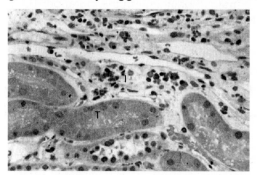

FIGURE 12-3. **Renal biopsy demonstrating interstitial eosinophils.** Tubules are indicated by "T," and the interstitium by "I." (Reproduced, with permission, from Fauci AS, et al. *Harrison's Principles of Internal Medicine*, 17th ed. New York: McGraw-Hill, 2008: Figure e9-25.)

What is the appropriate treatment for this condition?

Withdrawal of the offending agent is the primary therapy. The effectiveness of corticosteroid treatment has not been proven by a prospective, randomized controlled trial, but prednisone is often used empirically, especially in cases of failure to induce remission after withdrawal of drug therapy or advanced renal failure.

■ CASE 5

A 70-year-old African-American man returns to his physician for his annual follow-up visit after prior diagnosis of monoclonal gammopathy of undetermined significance (MGUS). He reports he continues to have mild lower back pain and proximal extremity weakness and notes that he has had polydipsia and polyuria in the past several months. Physical examination is unremarkable. Urinalysis is notable for aminoaciduria, glucosuria, and phosphaturia. Relevant laboratory results are as follows:

Sodium: 133 mEq/L   Bicarbonate: 18 mEq/L   Phosphate: 2.1 mg/dL
Potassium: 3.3 mEq/L   Glucose: 85 mg/dL   Uric acid: 2.0 mg/dL
Chloride: 110 mEq/L   Calcium: 8.3 mg/dL

What is the most likely diagnosis?

This patient has likely developed Fanconi syndrome (FS), which is characterized by a generalized transport defect in the proximal tubules, thus representing a proximal (type II) renal tubular acidosis (RTA). FS is either acquired or inherited. It can be acquired as a rare complication of plasma cell dyscrasias, including multiple myeloma, MGUS, Waldenström macroglobulinemia, and primary amyloidosis. FS may also result from Sjögren syndrome, heavy metal poisoning, and drug reactions. If inherited, FS is mostly transmitted as an autosomal recessive trait.

Although all of the urinalysis and laboratory findings support the diagnosis of FS, in a patient with MGUS and back pain, multiple myeloma should be on the differential.

What are the functions of the proximal convoluted tubules?

The proximal convoluted tubules are the "workhorses of the nephron" and reabsorb all glucose and amino acids and the majority of filtered sodium, potassium, phosphate, bicarbonate, and water. Ammonia is also secreted to buffer distally secreted H^+.

What is the pathogenesis of this condition?

FS is characterized by multiple proximal tubular transport defects. The exact mechanism varies with the etiology of FS. In FS associated with monoclonal gammopathies, kappa-type Bence Jones proteins have been found to be reabsorbed by proximal tubular cells. Subsequent failure to complete proteolysis of these light chains results in cytoplasmic crystalline inclusions, which may eventually compromise tubular function.

What medication can mimic the presentation of this condition?

Acetazolamide works by inhibiting bicarbonate in the proximal tubule and thus can cause proximal RTA.

What is glomerular filtration rate (GFR)?

The glomerulus filters plasma predominantly by molecular size and net charge. GFR measures the amount of plasma that is filtered into the Bowman's capsule from the glomerular capillaries within the glomeruli per unit time (milliliters per minute) and is a marker of renal function. Infusion of inulin is necessary for an accurate assessment of GFR because it is fully filtered but is not reabsorbed, secreted, metabolized, or produced endogenously. GFR, however, is more conveniently approximated by creatinine clearance (C_{Cr}), as represented by the formula:

$$GFR = U_{Cr} \times V/P_{Cr} = C_{Cr}$$

(P_{Cr}, plasma concentration of creatine; U_{Cr}, urine concentration of creatine; V, volume of urine per unit time.)

Since creatinine, unlike inulin, is secreted in the kidney, a creatinine-based GFR results in an overestimate of the true GFR. In FS, GFR is normal.

What is the mechanism of the observed hypokalemia?

The primary function of the kidneys is to preserve volume though the reabsorption of sodium and free water. In FS, there is an increased distal delivery of sodium due to the incompetent proximal tubules. The principal cells within the collecting ducts will compensate by increasing sodium reabsorption through an exchange for potassium. This results in potassium clearance rates that may be more than twice the GFR, indicating net tubular secretion. Metabolic acidosis secondary to defective proximal tubule bicarbonate reabsorption may also contribute to potassium loss, as cells tend to remove H^+ from circulation through an exchange for potassium, thereby increasing the filtered load of potassium.

■ CASE 6

A 42-year-old woman presents to her physician after coughing up blood several times in the past week. She reports she has been coughing more frequently and experiencing difficulty finishing her daily walks despite the fact that she recently stopped smoking. She has not noticed any significant changes in her urinary habits. Physical examination is notable for a blood pressure of 144/82 mm Hg and an absence of fever and dyspnea. X-ray of the chest demonstrates fluffy infiltrates bilaterally. Urinalysis reveals proteinuria, hematuria, and RBC casts. A spot protein/creatinine ratio shows significant but subnephrotic-range proteinuria.

What conditions should be considered in the differential diagnosis?

Acute glomerulonephritis and alveolar hemorrhage suggest Goodpasture syndrome (GP) or a systemic vasculitis, such as Wegener granulomatosis or microscopic polyangiitis. While vasculitis is more common, that would likely present with constitutional symptoms. Lupus and other forms of acute glomerulonephritis that are related to pulmonary infection or result in pulmonary edema should also be considered.

To aid in the diagnosis, which antibodies should be tested for by serology?

- Anti–glomerular basement membrane (anti-GBM) antibody
- Anti–neutrophilic cytoplasmic antibody (vasculitides)
- Anti-Smith antibody and anti–double-stranded DNA (lupus)

Only anti-GBM antibodies are subsequently isolated from the patient's serum. What is the epidemiology of the associated condition?

Isolation of anti-GBM antibodies suggests GP, which is a form of anti-GBM disease characterized by rapidly progressive glomerulonephritis, alveolar hemorrhage, and autoantibodies to type IV collagen. GP has a prevalence of 1:1 million. GP occurs with alveolar hemorrhage in 60%–70% of cases. Males 5–40 years of age are most commonly affected. Both genders are affected equally in older adults. Patients younger than 30 years of age are more likely to be severely affected. Untreated, GP has a fatality rate of 50%.

What is the pathogenesis of this condition?

IgG (rarely IgA or IgM) autoantibodies against type IV collagen are the distinguishing feature of GP, and they also correlate with the severity of disease. The α_3 chains of type IV collagen are present in the basement membranes of glomeruli, alveoli, and several other organs. The antigen targets of GP autoantibodies are normally inaccessible because of the presence of endothelial cells. The exposure of these antigens to circulating antibodies is more likely in the kidneys and lungs because of the fenestrated nature of the endothelial lining of glomerular capillaries and the increased susceptibility of the lungs to injury (eg, from smoking, toxin inhalation, or infection).

What type of hypersensitivity reaction is responsible for this patient's disease process?

A type II hypersensitivity reaction is responsible. Fixation of complement to the anti-GBM antibodies activates the classic complement pathway that results in the recruitment of neutrophils and monocytes. Type II hypersensitivity is also seen in myasthenia gravis, pernicious anemia, Graves disease, pemphigus vulgaris, and other conditions.

What are the typical kidney biopsy microscopy findings in this condition?

Light microscopy typically shows crescentic glomerulonephritis (see Figure 12-8). Immunofluorescence microscopy (Figure 12-4) demonstrates the nearly pathognomonic finding of a smooth linear deposition of IgG along the glomerular capillaries.

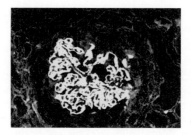

FIGURE 12-4. **Immunofluorescence microscopy of a kidney biopsy specimen from a patient with a linear ribbon-like pattern when stained for immunoglobulin.** (Reproduced, with permission, from Kasper DL, et al. *Harrison's Principles of Internal Medicine,* 16th ed. New York: McGraw-Hill, 2005: 1681.)

■ CASE 7

A 4-year-old boy presents with a 2-day history of rash that has spread from his legs to his buttocks. He is afebrile and has no sick contacts or other pertinent exposures. The rash consists of nonclustering, nonblanching, raised spots > 2 mm in size spread over his buttocks and posterior surfaces of his lower extremities. The boy also complains of knee and ankle stiffness and acute abdominal pain. His vital signs are stable, and urinalysis is unremarkable. His laboratory findings are as follows:

Hematocrit: 35%
International Normalized Ratio (INR): 1.0
WBC count: 7000/mm³
Prothrombin time: 12 sec
Platelet count: 200,000/mm³
Partial thromboplastin time: 25.2 sec

What is the most likely diagnosis?

Henoch-Schönlein purpura (HSP). In children, the combination of rash (as described above), arthralgias, abdominal pain, and renal disease is pathognomonic for HSP. However, only 63% of patients with HSP actually present with abdominal pain and only 40% with renal disease. An additional 33% of patients also have evidence of gastrointestinal bleeding. Less common symptoms include testicular torsion, intussusception, pancreatitis, cholecystitis, and protein-losing enteropathy. Approximately 1% of children with HSP progress to end-stage renal disease, and approximately 10% of HSP cases are seen in adults.

What are the dermatologic findings for this condition?

Both **purpura and petechiae** may be seen in HSP. Purpura is characterized by nonblanching, flat lesions measuring > 2 mm in diameter. Petechiae are non-blanching, flat lesions measuring < 2 mm in diameter. Both are signs of bleeding occurring in the skin.

What is the pathophysiology of this condition?

HSP is a small-vessel vasculitis. Although the precipitating factor is unknown, anecdotal evidence suggests upper respiratory infection for children. With HSP, IgA deposition in blood vessels causes leaking, which leads to purpura and petechiae. This is pathophysiologically similar to IgA nephropathy.

Which conditions should be considered in the differential diagnosis of this patient's rash?

The main concerns, in addition to HSP, are clotting disorders and sepsis; as a result, coagulation studies should be performed. A similar rash can be caused by rickettsial infections, although this patient is afebrile. It is important to distinguish HSP from **hemolytic-uremic syndrome** (HUS), as the two conditions present similarly and can both cause extensive renal disease. However, HUS is not likely in this patient, as there are no signs of hemolytic anemia such as schistocytes on blood smear. In adults, HSP must be distinguished from systemic diseases such as hypersensitivity vasculitis and systemic lupus erythematosus.

What are the appropriate treatments for this condition?

Treatment is based on the severity of symptoms, as the disease is typically self-limiting. An asymptomatic patient requires no treatment. However, severe symptoms, including signs of renal involvement, may require renal biopsy and steroids. Regardless of the severity of symptoms, patients with HSP require urinalysis every 3 months for 1 year, as HSP has a high rate of recurrence. Recurrence or flares typically occur within 4 months of the initial diagnosis.

■ CASE 8

A 45-year-old man is brought to the emergency department by his mother after 2 days of worsening confusion, polyuria, polydipsia, and constipation. His past medical history is significant only for chronic osteomyelitis of the right arm secondary to a burn injury sustained in a house fire 5 years ago. Physical examination is unremarkable except for uniformly depressed deep tendon reflexes. The patient is also visibly uncomfortable and disoriented and is uncooperative during much of the examination. Electrocardiogram (EKG) reveals a QTc interval of 390 msec. Relevant laboratory findings are as follows:

Serum calcium: 11.88 mEq/L
Serum albumin: 1.45 mEq/L
BUN: 21mg/dL
Serum creatinine: 1.4 mg/dL
Parathyroid hormone (PTH): 12 pg/mL
Alkaline phosphatase: 980 U/L

What is the most likely diagnosis?

Hypercalcemia. Symptoms include lethargy, hyporeflexia, confusion, depression, headaches, psychosis, bradycardia, a shortened QT interval, nausea, vomiting, constipation, muscle weakness, polyuria, polydipsia, and gastroduodenal ulcer disease (secondary to calcium-induced gastrin release).

How are ionized calcium and albumin used in the diagnosis of this condition?

Ionized calcium is the primary determinant of cellular and membrane activity. However, routine reporting of serum calcium levels includes calcium that is bound to proteins. Approximately 45% of calcium circulates in the free or ionized form, and another 40% is bound to albumin (the remainder is bound to various anions). Accurate assessment of calcium levels therefore requires the simultaneous measurement of albumin and serum calcium levels.

How does hypoalbuminemia affect this condition?

Hypoalbuminemia can decrease measured serum calcium levels independently of any net change in ionized calcium levels. For each decrease of 1.0 g/dL in serum albumin below the laboratory's reference normal value, 0.8 mg/dL should be added to the total calcium measured (the opposite is done in cases of hyperalbuminemia). Given the patient's hypoalbuminemia, the actual total serum calcium level is even greater than the already elevated total calcium observed.

What are the two most common causes of hypercalcemia?

Hyperparathyroidism (thus the importance of checking PTH levels) and malignancy are the leading causes of hypercalcemia.

What are the appropriate treatments for this condition?

Symptomatic hypercalcemia, as seen in this patient, should first be treated with a saline infusion to expedite renal calcium excretion. Furosemide may be initiated to promote calciuresis only after the patient is volume replete. Furosemide promotes natriuresis and increases calcium excretion. Bisphosphonates inhibit osteoclast activity and are also used to treat hypercalcemia. Given this patient's history of chronic osteomyelitis, suppressed PTH, and dramatically elevated alkaline phosphatase levels, there is a high clinical suspicion for underlying malignancy.

■ CASE 9

A 58-year-old man presents to the emergency department with a 1-week history of progressive weakness, fatigue, and shortness of breath on exertion. On physical examination, the man's heart rate is irregularly irregular, and his lung examination is notable for bilateral crackles that are most pronounced at the bases. X-ray of the chest demonstrates pulmonary edema. The patient is started on digoxin and furosemide. Three days later, he complains of light-headedness with progressive weakness. Laboratory values are significant for a serum sodium level of 142 mEq/L and a serum potassium level of 2.7 mEq/L. An EKG demonstrates torsades de pointes.

What is the most likely diagnosis?

Hypokalemia.

What two main factors predisposed the patient to torsades de pointes?

The patient was started on digoxin to increase cardiac output and to treat the atrial fibrillation; furosemide was added to treat the pulmonary edema. However, furosemide in the setting of congestive heart failure can lead to severe hypokalemia (serum potassium level < 2.5 mEq/L). Hypokalemia has been shown to promote digitalis induced arrhythmias, even when digitalis levels are in the therapeutic range. Digitalis toxicity can induce fatal arrhythmias.

What are the most common causes of this condition?

There are three broad etiologies of hypokalemia: decreased intake, increased losses, and increased translocation into cells.

- Decreased intake is a rare cause of hypokalemia.
- Increased losses can be:
  - Gastrointestinal, from diarrhea, laxative abuse, VIPomas, nasogastric suctioning, and/or vomiting.
  - Urinary, as from diuretic use, polyuria and other salt-wasting conditions, hyperaldosteronism, loss of gastric secretions, or metabolic acidosis.
  - Due to excessive sweating.
- Increased translocation into cells occurs with hypothermia, alkalosis, increased insulin availability, and β-adrenergic activity.

How does alkalosis lead to this condition?

The Na^+-K^+-ATPase pump keeps intracellular potassium levels much higher than the serum/extracellular level. However, in the setting of alkalosis, hydrogen ions leave cells to minimize pH change. In the process, hydrogen ions function in an apparent exchange for potassium that can lead to hypokalemia.

How is metabolic acidosis associated with this condition?

Metabolic acidosis causes an exchange of hydrogen ions into the cells for potassium ions into the plasma, leading to hyperkalemia. However, in the setting of metabolic acidosis (notably diabetic ketoacidosis), urinary potassium excretion is also increased. This leads to a situation in which potassium is being moved from the cells and then excreted in the urine. As a result, although the serum potassium level is normal or even high in metabolic acidosis, the total body stores are actually low. The hypokalemia often reveals itself once the acidosis is corrected.

What are the appropriate treatments for this condition?

Potassium can be repleted either directly (ie, with potassium chloride) or through the use of a potassium-sparing diuretic such as amiloride, spironolactone, or triamterene. Amiloride is often the diuretic of choice, as it lacks the hormonal adverse effects of spironolactone (gynecomastia and amenorrhea).

■ CASE 10

An 86-year-old woman living in a nursing home is brought to the attention of the medical staff because of her lethargy. Relatives note that she has been unable to recognize family members in the past week. Her past medical history is notable for Alzheimer disease, osteoporosis, and hypertension. Her medications include memantine, donepezil, alendronate, and hydrochlorothiazide, the dose of which was recently increased. Physical examination reveals a blood pressure of 139/80 mm Hg. The patient is sleepy and oriented only to person. CT scan of the head is unremarkable. Laboratory testing is notable for a sodium concentration of 122 mEq/L and normal glucose levels, renal function, and hematocrit.

What is the most likely diagnosis?

Hyponatremia, which is commonly defined as a serum sodium concentration ≤ 135 mEq/L. Hyponatremia is more prevalent in the hospital setting or in nursing homes.

What are the common causes of this condition?

Most cases of hyponatremia can be thought of as arising from three general mechanisms:

- Too much water, such as in the syndrome of inappropriate secretion of antidiuretic hormone (SIADH), nephrotic syndrome, congestive heart failure, cirrhosis, or excessive fluids (iatrogenic or marathon runners).
- Too little salt, such as in salt-wasting conditions (eg, aldosterone resistance or deficiency), diuretic abuse, dehydration, or vomiting.
- High serum osmolality, which most often occurs in the setting of hyperglycemia. This is a form of pseudohyponatremia where you correct for Na according to the glucose level.

What symptoms are typically associated with this condition?

The decreased osmolarity (for most cases of hyponatremia) causes an osmotic water shift that increases intracellular fluid volume. Clinical manifestations are typically neurologic in nature secondary to cerebral edema within the confines of the cranial vault. Nonspecific symptoms, such as malaise or nausea, are common. Headache, lethargy, confusion, and obtundation may appear as sodium levels fall further. Stupor, seizures, and coma can occur if progression is rapid or concentrations fall below 120 mEq/L.

What is the pathogenesis of this condition in this particular patient?

This patient is likely suffering from diuretic-induced hyponatremia. Thiazides deplete serum sodium and potassium levels and stimulate ADH-mediated water retention. It should be noted, though, that loop diuretics are unlikely to cause hyponatremia, as the maximal urine concentrating ability, and thereby water retention, is reduced with the decrease in medullary interstitial tonicity. If hyponatremia develops over a period of days rather than acutely, the brain cells react to hyponatremia by secreting salts and, over time, organic osmolyte to prevent excess water entry and swelling. This may explain why no significant swelling can be seen on CT scan of the head.

What other laboratory test will help identify the etiology of this condition in this patient?

Plasma osmolality, urine osmolality, fractional excretion of sodium, urine sodium concentration, and urine potassium concentration are helpful. If diuretics are responsible, as in this case, the plasma osmolality may be slightly low. Urine osmolality is elevated, as thiazides stimulate antidiuretic hormone (ADH). Urine sodium is elevated because of a thiazide-mediated decrease in reabsorption. However, some of the excess sodium delivered to the collecting duct is reabsorbed at the expense of potassium. Urine potassium therefore would also be elevated.

What is the most appropriate treatment for this condition?

Rapid correction of chronic hyponatremia can result in **central pontine myelinolysis,** a diffuse (not limited to the pons) demyelination syndrome. A rapid increase in serum osmolarity leads to brain cell shrinkage, and this is believed to result in demyelination. If hyponatremia occurs suddenly, over a few hours, then rapid correction is unlikely to cause demyelination as the brain will not have time to undergo compensatory measures as discussed above.

■ CASE 11

The parents of a 5-year-old boy bring their son to a physician seeking a second opinion on his short stature and the bowing of his legs that has existed since he was 2 years of age. The family history is notable for bowed legs in the maternal grandfather and poor dentition in the mother. Physical examination is remarkable for frontal bossing, dental abnormalities, and tibia vara. Urine electrolyte analysis reveals elevated phosphate. Serum calcidiol is within normal limits, but calcitriol is low. Other relevant laboratory values are as follows:

Blood urea nitrogen: 16 mg/dL
Serum creatinine: 0.4 mg/dL (normal for age)
Parathyroid hormone (PTH): 54 pg/mL (normal: 10–55 pg/mL)
Serum albumin: 4.5 g/dL
Serum phosphate: 1.3 mg/dL
Alkaline phosphatase: 450 U/L
Total calcium: 8.7 mg/dL

What is the most likely diagnosis?

Hypophosphatemic (previously vitamin D–resistant) rickets is suggested by the patient's slow growth and skeletal findings as well as by his laboratory values: upper normal PTH, normal calcidiol and calcium levels with low calcitriol (which would normally be elevated in the setting of hypophosphatemia), and phosphaturia in the setting of normal renal function. Two inheritable forms exist. X-linked hypophosphatemic (XLH) rickets is more likely in this case, as it generally affects males and presents in childhood. The grandfather likely was similarly affected, whereas the heterozygous mother is only mildly affected with dentition problems. Less common autosomal dominant and recessive forms also exist, which affect both genders equally and present later in life.

What is the pathogenesis of this condition?

XLH is associated with a loss-of-function mutation in a gene on the X chromosome responsible for the clearance of fibroblast growth factor-23. Failure to clear this growth factor leads to phosphaturia and decreased 1α-hydroxylase activity in the kidney. Increased excretion of phosphate, decreased calcitriol, and bone deformities result.

What are the typical radiologic findings in this condition?

Figure 12-5 shows the widened diaphyses, funnel-like beaking of the metaphyses, and increased curvature of the femoral and tibial shafts. Enthesopathy (calcification of tendons, ligaments, and joint capsules) is also often seen. Lower-extremity deformities develop as the child begins to bear weight with ambulation.

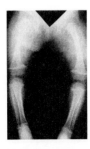

FIGURE 12-5. **Bowed long bones and irregular, flared physes.** (Reproduced, with permission, from Skinner HB. *Current Diagnosis & Treatment in Orthopedics*, 4th ed. New York: McGraw-Hill, 2006: 603.)

How is phosphate regulated in the body?

Calcium and phosphate regulation are linked. Phosphate is primarily reabsorbed in the proximal renal tubules. **PTH** release is stimulated by low serum calcium, high phosphate, and low vitamin D. PTH decreases phosphate levels by inhibiting phosphate reabsorption in the proximal tubules.

Calcitriol formation is stimulated by low serum calcium and phosphate levels and high PTH levels. It enhances gut absorption of both calcium and phosphate. It also decreases PTH secretion.

What is the appropriate treatment for this condition?

A combination of phosphorus and calcitriol is required to restore age-appropriate growth velocity. Administration of either substance alone is insufficient. Phosphorus by itself decreases ionized calcium levels, which results in PTH release and secondary hyperparathyroidism. Serum phosphorus normalization also simultaneously decreases calcitriol formation. This removes the inhibitory effect of calcitriol on PTH synthesis and its stimulatory effect on intestinal reabsorption of calcium and calcium deposition in bone.

■ CASE 12

A 24-year-old woman presents to the emergency department with nausea, vomiting, tachypnea, sweating, and tinnitus. Her mother reports that she found an empty bottle of aspirin in the patient's bedroom. Physical examination reveals a temperature of 38.6°C (101.5°F), a heart rate of 100/min, a respiratory rate of 40/min, and altered mental status. Arterial blood gas is notable for a pH of 7.28, partial carbon dioxide pressure (P_{CO_2}) of 25 mm Hg, and bicarbonate of 17 mEq/L. Her anion gap is 22 mEq/L. Salicylate levels are pending. Intravenous fluids are initiated, and charcoal and sodium bicarbonate are administered orally. The patient is transferred to the intensive care unit for further stabilization.

What is the acid-base disturbance in this patient?

A mixed metabolic acidosis and respiratory alkalosis. The pH < 7.35 indicates acidemia. Respiratory acidosis is unlikely given the below-normal P_{CO_2} and the high anion gap. In this setting the low bicarbonate indicates metabolic acidosis. Applying Winter's formula ($P_{CO_2} = (1.5 \times [HCO_3^-]) + 8 \pm 2$), the appropriate respiratory compensation is $P_{CO_2} = 1.5(17) + 8 = 33.5 \pm 2$. The "compensation" in this case is therefore excessive, suggesting an independent respiratory alkalotic process, which is consistent with a respiratory rate of 40/min.

What are the causes and two main types of metabolic acidosis?

Metabolic acidosis derives from the loss of bicarbonate or the retention of acid, leading to a non–anion gap acidosis in the former, and an anion gap acidosis in the latter. A non–anion gap acidosis is always the result of conditions that result in hyperchloremia ($Cl^- > 109$ mEq/L), such as renal tubular acidosis. The excess chloride suppresses bicarbonate reabsorption. Metabolic acidosis that is caused by retention of acid results in an anion gap metabolic acidosis because unmeasured acidic anions are retained. To recall the major causes of anion gap metabolic acidosis, the mnemonic **MUD PILES** is useful (**M**ethanol, **U**remia, **D**iabetic ketoacidosis, **P**araldehyde or **P**henformin, **I**ron tablets or **I**soniazid, **L**actic acidosis, **E**thylene glycol, **S**alicylates.)

What are the causes of respiratory alkalosis?

Anything that stimulates the central respiratory drive and causes hyperventilation, such as cerebrovascular accidents or neurologic disease, can cause respiratory alkalosis. Hypoxia, such as that caused by anemia, high altitudes, and pulmonary disease, can likewise increase respiratory rate and respiratory alkalosis. Other hyperventilatory states such as mechanical overventilation or voluntary hyperventilation, such as in cases of anxiety, can also be causative.

How is anion gap calculated?

The equation $Na^+ - (Cl^- + HCO_3^-)$ is typically used. K^+ is typically not included because of its small contribution as a predominantly intracellular cation. A normal anion gap is 6–12 mEq/L. The presence of unmeasured anions, such as salicylates, displaces and reduces serum bicarbonate, thereby producing an apparently larger gap.

What is the pathogenesis of this patient's condition?

Aspirin is hydrolyzed to salicylate once ingested. At toxic levels, salicylates cause a primary respiratory alkalosis by stimulating the medullary respiratory center to hyperventilate. Salicylates also stimulate skeletal muscle metabolism, increasing oxygen consumption and carbon dioxide production. This further stimulates hyperventilation. The metabolic acidosis component occurs because salicylates cause both lipolysis and uncoupling of oxidative phosphorylation, resulting in the production of organic acids, pyruvate, and ketones.

■ CASE 13

A 19-year-old man on his first postoperative day after an appendectomy develops nausea and vomiting that is unresponsive to antiemetic therapy. He is unable to retain any fluids and has not consumed anything by mouth. Physical examination is notable for orthostatic hypotension. His arterial blood gas is notable for a pH of 7.48, partial pressure of carbon dioxide (Pco_2) of 42 mm Hg, and bicarbonate of 28 mEq/L.

What acid-base disturbance is seen in this patient?

Metabolic alkalosis. The pH of the arterial blood is > 7.45, which indicates alkalemia. Metabolic alkalosis can be distinguished from respiratory alkalosis by examining the Pco_2. Normal or increased Pco_2 with increased bicarbonate indicates that the alkalosis is metabolic.

What does the body do to partially compensate for this condition?

A patient may hypoventilate to cause respiratory acidosis, which reduces pH as a compensatory measure. Pco_2 is increased by 0.7 mm Hg for every 1 mEq/L increase in bicarbonate. In this case, the bicarbonate is approximately 3 mEq/L above normal, which translates into an expected Pco_2 of 40 + 0.7(3) = 42.1 mm Hg. Therefore, the metabolic alkalosis here is appropriately compensated.

How is this condition further classified?

Metabolic alkalosis usually reflects chloride losses. It can be caused by a number of conditions. **Saline-responsive** conditions are characterized by hypochloremia (Cl^- < 95 mEq/L) and low urinary chloride (Cl^- < 10 mEq/L). Saline-responsive metabolic alkalosis is caused by chloride losses and volume depletion, such as from persistent vomiting, cystic fibrosis, hypokalemia secondary to diuretic use, congenital familial chloridorrhea, and hypercapnia.

Saline-unresponsive conditions are associated with low serum chloride and high urinary chloride (Cl^- > 10 mEq/L). Saline-unresponsive metabolic alkalosis can be caused by hyperaldosteronism, Cushing syndrome, alkali administration, and exogenous stimulation of mineralocorticoid production (eg, from licorice).

What is the pathogenesis of this patient's condition?

This patient is volume depleted because he stopped his intravenous fluids. In addition, he has been vomiting, which removes further fluid and chloride (from HCl). His alkalemia is therefore likely saline responsive. His dehydration stimulates the renin-angiotensin-aldosterone system. Elevated aldosterone causes reabsorption of Na^+ in exchange for K^+ and H^+. This further exacerbates the alkalemia and also leads to hypokalemia. Treatment involves restoration of volume status to prevent further exacerbation of the alkalemia and the complications of hypokalemia.

How does aciduria occur in this condition?

Aciduria is paradoxical in the setting of alkalemia. It can occur, however, in the setting of an extended period of volume depletion. The activated renin-angiotensin-aldosterone system exchanges Na+ for K^+ and H^+. Over time, the pool of available intracellular K^+ becomes depleted, resulting in the exchange of only H^+. The subsequent aciduria is an indication of a metabolic emergency with severe hypokalemia.

■ CASE 14

A 3-year-old boy is brought to his pediatrician after his mother notices that his limbs seem swollen and his stomach distended. She says the boy received an influenza shot 1 week ago. Physical examination reveals generalized pitting edema and shifting dullness of the abdomen suggestive of ascites. Urinalysis reveals 4+ proteinuria, and laboratory findings show decreased serum albumin, hypertriglyceridemia, and normal serum ionized calcium. The total calcium may be low because of the hypoalbuminemia. Blood pressure, blood urea nitrogen (BUN), and serum creatinine values are within normal limits.

What is the most likely diagnosis?

The boy likely has nephrotic syndrome in the form of minimal change disease (lipoid nephrosis). This is the most common manifestation of nephrotic syndrome in children (approximately 90% of cases occur in children younger than 10 years of age). Age younger than 6 years, normal renal function, and absence of hypertension are strong indicators for this diagnosis.

What are the four classic symptoms of this condition?

Nephrotic syndrome classically presents with proteinuria, hypoalbuminemia, edema, and hypercholesterolemia (Table 12-1).

TABLE 12-1	Findings in Nephrotic Versus Nephritic Syndrome	
	NEPHROTIC SYNDROME	NEPHRITIC SYNDROME
Clinical findings	Edema (often periorbital) Minimal hematuria	Hypertension Gross hematuria Decreased urine output
Laboratory findings	Hypoalbuminemia Hypercholesterolemia Proteinuria	Red cells/casts in urine Elevated creatinine Mild proteinuria

What pathologic changes at the glomerular level are associated with this condition?

The glomerular basement membrane contains heparan sulfate, which acts as a negative charge barrier that keeps small and negatively charged proteins such as albumin from crossing the membrane. Minimal change disease can be preceded by a recent infection or vaccination. It is believed that T cells release cytokines that injure glomerular epithelial cells. Consequently, the negative charge barrier is lost, whereas the size filter provided by the slit diaphragm proteins may remain intact. This leads to renal albumin wasting since albumin has a negative charge at neutral pH.

What are the likely histology findings?

Glomeruli appear normal on light microscopy, leading to the name *minimal change*. However, when the glomeruli are viewed under electron microscopy, effacement or flattening of foot processes can be seen. The electron micrograph in Figure 12-6 shows effacement of the foot processes (arrowhead).

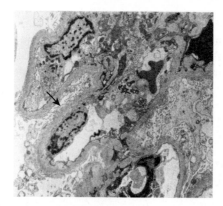

FIGURE 12-6. **Electron micrograph showing effacement of the foot processes in minimal change disease.** (Reproduced, with permission, from Le T, et al. *First Aid for the USMLE Step 1: 2008.* New York: McGraw-Hill, 2008: Color Image 93.)

What is the appropriate treatment for this condition?

Given the high incidence of minimal change disease in children with nephrotic syndrome, this can be presumed to be the diagnosis until proven otherwise. Corticosteroids are given both as treatment and as a diagnostic tool because the majority of patients with minimal change disease respond promptly (thus avoiding biopsy).

■ CASE 15

A 7-year-old boy is sent to his school nurse after his gym teacher notes that he was unusually short of breath while playing basketball. After noticing that the boy's socks left deep indentations in his calves and shins bilaterally and that there is swelling around his eyes, the nurse obtains a urine sample that demonstrates proteinuria but not glucose, RBCs, or WBCs. The boy is then brought to the emergency department for further workup. Relevant laboratory test results are as follows:

Serum:
  Sodium: 129 mEq/L
  Potassium: 2.9 mEq/L
  Albumin: 2.3 g/dL
Cholesterol levels: Elevated

What is the most likely diagnosis?

The boy's presentation suggests nephrotic syndrome, which is characterized by the triad of high urine protein losses, hypoalbuminemia, and hypercholesterolemia. Patients often present with periorbital edema, peripheral edema, and/or ascites secondary to decreased plasma protein. This results in decreased plasma oncotic pressure, which, in turn, leads to sodium and free water retention.

What is the most likely cause of this patient's proteinuria?

The likely mechanism of action is loss of charge barrier at the glomerular membrane due to effacement of foot processes (which would be seen on electron microscopy; no changes would be seen on light microscopy).

What are the typical laboratory findings in this condition?

Serum albumin levels are low, and 24-hour urine protein excretion is high secondary to the massive loss of albumin at the glomerulus. Patients also often demonstrate severe hyperlipidemia. Less than one-half of patients have microscopic hematuria.

What are the appropriate treatments for this condition?

Nephrotic syndrome is treated with prednisone. Although the etiology of minimal change disease is unknown, it is thought to be due to an immune system abnormality. Therefore, corticosteroids (prednisone) and other immune suppressants are commonly used. Symptomatic treatment should also be initiated for edema, hypercoagulability, infection, decreased intravascular volume, and other clinical manifestations.

After 2 months of steroid treatment, the patient shows no decrease in his proteinuria, and a renal biopsy is obtained. What is the most likely diagnosis?

The boy likely has developed **focal segmental glomerular sclerosis** (Figure 12-7), which can be resistant to steroid treatment. Light microscopy of the biopsy specimen may demonstrate focal areas of glomeruli with segmental sclerosis. Electron microscopy demonstrates foot process derangement.

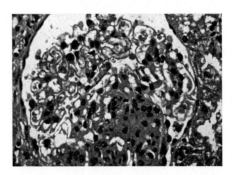

FIGURE 12-7. **Focal segmental glomerulosclerosis.** Note the well-defined segmental increase in matrix and obliteration of capillary loops, the sine qua non of segmental sclerosis. (Reproduced, with permission, from Fauci AS, et al. *Harrison's Principles of Internal Medicine*, 17th ed. New York: McGraw-Hill, 2008: Figure 9-1.)

■ CASE 16

A 16-year-old previously healthy girl visits her doctor with recent-onset flank pain. She is given ibuprofen and sent home. A day later, she develops a fever accompanied by nausea, emesis, and worsening flank pain. Upon questioning, she recalls episodes of urgency as well as decreased urine output. Physical examination is notable for a temperature of 38.9°C (102.0°F) and costovertebral angle tenderness. Laboratory findings are as follows:

WBC count: 13,900/mm³
Neutrophils: 74%
Hematocrit: 33%
Blood urea nitrogen (BUN): 10 mg/dL
Serum creatinine: 1.1 mg/dL
Urinalysis: 2+ protein, small leukocyte esterase, many WBCs, 2–5 RBCs/hpf, few bacteria, and WBC casts

What is the most likely diagnosis?

The presence of flank pain, emesis, high fever, and costovertebral angle tenderness indicate acute pyelonephritis. Pyelonephritis is a urinary tract infection (UTI) that has progressed from the lower urinary tract (bladder/urethra) to the upper urinary tract. It is most common in young children and sexually active women. Men are less likely to develop pyelonephritis or acute cystitis, in part because of their longer, less exposed urethras. Other predisposing factors include vesicoureteric reflux (congenital), flow obstruction, catheterization, gynecologic abnormalities, diabetes, and pregnancy.

What are the most likely pathogens in UTIs?

Escherichia coli is the most common cause of UTIs (50%–80% of cases). *Staphylococcus saprophyticus* is the second most common cause of UTIs in young, sexually active women. Other common causative organisms include *Proteus mirabilis*, *Klebsiella* (second most common cause overall), *Serratia*, *Enterobacter*, and *Pseudomonas*. Group B β-hemolytic streptococcal infection can cause UTIs in infants as part of the sepsis they develop.

How can this patient's symptoms be distinguished from those associated with cystitis, urethritis, or vaginitis?

Pyelonephritis classically manifests as flank pain, costovertebral angle tenderness, nausea, and vomiting with high fever. By contrast, the classic primary complaint in cystitis is dysuria accompanied by frequency, urgency, suprapubic pain, and hematuria. Urethritis and vaginitis present with dysuria, discharge, pruritus, dyspareunia, and an **absence** of frequency or urgency.

What are the characteristic laboratory findings in this condition?

Pyuria is an essential finding in UTIs. Urinalysis typically shows >10 WBCs/HPF. Hematuria is also common in women with UTI but not in women with urethritis or vaginitis. Leukocyte casts in the urine is pathognomonic for pyelonephritis. Additionally, serum tests show leukocytosis, an elevated erythrocyte sedimentation rate, and an elevated C-reactive protein level.

What are the appropriate treatments for this condition?

The goal of empiric therapy is to use drugs that achieve high concentrations in the renal medulla. Oral medications include the fluoroquinolones (especially ciprofloxacin) and trimethoprim-sulfamethoxazole. Intravenous options include ceftriaxone, ciprofloxacin, ampicillin and gentamicin, and piperacillin/tazobactam.

■ CASE 17

A 37-year-old woman presents to her rheumatologist complaining of increased fatigue, periorbital edema, and swelling of her lower extremities of 3 days' duration. One month earlier she started on prednisone and hydroxychloroquine for her newly diagnosed lupus. Her previously normal urinalysis now reveals hematuria, proteinuria, dysmorphic RBCs, and RBC casts. Her serum creatinine is 2.5 mg/dL. Physical examination at this visit reveals a temperature of 38.3°C (100.9°F), a blood pressure of 150/90 mm Hg, and a weight increase of 5 kg (11 lb). Moderate ascites and lower-extremity pitting edema up to her thighs are present.

What classification of renal disorders do these symptoms represent?

Hematuria with RBC casts, dysmorphic RBCs, and proteinuria on urinalysis in the setting of hypertension and edema indicate a nephritic syndrome. Causes of nephritic syndrome include rapidly progressive glomerulonephritis (RPGN), poststreptococcal GN, IgA nephropathy, lupus nephritis, and mesangial proliferative GN.

The next day, the patient is oligo-anuric, and her serum creatinine rises to 3.2 mg/dL. What is the most likely diagnosis?

This patient most likely has RPGN, a clinical diagnosis characterized by a doubling of serum creatinine in a 3-month period and rapid progression to acute renal failure. RPGN can result from a primary glomerulopathy or a secondary glomerulopathy mediated by a systemic disease, such as lupus in this case, or a streptococcal infection.

Kidney biopsy is also performed the next day (Figure 12-8). How does it aid in the diagnosis of this condition?

Kidney biopsy remains the gold standard for diagnosis. Light microscopy (LM) demonstrates the typical crescent formation of RPGN (Figure 12-8). Immunofluorescence microscopy of a renal specimen distinguishes three major patterns of immunoglobulin deposition, representing three diagnostic categories:

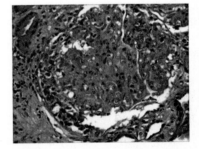

- Immune-complex glomerulonephritis is categorized by scattered granular deposits of immune complexes. This is the typical "lumpy bumpy" pattern. It can be seen in Henoch-Schönlein purpura and lupus among others.
- Anti–glomerular basement membrane disease shows smooth, linear deposition of immunoglobulin as seen in Figure 12-4.
- Pauci-immune glomerulonephritis (the most common type) manifests sparse or absent immunoglobulins. It can be seen idiopathically or in the setting of anti–neutrophilic cytoplasmic antibody vasculitides.

FIGURE12-8. (Reproduced, with permission, from USMLERx.com.)

What is the pathogenesis of this condition?

RPGN is on the spectrum of immunologically mediated PGN. Lupus-associated RPGN is rare but likely shares a mechanism similar to other types of lupus renal diseases. Mesangial and subendothelial deposition of immune complexes, primarily composed of DNA-anti-DNA, are present. Subsequent activation of complement initiates the immune response.

How does the morphology of urine erythrocytes distinguish upper and lower urinary tract disorders?

Dysmorphic RBCs suggest upper tract bleeding or inflammatory glomerular or tubulointerstitial disease. RBC casts are also an indication of a glomerular disorder. Normal erythrocytes or eumorphic RBCs suggest lower urinary tract bleeding.

Should this patient receive treatment or will the condition self-resolve?

Untreated RPGN typically progresses to end-stage renal disease over weeks to months; therefore, prompt treatment is essential. Although treatment varies based on underlying etiology, empiric steroids should be given to all RPGN patients, sometimes with cyclophosphamide.

■ CASE 18

A 70-year-old man visits his primary care physician after going to a health fair and discovering that his blood pressure is 170/100 mm Hg. The previous year, his blood pressure was 135/85 mm Hg. The man also has a history of hypercholesterolemia. At the physician's office, his blood pressure is 150/100 mm Hg and heart rate is 80/min. An abdominal bruit is detected in the epigastric region to the right of midline. Laboratory findings are significant for a serum sodium level of 147 mEq/L and a serum potassium level of 3.3 mEq/L.

What is the most likely diagnosis?

The man most likely suffers from renal artery stenosis. The bruit described is in the region of the renal artery; this finding, in addition to the sudden increase in blood pressure and hypokalemia supports the diagnosis of renal artery stenosis. Imaging confirms the diagnosis.

What is the pathogenesis of this condition in this patient and how would it differ in a young woman?

In the elderly population, renal artery stenosis is seen more often in men and is mostly caused by atherosclerotic plaques (secondary to hypercholesterolemia). For younger patients, fibromuscular dysplasia of the renal arteries, seen more in females, would be the likely cause.

What changes in renin secretion from each kidney are likely?

The kidney ipsilateral to the stenosis will increase renin secretion in response to a perceived decrease in arterial pressure due to decreased flow to the juxtaglomerular apparatus. The contralateral kidney will respond to the patient's resulting hypertension by decreasing its renin secretion (Figure 12-9).

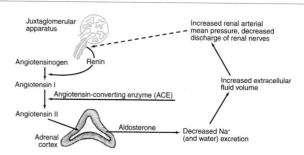

FIGURE 12-9. **Renin-angiotensin system.** (Reproduced, with permission, from McPhee SJ, Hammer GD. *Pathophysiology of Disease: An Introduction to Clinical Medicine*, 6th ed. New York: McGraw-Hill, 2010: Figure 21-9.)

How does elevated plasma renin lead to hypertension?

In the plasma, renin converts angiotensinogen (produced in the liver) to angiotensin I. This is converted to angiotensin II by angiotensin-converting enzyme (ACE), which is secreted by pulmonary and renal endothelial cells. **Angiotensin II** acts on vascular smooth muscle to increase blood pressure. Angiotensin II also acts on the adrenal cortex to stimulate the release of aldosterone, which increases renal absorption of sodium to increase blood volume and thus blood pressure.

What electrolyte abnormalities are associated with this condition?

As seen in hyperaldosteronism, the sodium reabsorption is isotonic; therefore, the serum sodium is normal but hypertension ensues, and hypokalemia is expected as a consequence of renal potassium losses.

What is the medication of choice for this condition?

To correct the increased angiotensin II, an ACE inhibitor (such as captopril) or an angiotensin II receptor blocker (such as losartan) would be the medication of choice. Caution should be used with these drugs when renal artery stenosis is bilateral.

What four classes of antihypertensive drugs directly target the effects of renin?

- ACE inhibitors (captopril, enalapril, and lisinopril).
- Angiotensin II receptor blockers (losartan).
- Aldosterone-antagonizing diuretics (spironolactone).
- Renin inhibitors (aliskiren).

CASE 19

A 64-year-old woman presents to her physician with sudden onset of nausea and severe back pain on her right side. The patient is in acute distress and is unable to find a comfortable position. She has no prior history of back pain. Her temperature is 36.9°C (98.4°F), her heart rate is 90/min, and her blood pressure is 130/80 mm Hg. Relevant laboratory findings are as follows:

Serum:
Sodium: 140 mEq/L
Chloride: 100 mEq/L
Potassium: 4 mEq/L
Phosphoric acid: 2.1 mEq/L
Magnesium: 1.8 mg/dL
Glucose: 100 mg/dL
Calcium: 13 mg/dL
Bicarbonate: 25 mEq/L
BUN: 15 mg/dL
Creatinine: 1 mg/dL
Urinary pH: 5.85
Urinalysis shows RBCs

What is the most likely diagnosis?

Nephrolithiasis (kidney stones). Acute back/side pain (especially related to movement or that waxes and wanes) with elevated calcium and RBCs in the urine indicates kidney stones.

How is this condition classified?

Approximately 85% of renal calculi are **calcium oxalate stones** (Figure 12-10), which are strongly radiopaque. The second most common kidney stones are **struvite** (ammonium magnesium phosphate), which are radiopaque and associated with *Proteus vulgaris* and *Staphylococcus aureus* infection. Other, less common stones include **uric acid stones** (radiolucent) and **cystine stones** (moderately radiopaque). This patient most likely has calcium oxalate stones given her hypercalcemia and normal temperature.

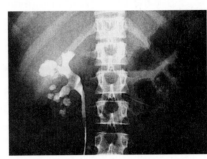

FIGURE12-10. **Kidney stones.** (Reproduced, with permission, from Tanagho EA, McAninch JW. *Smith's General Urology*, 16th ed. New York: McGraw-Hill, 2004: 259.)

What is the pathogenesis of this condition?

Calcium oxalate stones can be caused by hypercalciuria, hyperoxaluria, or hypocitraturia (citrate is a potent inhibitor of calcium precipitation/stone formation).

What is the pathogenesis of the other three classifications of this condition?

Struvite stones form in the presence of alkaline urine, created by urease-splitting organisms such as *Proteus vulgaris*, *Klebsiella*, or *Staphylococcus aureus*. Uric acid stones are associated with hyperuricemia, which is seen in gout and conditions with high cell turnover such as leukemia or myeloproliferative disease. Cystine stones are observed in congenital cystinuria.

What is the appropriate treatment for this patient's condition?

Treatment consists of analgesics, hydration, and if obstructed or infected, antibiotics ± stenting. Thiazide diuretics are contraindicated in this patient because of her hypercalcemia. Extracorporeal shockwave lithotripsy may be necessary for stones that do not pass spontaneously as a minimally invasive surgical intervention is usually indicated for stones > 5 mm.

What hormonal imbalance can cause the electrolyte abnormalities seen in this condition?

Hyperparathyroidism should always be considered in a patient with calcium stones. The high calcium concentration and low phosphate concentration may be a result of excess parathyroid hormone (PTH). High PTH level increases renal reabsorption of calcium and decreases renal reabsorption of phosphate. It also stimulates renal activation of vitamin D, which increases calcium and phosphate absorption from the gastrointestinal tract.

■ CASE 20

A 60-year-old man with a 30-year smoking history presents to his physician with complaints of cough, fatigue, and a recent 9.1-kg (20-lb) weight loss. X-ray of the chest reveals a 2-cm hilar mass that is identified on biopsy as small cell lung cancer. On physical examination, the patient has some cachexia but normal skin turgor, no edema or jugular venous distention, and no orthostatic hypotension. Relevant laboratory findings are as follows:

Serum:
  Sodium: 128 mEq/L
  Potassium: 4 mEq/L
  Blood urea nitrogen (BUN):
   8 mg/dL
  Glucose: 90 mg/dL

Urine:
  Sodium: Normal
  Osmolality: 610 mOsm/kg H_2O

What is the most likely diagnosis?
Hyponatremia.

How is the etiology of this condition determined?
Volume status is assessed first. Although sodium loss can cause hyponatremia, excessive retention of water is usually the cause. A thorough history and physical examination can help correlate the patient's volume status to a cause of hyponatremia, and laboratory values can be used to confirm volume status. The cause of fluid loss can be determined by history (eg, vomiting, diuretics, diarrhea) and physical findings of low volume (eg, decreased skin turgor, low jugular venous pressure). Signs of excessive fluid retention include peripheral edema.

What laboratory findings can help determine a patient's volume status?
Serum and urine osmolarity and sodium concentration can help confirm a patient's volume status. Most hyponatremic patients have a decreased serum osmolarity; however, renal failure and hyperglycemia are two important causes of hyponatremia that accompany normal or increased serum osmolarity.

In patients with low plasma osmolarity, urine osmolarity can differentiate primary polydipsia (low/normal urine osmolarity) from impaired water excretion (high urine osmolarity, as in the majority of patients).

In patients with hypo-osmolar serum and hyperosmolar urine, urinary sodium can then distinguish between hyponatremia caused by circulating volume depletion (eg, from heart failure, cirrhosis, hypovolemia leading to decreased urinary sodium) and euvolemic hyponatremia (eg, **syndrome of inappropriate secretion of antidiuretic hormone** [SIADH] leading to normal urinary sodium).

In this case, what is the most likely etiology of the patient's volume status?
This patient's small cell lung tumor raises the likelihood of SIADH (a paraneoplastic syndrome for small cell lung cancer). Physical findings and lab values are also consistent with SIADH.

What are the major causes of this condition?
- Ectopic ADH production by a tumor, particularly small cell (oat cell) carcinoma of the lung.
- Intracranial pathology, such as trauma, stroke, tumors, or infection.
- A wide range of drugs.
- Major surgery, pain.
- HIV infection.
- SIADH may also be idiopathic.

What is the mechanism of action of ADH?
ADH is the main regulator of serum osmolality. ADH causes water channels (eg, aquaporin-2) of the principal cells of the kidney's collecting ducts to translocate to the cell membrane, thereby allowing more water to be reabsorbed. Its release from the posterior pituitary is stimulated by hyperosmolarity and by decreased effective circulating volume.

What are the appropriate treatments for this condition?
Treatment consists of tumor resection. If evidence of SIADH persists or resection is not possible, treatment involves restriction of free water intake or use of hypertonic saline with loop diuretics or demeclocycline.

■ CASE 21

A 5-year-old girl develops a fever of 39°C (102.2°F) 25 days after receiving a well-matched deceased donor renal transplant for focal segmental glomerulosclerosis. Her immunosuppression consists of basiliximab (anti-interleukin-2), prednisone, mycophenolate, and tacrolimus. Blood cultures and viral titers including cytomegalovirus (CMV) are pending.

What is cross-matching?

In transplantation, the process of cross-matching determines whether the recipient has antibodies to the donor's WBCs. This measure prevents hyper acute rejection due to preformed antibodies.

If CMV is present, what fraction of a blood sample will have the highest yield for the virus?

Because CMV invades WBCs, these cells contain the highest titer of the virus. Upon centrifuging a blood sample, a "buffy coat," representing < 1% of blood and seen between the plasma and hematocrit, will separate out most of the WBCs and platelets. Figure 12-11 shows a CMV giant cell with multiple hyaline inclusions.

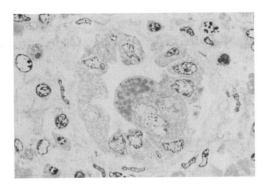

FIGURE 12-11. **Photomicrograph of CMV.** (Reproduced, with permission, from Le T, et al. *First Aid for the USMLE Step 1: 2008.* New York: McGraw-Hill, 2008: Color Image 6.)

Why is CMV of particular concern in this patient?

The girl is immunosuppressed, and there is a significant probability that she has been exposed to CMV. Approximately 80% of normal adults are infected with CMV yet remain asymptomatic because of their functional immune systems. Therefore, there is a high likelihood that the donor may have been CMV positive. As with other members of the herpes virus family, CMV is more likely to activate in an immunosuppressed host. In the immunocompromised host CMV can cause a variety of syndromes, including a mildly febrile upper respiratory illness, severe gastrointestinal syndrome with mild hepatitis, marked pancytopenia, or pneumonitis. CMV can also directly cause graft dysfunction.

What is the mechanism of action of ganciclovir against CMV?

Ganciclovir is a guanosine derivative that inhibits CMV DNA polymerase. The most common side effects of ganciclovir are hematologic thrombocytopenia (57%) and leukopenia (41%).

How does infection lead to fever in a normal individual?

Pyrogenic cytokines released by phagocytic cells of the immune system trigger the release of cytokines, including tumor necrosis factor-α and interleukin-1, which causes the hypothalamus to increase the set point of core body temperature. A key factor in the ability to mount a fever is the presence of an intact immune system. Infection is often difficult to detect in patients with poor immune function, as their ability to mount a fever is severely blunted.

CASE 22

An 18-month-old boy is brought to the pediatrician with symptoms of his third urinary tract infection (UTI) since birth. His mother reports the child has malodorous urine, a low-grade fever, and poor appetite. Urinalysis reveals bacteria on Gram stain.

What is the most likely diagnosis?

This boy most likely has vesicoureteral reflux (VUR), which is the most common urologic finding in children. It is seen in 1% of all newborns and almost 50% of young children presenting with a UTI.

Where is the bladder located in men and women?

The bladder sits behind the pubic symphysis and anterior to the rectum in both men and women. In men, the bladder lies anterior to the seminal vesicles above the prostate gland and is anterior to the uterus in women.

What are the two regions of the bladder?

The lower region is the trigone or the base of the bladder. The entry of the ureters marks the base of the trigone. The apex of the trigone is where the urethral orifice is surrounded by the internal urethral sphincter. The upper region of the bladder holds urine that enters the bladder via the ureteral orifices. The bladder can expand vertically and horizontally to hold up to 300–400 mL (~ 20-30 mL/kg) of urine before voiding.

What is the innervation of the bladder?

Afferent innervation involves afferent branches of the visceral nervous system, stretch receptors via parasympathetic nerves, and pain receptors via sympathetic nerves.

Efferent innervation is subdivided into parasympathetic and sympathetic innervation.

- Parasympathetic innervation involves pelvic splanchnic nerves. The preganglionic axons arise from the lateral horn cells at the S2–S4 levels; postganglionic cell bodies are in the bladder wall. These efferent nerves cause detrusor contraction and internal sphincter relaxation during micturition.
- Sympathetic innervation involves the sacral splanchnic nerves. The preganglionic axons arise from lateral horn cell bodies at the T10–T12 and L1–L2 levels. The postganglionic cell bodies are in the inferior mesenteric and hypogastric ganglia. These efferent nerves relax the detrusor and increase the tone of the internal sphincter during bladder filling and prevent reflux of urine into the ureters. In the adult male these efferents also prevent reflux of semen into the bladder at the ureterovesical junction.

13

Reproductive

■ CASE 1

A 29-year-old woman in week 28 of her third pregnancy is involved in a motor vehicle accident but does not immediately seek medical attention. Four hours after the accident, she notes lower abdominal pain and vaginal bleeding, so she goes to the emergency department. Upon presentation, the patient appears uncomfortable and says she thinks she is having prolonged contractions. Her vital signs are notable for mild hypotension. Relevant laboratory findings are as follows:

Hematocrit: 34%
Platelet count: 80,000/mm³
Plasma fibrinogen: 180 mg/dL

What is the most likely diagnosis?

Abruptio placentae. The presence of painful vaginal bleeding in the second or third trimester suggests abruption, and the presence of contractions is an additional clinical hint. The laboratory values, particularly the mild thrombocytopenia (normal platelet count in pregnancy is > 100,000/mm³) and decreased plasma fibrinogen (normal fibrinogen is > 400 mg/dL in pregnancy), also suggest placental abruption with developing consumptive coagulopathy.

What is the differential diagnosis of painful vaginal bleeding in the third trimester?

Abruption often presents as painful vaginal bleeding, whereas placenta previa (a complication of pregnancy in which placental tissue either partially or fully covers the cervical os) presents as painless vaginal bleeding. Other causes of third-trimester painful bleeding include labor, genital laceration, and uterine rupture (typically seen during labor in women who attempt vaginal delivery after cesarean section).

What is the pathophysiology of this condition?

Abruptio placentae is the premature separation of a normal placenta from the uterus occurring after 20 weeks' gestation and before delivery. The rupture of maternal blood vessels at the anchoring villi of the placenta causes a separation from the endometrium in which blood can accumulate. The hemorrhage can be external or concealed (Figure 13-1). This in turn disrupts the fetal blood supply and in severe cases can lead to fetal death.

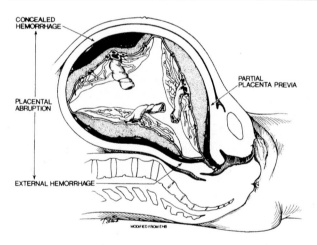

FIGURE 13-1. **Layers in abruptio placentae.** (Reproduced, with permission, from Cunningham FG, et al. *Williams Obstetrics*, 22nd ed. New York: McGraw-Hill, 2005: 812.)

What risk factors are associated with this condition?

Risk factors that can increase disruption or weakening of the maternal blood vessels include trauma, maternal hypertension, cigarette smoking, cocaine use, thrombophilia, increased parity, direct abdominal trauma, amniocentesis, and multifetal gestation.

What complication is the patient at greatly increased risk for developing?

Disseminated intravascular coagulation (DIC) occurs in approximately 10%–20% of cases of serious abruption with fetal death. In these cases, it is thought that the death of the fetus releases procoagulants into the mother's circulation, triggering DIC. This initiates intravascular activation of coagulation and results in consumption of platelets and clotting factors. Fibrin may deposit in the microcirculation, causing ischemic organ damage and hemolytic anemia and then fibrinolysis of the fibrin deposition. Ultimately, this can cause a bleeding diathesis along with clinical manifestations of thrombosis.

CASE 2

A 17-year-old girl presents to the clinic for primary amenorrhea. She reports that she has never had a period. Physical examination reveals normally developed breasts, the lack of axillary and pubic hair, and a small right inguinal mass.

What is the most likely diagnosis?

Androgen insensitivity syndrome (also known as testicular feminization syndrome) should be suspected in a woman with primary amenorrhea, little or no axillary/pubic hair, and an inguinal mass. The disease affects approximately 1:100,000 chromosomal males.

What is the clinical presentation of this condition?

There are two main presentations of this disorder:

- In newborns it presents as an inguinal mass.
- In adolescents it presents as primary amenorrhea.

The inguinal mass seen in newborns is caused by aberrant descent of the testes, which usually remain in the abdomen.

What is the pathophysiology of this condition?

This disorder results from dysfunction of the androgen receptors in a genetically male patient. The testes are present and secrete testosterone and müllerian inhibiting factor (MIF). However, the person cannot respond to this testosterone because the peripheral receptors are nonfunctional. Instead, the testosterone is converted into estradiol in peripheral tissues (especially adipose tissue), which initiates breast development. The vagina is often present but may be short and blind-ending. The MIF secretion inhibits normal development of the ovaries and uterus. Figure 13-2 illustrates genetic regulation of gonadal development.

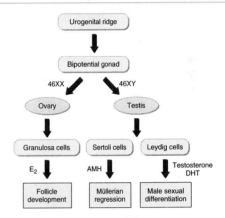

FIGURE 13-2. Transcription factors and cell types responsible for sexual differentiation. AMH = anti-müllerian hormone (müllerian-inhibiting factor); DHT = dihydrotestosterone. (Reproduced, with permission, from Fauci AS, et al. *Harrison's Principles of Internal Medicine*, 17th ed. New York: McGraw-Hill, 2008: Figure 343-2.)

What would confirmatory testing show in this condition?

- On karyotype, these patients are 46,XY.
- Pelvic ultrasound can show testes and the absence of a uterus and ovaries.
- Polymerase chain reaction assay can show mutations of the androgen receptor.
- Testosterone and dihydrotestosterone (DHT) levels should also be measured. Both should be normal or high. Low testosterone may indicate testicular dysgenesis or Leydig cell aplasia/hypoplasia. If testosterone levels are normal but DHT levels are low, 5α-reductase deficiency is suspected because testosterone is converted to DHT by 5α-reductase.

What is the appropriate treatment for this condition?

Initially, removal of the testes is performed because of the high risk of cancer development without such a procedure. Thereafter, treatments are mainly hormone replacement therapy and psychological support. Estrogen, but not progesterone, is given because no uterus is present. Estrogen is given to replace the loss of sex hormone production with the removal of the testes. Psychological therapy is given because of the potential for gender confusion. Surgical reconstruction may be needed to create a "functional" vagina, although if found earlier the use of dilators may obviate surgical intervention.

■ CASE 3

A 35-year-old woman presents to the clinic with complaints of increased fishy-smelling vaginal discharge. She is married, in a monogamous relationship. A wet smear of the discharge reveals stippled squamous epithelial cells with smudged borders (Figure 13-3).

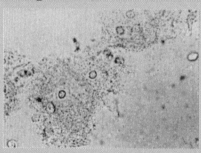

FIGURE 13-3. (Reproduced, with permission, from Kasper DL, et al. *Harrison's Principles of Internal Medicine*, 16th ed. New York: McGraw-Hill, 2005: 767.)

What is the most likely diagnosis?

Bacterial vaginosis (BV). The presence of **clue cells**, which are squamous epithelial cells with smudged borders (Figure 13-3), is strong evidence that the infection is bacterial in origin. An elevated pH (> 4.5) and a positive **whiff test** (amine release with potassium hydroxide results in a fishy smell) may aid in the diagnosis.

What organism causes this condition?

BV is not generally considered a sexually transmitted infection (STI), and it can also occur in women who have not had intercourse. It is caused by an imbalance of naturally occurring bacterial flora within the vagina, with a decrease in favorable bacteria (lactobacilli) and an overgrowth of existing commensal bacteria (eg, *Gardnerella vaginalis*).

What other conditions should be considered in the differential diagnosis?

As this woman is in a monogamous relationship she is not at high risk for STIs such as *Trichomonas*, *Neisseria gonorrhoeae*, or *Chlamydia*. Most women with chlamydia and gonorrhea are asymptomatic, although they can have cervical motion tenderness on pelvic exam. *Trichomonas* often causes a frothy discharge. *Candida* is another common cause of vaginitis, which is not sexually transmitted. Women with candida often present with vaginal itching and increased white, curdlike discharge.

What is the appropriate treatment for this condition?

Metronidazole (oral or vaginal gel) is used to treat bacterial vaginosis (BV). Chlamydia is treated with azithromycin. Gonorrhea is treated with ceftriaxone. Candida is treated with fluconazole.

CASE 4

A 64-year-old man goes to his provider's office complaining of difficulty urinating. He says he has trouble initiating his stream of urine. After it begins, the flow is hard to maintain, and afterward his bladder still feels full. He often has to rush to the bathroom to make it in time, and the need to urinate awakens him several times each night.

What is the most likely diagnosis?

Benign prostatic hyperplasia (BPH). BPH increases with age and is found in approximately one half of men 51–60 years of age.

What are the typical signs and symptoms of this condition?

Classic symptoms of BPH include the following:

- Frequency.
- Urinary urgency.
- Nocturia.
- Difficulty initiating and maintaining a stream.
- A feeling of fullness in the bladder after voiding.
- Dribbling.

Classic signs and laboratory findings in BPH include the following:

- Enlarged prostate on digital rectal exam.
- Elevated prostate-specific antigen (PSA) levels of 4–10 ng/mL. A markedly elevated PSA (especially values > 10 ng/mL) raises suspicion for prostate cancer.

What is the pathophysiology of this condition?

The prostate gland has a central region surrounding the urethra and a peripheral region. In BPH the central region hypertrophies in response to stimulation from the growth hormone dihydrotestosterone (DHT). In prostate cancer, it is often the peripheral region that grows.

What are the potential complications of this condition?

Complications of BPH include the following:

- UTI secondary to urine stasis.
- Bladder stone formation secondary to urine stasis.
- Daytime sleepiness and exhaustion due to repeated nighttime awakenings from nocturia.
- Acute urinary retention, which presents with symptoms such as abdominal pain and a suprapubic mass (the filled bladder). This can be spontaneous or secondary to triggers such as anticholinergics, antihistamines, or α-receptor agonists (eg, cold medications), all of which decrease bladder contractility.

What is the appropriate treatment for this condition?

Medical options include cholinergics (eg, bethanechol), α-blockers (eg, prazosin), and 5α-reductase inhibitors (eg, finasteride). Cholinergics help increase bladder contractility, whereas α-blockers relax the bladder neck so that urine flows more easily. The 5α-reductase inhibitors prevent the formation of DHT so that prostate growth is retarded. Side effects of finasteride include sexual dysfunction and postural hypotension. Surgery is also an option.

■ CASE 5

A 24-year-old woman presents to her physician after noticing a lump in her left breast that is associated with some discomfort. It seems to change sizes over the course of her menstrual cycle. The lump moves with touch, and she is concerned about cancer. On physical examination, the lump feels firm, has well-defined borders, and is mobile. There are no changes in the skin or nipple, and no discharge is present or expressible. No axillary lymph nodes are palpable.

What is the most likely diagnosis?

Approximately 90% of breast lumps discovered in women between 20 and 50 years of age are benign. **Fibroadenomas** are the most common breast tumors seen in young women. They are benign, often arise quickly, and reabsorb within several weeks to months. Fibroadenomas do not carry an increased risk of breast cancer. Approximately 20% of fibroadenomas are bilateral or multiple. The risk associated with having a first-degree relative with breast cancer is higher the younger the relative is at diagnosis.

What are Cooper ligaments?

The superficial and deep pectoral fascia surrounding the breast are connected by fibrous bands known as **Cooper suspensory ligaments.**

What is the structure of breast tissue?

Breast tissue is found between the second and sixth ribs and is made of parenchyma and stroma (Figure 13-4). The parenchyma has 15–25 lobes, each of which has 20–40 lobules composed of alveoli. Lactiferous ducts offer drainage to the corresponding lobe. The ducts are dilated immediately before the nipple, forming the lactiferous sinuses.

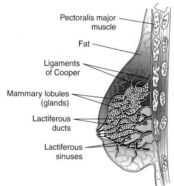

FIGURE 13-4. Normal breast tissue. (Reproduced, with permission, from DeCherney AH, Nathan L. *Current Obstetric & Gynecologic Diagnosis and Treatment*, 10th ed. New York: McGraw-Hill, 2007: 1032.)

What are the muscles of the breast tissue, and how are they innervated?

- The serratus anterior is innervated by the long thoracic nerve.
- The latissimus dorsi is innervated by the thoracodorsal nerve.
- The pectoralis minor is innervated by the medial pectoral nerve.
- The pectoralis major is innervated by the pectoral nerve.

What is the appropriate treatment for this condition?

Because of their benign nature, no treatment is necessary. The patient should be followed up in 1–2 months to assess for reabsorption. If there remains concern for breast cancer, a needle or excision biopsy is indicated.

CASE 6

A 17-year-old girl is brought to the emergency department complaining of a 3-day history of nausea, vomiting, and intense abdominal pain. Her last menstrual period was 6 weeks ago, but she has a history of irregular cycles. She is not taking oral contraceptives. Her past medical history is significant for an appendectomy at 13 years of age. Physical examination reveals a tenderness in the right lower quadrant. Laboratory tests show that the β-human chorionic gonadotropin (β-hCG) level is 1500 mIU/L. Transvaginal ultrasonography reveals no uterine pregnancy.

What is the most likely diagnosis?

Ectopic pregnancy. Ectopic pregnancy occurs at a rate of 17:1000 pregnancies. The majority (98%) of cases occur in the fallopian tubes, most often (90%) in the ampulla.

What signs and symptoms are commonly associated with this condition?

- Nonruptured ectopic pregnancy:
  - Abnormal bleeding.
  - Abdominal/pelvic pain.
  - Nausea/vomiting.
  - Pelvic mass.
- Ruptured ectopic pregnancy:
  - Local or generalized abdominal tenderness.
  - Orthostatic hypotension.
  - Shock.
  - Shoulder pain (blood in the abdominal cavity irritates the diaphragm and causes referred pain in the distribution of the phrenic nerve).
  - Tachycardia.

What risk factors are associated with this condition?

Risk factors include conditions causing structural or functional damage to the fallopian tubes:

- Diethylstilbestrol exposure in utero.
- In vitro fertilization.
- Pelvic inflammatory disease.
- Pelvic surgery.
- Previous ectopic pregnancy.
- Tubal ligation.
- Tuboplasty.

What are the typical laboratory findings in this condition?

The β-hCG level in an ectopic pregnancy is typically < 6500 IU/L, which is markedly lower than in a uterine pregnancy. The serum progesterone level (typically < 15 ng/mL) is also much lower than in a uterine pregnancy. In a normal intrauterine pregnancy, the β-hCG level increases by 50% every 48 hours. If this trend does not occur on serial laboratory results, then an ectopic pregnancy is suspected.

What are the appropriate treatments for this condition?

Treatment may be medical or surgical depending on the clinical situation. The usual medical treatment is methotrexate, which may be given if the ectopic pregnancy is < 3 cm, the β-hCG level is < 12,000 IU/L, no fetal heart rate is present, and the mother's liver and renal tests are normal. β-hCG levels must be checked serially after administration of methotrexate to ensure the proper decline in β-hCG, indicating ectopic demise. Surgery is indicated if the criteria for medical intervention are not met. Surgery may remove part or all of the fallopian tube. Segmental resection might be necessary for an ischemic ectopic pregnancy. Salpingectomy is usually reserved for a ruptured ectopic pregnancy.

■ CASE 7

A 26-year-old woman presents to her physician complaining of intense abdominal pain associated with the start of her menstrual periods. She has been trying unsuccessfully to get pregnant for the past 2 years. On questioning, she reports pain with intercourse, especially on deep penetration. Her older sister has a similar history.

What is the most likely diagnosis?

Endometriosis.

What signs and symptoms are commonly associated with this condition?

Symptoms of endometriosis include the following:

- Cyclic pelvic pain starting 1–2 days before menses and continuing through the first few days of the cycle.
- Dysmenorrhea.
- Dyspareunia.
- Abnormal bleeding.
- Infertility.

Signs of endometriosis include the following:

- Uterosacral nodularity.
- Palpable adnexal mass.
- Definitive laparoscopic evaluation:
  - Endometrial implants appear as raspberry lesions or **"powder burns."** These raised, blue or dark brown lesions lead to adhesions.
  - Ovarian cysts can have large collections of old blood called **endometriomas** or **"chocolate cysts."**

What is the pathophysiology of this condition?

In endometriosis, endometrial tissue is found outside the endometrial cavity, usually in the ovary and pelvic peritoneum. It is thought that this endometrial tissue is either transported via the lymphatic system, causing peritoneal tissue to undergo metastatic change to become functional endometrial tissue, or that it is transported through the fallopian tubes in retrograde menstruation. Endometrial tissue causes adhesions, fibrosis, and severe inflammation.

What risk factors are associated with this condition?

Endometriosis occurs in 10%–15% of women overall but is more common (30%–40%) in women with infertility. The risk of endometriosis is seven-fold higher in women who have a first-degree relative with the condition. Endometriosis has also been linked to autoimmune disorders such as lupus. It is less commonly identified in African-American women.

What are the appropriate treatments for this condition?

Medical treatment includes alleviating symptoms (with nonsteroidal anti-inflammatory drugs) and suppressing menstrual cycles to allow the lesions to involute. This is done with continuous oral contraceptive pills, medroxyprogesterone (inducing "pseudopregnancy"), androgen derivatives, or gonadotropin-releasing hormone agonists (inducing "pseudomenopause"). Surgical treatment may be necessary in refractory cases.

■ CASE 8

A 66-year-old man presents to clinic for follow-up on his hypertension. At the end of the visit, he mentions that he has recently had trouble maintaining an erection. He wants to know what the treatment options are for treating this condition in order to maintain a sexual relationship with his wife.

What is the most likely diagnosis?

Erectile dysfunction (ED) affects up to 50% of men 40–70 years of age.

What physiologic factors are necessary to maintain an erection?

Developing and maintaining an erection depends on neurologic, vascular, and hormonal factors (Figure 13-5). Neurologic control of erectile function is via the dorsal nerve of the penis, a branch of the pudendal nerve which provides autonomic innervation to the pelvis. Vascularly, significant arterial flow into the penis (specifically into the corpora cavernosa and corpora spongiosum) must be maintained and venous outflow prevented. Adequate blood flow is achieved through cyclic guanosine monophosphate (cGMP)-mediated relaxation of the smooth muscle of the corporae, which requires nitric oxide. Hormonally, adequate production of testosterone is required.

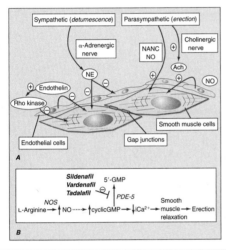

FIGURE 13-5. Innervation and neurotransmitters of penile tumescence and erection. Cyclic GMP = cyclic 3′,5′-guanosine monophosphate; iCa²⁺ = intracellular calcium; NANC = non-adrenergic, noncholinergic pathways; NO = nitric oxide; NOS = nitric oxide synthase; PDE-5 = phosphodiesterase type 5. (Reproduced, with permission, from Fauci AS, et al. *Harrison's Principles of Internal Medicine,* 17th ed. New York: McGraw-Hill, 2008: Figure 49-1.)

What risk factors are associated with this condition?

The main risk factors for developing ED are primarily vascular (hypertension, cardiovascular disease, and diabetes mellitus).

Other risk factors include obesity, sedentary lifestyle, nerve injury, pelvic trauma/radiation, spinal cord injury, prostate surgery, and psychiatric disorders (eg, depression, performance anxiety, fear of sudden death).

What drugs most commonly cause this condition?

- Selective serotonin reuptake inhibitors (SSRIs).
- Spironolactone.
- Sympathetic blockers (clonidine, guanethidine, methyldopa).
- Thiazide diuretics.
- Ketoconazole.
- Cimetidine (but not ranitidine).
- Antipsychotics.
- Cholesterol-lowering drugs.
- Alcohol.
- Nicotine.

What is the appropriate treatment for this condition?

The main treatment for ED is phosphodiesterase inhibitors, such as sildenafil and vardenafil. These work by preventing the degradation of cGMP, thereby allowing dilatation of the corpora and adequate blood flow into the penis. Other treatments include vacuum pumps, penile prosthesis, and direct injection of α-blockers (eg, phentolamine) into the penis. Depression should be treated as appropriate. SSRIs and behavioral therapy are helpful in the treatment of performance anxiety.

▮ CASE 9

A 22-year-old woman presents to the emergency department with a 3-day history of fever, abdominal pain, and vaginal discharge. Her temperature at presentation is 38°C (100.4°F). The patient reports that she is sexually active but does not always use protection. Her last menstrual period ended 5 days ago. She has been with her most recent partner for approximately 1 month. On physical examination, her abdomen is diffusely tender without rebound or guarding. Cervical motion tenderness is present, as is right-sided adnexal tenderness. Relevant laboratory findings are as follows:

WBC count: 11,000/mm³
β-hCG: Negative

What is the most likely diagnosis?

Pelvic inflammatory disease (PID) is the most likely diagnosis. This condition occurs as a complication of ascending gonococcal or chlamydial infection. Ascending infection by these agents can also cause tubo-ovarian abscess or Fitz-Hugh–Curtis syndrome (perihepatitis resulting in right upper quadrant pain).

What signs and symptoms are commonly associated with this condition?

- Fever.
- Pelvic pain.
- Cervical motion tenderness.
- Adnexal tenderness.
- WBC elevation.
- ESR >15.

What is the pathophysiology of this condition?

Chlamydia is the most common cause of PID. *Neisseria gonorrhoeae* also causes PID.

What risk factors are associated with this condition?

- Cigarette smoking.
- High frequency of intercourse.
- Multiple partners.
- New sexual partner within 1 month of symptom onset.
- Recent history of douching.
- Use of an intrauterine device.
- Young age at first intercourse.

What are the likely Gram stain and culture findings?

PCR is the gold standard to detect *Chlamydia* or *N gonorrhoeae*. The sample can be done with a first-catch urine or a cervical swab. Urine PCR is as specific, but less sensitive than a cervical swab.

What are the appropriate treatments for this condition?

Uncomplicated PID is treated as an outpatient with ceftriaxone and doxycycline. If the patient is pregnant, has a tubo-ovarian abscess, or is nauseous and cannot tolerate oral medications, she must be hospitalized for administration of intravenous antibiotics. Surgery is indicated in cases of tubo-ovarian abscess.

CASE 10

A 36-year-old woman at 24 weeks' gestation presents to the clinic for a routine prenatal visit. Her fetus is large for gestational age, and she is scheduled for an oral glucose tolerance test (OGTT). She had one previous pregnancy with no complications and is obese but otherwise healthy. Results of the OGTT are as follows:

1-hour OGTT: glucose level 144 mg/dL
3-hour OGTT: fasting glucose level 97 mg/dL
Glucose level at 1 hour: 210 mg/dL
Glucose level at 2 hours: 190 mg/dL
Glucose level at 3 hours: 143 mg/dL

What is the most likely diagnosis?

Gestational diabetes mellitus (DM) is defined as glucose intolerance first documented in pregnancy.

What is the pathophysiology of this condition?

Gestational DM occurs in approximately 4% of all pregnancies. Normal pregnancy is a diabetogenic (pro-diabetic) state characterized by insulin resistance and decreased peripheral uptake of glucose. This is mediated by the production of counterregulatory (anti-insulin) hormones by the placenta, including human placental lactogen, cortisol, and placental growth hormone.

How is this condition diagnosed?

Gestational DM is most often asymptomatic and is usually detected at 24–28 weeks' gestation by a routine OGTT.

In gestational DM, any two of the following levels are diagnostic: 1-hour postprandial glucose > 190 mg/dL, 2-hour postprandial glucose > 165 mg/dL, and/or 3-hour postprandial glucose > 145 mg/dL. Other signs include glycosuria, hyperglycemia, and fetus large for gestational age.

What risk factors are associated with this condition?

Risk factors include age < 25 years, family or past history of gestational DM, fetus large for gestational age, glycosuria at first prenatal visit, obesity, polycystic ovarian syndrome, previous stillbirths or abortions, maternal birthweight > 4.1 kg (9 lb), and Hispanic or African American race.

What are the common fetal complications associated with this condition?

Common fetal complications include:

- Congenital defects.
- Macrosomia.
- Perinatal mortality (2%–5%).
- Shoulder dystocia.

What are the appropriate treatments for this condition?

Affected women should adhere to a diabetic diet. Fasting blood glucose and 2-hour postprandial glucose levels should be routinely monitored. If levels remain high for 2 weeks, insulin therapy, rather than oral hypoglycemics, should be instituted. Fetal growth should also be monitored.

■ CASE 11

A husband and wife present to a fertility clinic because for a year they have been trying to get pregnant without success. The husband is tall and thin. On physical examination, he has sparse axillary and pubic hair, decreased muscle mass, small testes, and gynecomastia. His urinary gonadotropin levels are elevated and analysis of his sperm reveals azoospermia.

What is the most likely diagnosis?

Klinefelter syndrome.

What is the pathogenesis of this condition?

Klinefelter syndrome is estimated to occur in men at a rate of approximately 1:1000 and is a chromosomal abnormality in which the genotype is **47,XXY.** Dysgenesis of the seminiferous tubules causes primary testicular failure with decreased androgen production.

Complications of Klinefelter include the following:

- Azoospermia and infertility.
- Gynecomastia.
- Small testes and penis.
- Loss of libido.
- Osteoporosis.
- Decreased muscle mass.
- Sparse axillary and pubic hair.

Risks of Klinefelter include the following:

- Increased risk of developing **breast cancer** 20 times that of the typical male.
- Decreased mental capacity.
- Increased risk of anxiety and depression.

All of these complications and risks worsen with an increasing number of X chromosomes.

What tests and/or imaging tools could be used to confirm the diagnosis?

- Elevated follicle-stimulating hormone (FSH) levels are a key finding in Klinefelter. Because the seminiferous tubules are unformed, there is a lack of Sertoli cells; therefore, no inhibin (made by Sertoli cells) is produced. Without inhibin, there is a loss of negative feedback on FSH, causing elevated levels (Figure 13-6). LH levels are also elevated as a result.
- Testosterone levels are low, whereas estradiol levels are high.
- The definitive diagnosis requires karyotype.

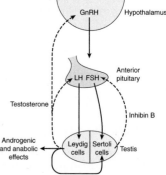

FIGURE 13-6. **Hypothalamic-pituitary-gonadal axis.** FSH = follicle-stimulating hormone; LH = luteinizing hormone. (Reproduced, with permission, from Barrett KE, et al. *Ganong's Review of Medical Physiology,* 23rd ed. New York: McGraw-Hill, 2010: Figure 25-20.)

What is the appropriate treatment for this condition?

Androgen replacement therapy should begin around puberty. Androgen replacement has been shown to help with virilization, psychosocial development, hair growth, muscle mass, libido, testicular size, and precocious osteoporosis. Also, the patient needs to be educated and counseled about the fact that he is infertile.

What can be done to increase the fertility of patients with this condition?

Most men with Klinefelter produce small amounts of sperm, but it is typically not found in the ejaculate. Since some sperm are produced, they can be extracted from the testicles for use in vitro fertilization.

■ CASE 12

A 42-year-old African-American woman visits her physician complaining of heavy menstrual periods that last for several days. This has been occurring for the past 3 months and is associated with pain and fatigue. Physical examination reveals an enlarged uterus with multiple palpable masses. Laboratory tests show that hemoglobin is 11.3 g/dL and hematocrit is 33.3%.

What is the most likely diagnosis?

The heavy vaginal bleeding and palpable masses suggest leiomyomas, or uterine fibroids.

What is the epidemiology of this condition?

Uterine fibroids can be found in 25% of all reproductive-aged women. The incidence of leiomyoma is greatly increased in African-American women (two to three times increased risk compared to white women). Leiomyoma is the most common benign neoplasm in females.

Which cells of the uterus are most commonly affected in this condition?

Smooth muscle cells of the myometrium are most commonly affected, although fibroids can also occur in subendometrial or subperitoneal areas (Figure 13-7). Fibroids within the uterus can be submucosal, subserosal, or intramural. **Submucosal fibroids** are most often associated with abnormal bleeding, whereas **subserosal fibroids** are most often the cause of pressure due to mass effect.

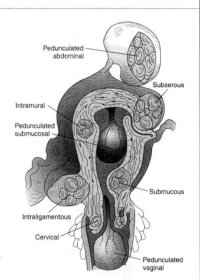

FIGURE 13-7. **Myomas of the uterus.** (Reproduced, with permission, from DeCherney AH, Nathan L. *Current Obstetric & Gynecologic Diagnosis & Treatment*, 10th ed. New York: McGraw-Hill, 2007: 640.)

How does the size of this neoplasm change with age?

The estrogen sensitivity of leiomyomas usually results in increased size during the first trimester of pregnancy and shrinkage after menopause.

Is this patient at increased risk for uterine malignancy?

Most leiomyosarcomas arise de novo and malignant transformation of leiomyomas into leiomyosarcoma is rare. Approximately 9% of uterine malignancies are leiomyosarcomas.

What uterine abnormality is associated with an increased risk of endometrial cancer?

Endometrial hyperplasia, which is characterized by abnormal glandular proliferation, is considered to be a premalignant lesion. This is caused by increased estrogen stimulation and, like uterine fibroids, often presents with abnormal vaginal bleeding. Therefore, its presence must be distinguished from abnormal vaginal bleeding secondary to uterine fibroids. This can be accomplished by histological examination of the endometrium obtained by endometrial biopsy.

What is the usual treatment for this condition?

Expectant management is often considered in mild cases. Hormonal therapies (oral contraceptive pills) are commonly prescribed for symptomatic treatment. For definitive treatment, surgery, including myomectomy or hysterectomy, can be performed. Other possibilities include uterine artery embolization and MRI-guided focused ultrasound surgery.

CASE 13

A 51-year-old woman presents to the clinic because her periods have become irregular. She says that sometimes there are 3 months between periods and that this irregularity began about 3 years ago. She complains of hot flashes that occur a few times each day and sometimes awaken her at night. She says she is also less interested in sex because she has begun to find it somewhat painful.

What is the most likely diagnosis?

The start of menopause. Menopause is defined as 12 months without a period (amenorrhea) in a woman older than 45 years of age without another cause for amenorrhea. The average age of menopause onset is 51 years. In women younger than 40 years of age, a full workup should be performed to evaluate the cause of what would be called premature ovarian failure.

What is the differential diagnosis for irregular vaginal bleeding, and how should it be evaluated?

Vaginal bleeding may be caused by the following:

- Uterine fibroids.
- Uterine polyps.
- Pregnancy complications.
- Menopause.
- Thyroid dysfunction.
- Endometrial hyperplasia (often secondary to anovulatory cycles and chronic estrogen exposure).
- Endometrial cancer.

The gold standard to evaluate these conditions is a uterine biopsy. Transvaginal ultrasound can also be diagnostic.

What are the signs, symptoms, and laboratory values associated with this condition?

Signs and symptoms of menopause include a change in menstrual cycle length, skipped periods, hot flashes, sleep disturbance, vaginal dryness (resulting in itching and dyspareunia), and an increase in urinary tract infections (due to increased vaginal pH).

Laboratory values in menopause include elevated follicle-stimulating hormone and, in early menopause, elevated estradiol levels.

What complications are associated with this condition?

One complication is morbidity from the symptoms of menopause, such as vasomotor flushing. Menopause also increases a woman's risk of developing osteoporosis. It is estimated that women can lose up to 20% of their bone density in the years surrounding menopause. This occurs because estrogen, which normally inhibits bone resorption, is decreased. Women undergoing menopause are also at risk for depression.

What are the appropriate treatments for this condition and its complications?

Short-term estrogen therapy (2–3 years and not more than 5 years) is recommended for moderate to severe vasomotor flushing. Long-term therapy is not recommended. The benefits of reducing hot flash symptoms must be weighed carefully with the increase in cardiovascular adverse events. Topical estrogen can be applied to treat vaginal dryness. For women with osteoporosis or at high risk for the disease, bisphosphonates, which prevent bone resorption, are the preferred first-line agent. The selective estrogen receptor modulator raloxifene is another alternative. These therapies should be used in addition to calcium/vitamin D, exercise, and smoking cessation. Selective serotonin reuptake inhibitors can be given for depressive symptoms.

■ CASE 14

A 17-year-old woman in her second trimester of pregnancy presents to a primary care clinic with painless vaginal bleeding and severe nausea and vomiting. She has not received medical care during her pregnancy. On physical examination, uterine enlargement is noted and grapelike clusters are found on pelvic examination. On ultrasound, a "snowstorm pattern" is seen.

What is the most likely diagnosis?

Hydatidiform mole or molar pregnancy. In North American and European countries, rates tend to be 1:1000–1500 pregnancies, whereas in Asian and Latin American countries the rates are higher, reaching 1:12–500 pregnancies.

What risk factors are associated with this condition?

The main risk factor is extremes of reproductive age (younger than 20 or older than 35 years). A history of molar pregnancy is also predictive.

How does this condition develop?

A **complete mole** develops when an enucleate egg is fertilized by a haploid sperm that then replicates. This results in 46 chromosomes (all paternal) but no fetal parts. A **partial mole** results from a haploid ovum and two sperm. The karyotype is typically triploid (69 chromosomes) and fetal parts may be present. There are some cases of recurrent moles that are due to a loss of maternal imprinting.

What are the typical signs, symptoms, and clinical presentation of this condition?

Classic presentation includes the following:

- Vaginal bleeding.
- Hyperemesis (due to high levels of β-hCG).
- Hyperthyroidism.

Patients usually present in the second trimester. Most patients do not develop symptoms because the mole is detected beforehand by the patient's OB/GYN.

The presence of a molar pregnancy is detected by an overly large uterus, lack of fetal heartbeat, lack of a fetus on ultrasound, very high levels of β-hCG (levels are often > 100,000 mIU/mL), and, occasionally, grapelike clusters exuding from the cervix. The diagnosis is typically made in early pregnancy with evidence of a "snowstorm pattern" on ultrasound, as seen in this patient.

What complications are associated with this condition?

- Increased risk for preeclampsia.
- Ovarian theca-lutein cysts (which are benign and resolve when the mole is removed).
- Respiratory distress (secondary to trophoblastic embolization).
- Choriocarcinoma (other causes of choriocarcinoma are spontaneous or induced abortion, ectopic pregnancy, and normal pregnancy).

What is the appropriate treatment for this condition?

This condition is highly sensitive to chemotherapy (usually methotrexate or actinomycin D) and has a low rate of recurrence. The most common site of metastasis is the lungs, and the metastases also resolve with chemotherapy. Patients who develop choriocarcinoma are asked not to get pregnant for a year so that they can be monitored for recurrence through serial β-hCG levels.

■ CASE 15

A 65-year-old-woman presents to the clinic with several months of abdominal and pelvic pain, vaginal bleeding, and a change in bowel habits. Her physical examination is normal and her cancer antigen–125 (CA-125) levels are within normal limits. However, malignancy is suspected, so a diagnostic laparotomy is recommended.

What is the most likely diagnosis?

Ovarian cancer is the second most common gynecologic malignancy. It is also the fifth most likely cause of cancer death in women.

What are the typical signs and symptoms of this condition?

Nonspecific symptoms are characteristic in ovarian cancer and include abdominal and pelvic pain, bloating, vaginal bleeding, and changes in bowel habits.

Physical signs are usually present only in advanced disease and include palpable ovarian or pelvic masses, ascites, pleural effusions, and bowel obstruction.

What are the different forms of this condition?

Most ovarian cancers (90%) are epithelial in origin. There are two types of epithelial ovarian cancer: serous and mucinous. The serous type is slightly more common and is often bilateral. The mucinous type can progress to pseudomyxoma peritonei. Pseudomyxoma peritonei is a condition in which the mucinous adenocarcinoma cells seed the peritoneum. These cells continue to produce mucous and fill the abdominal cavity, eventually obstructing the bowel.

Other types of ovarian cancers include sex cord stromal tumors, germ cell tumors, and metastatic cancer to the ovaries.

What risk factors are associated with this condition?

- Early menarche or late menopause.
- Nulligravidity.
- Infertility.
- Endometriosis.
- Family history of ovarian or breast cancer.
- *BRCA* mutation or Lynch syndrome.

Conversely, protective factors include multiple pregnancies and oral contraceptive pill use. It is theorized that protection against ovarian cancer results from a decreased number of ovulatory cycles.

What tests and/or imaging tools can be used to confirm the diagnosis?

Initial tests include transvaginal ultrasound, CT, and screening for the tumor marker CA-125. CT and ultrasound often miss cancers, however, and CA-125 is better able to detect recurrences than to establish an initial diagnosis. If suspicion remains high even with negative initial testing, exploratory surgery is usually recommended; findings are used to stage the disease.

What is the appropriate treatment for this condition?

Treatment is usually debulking surgery followed by chemotherapy, although choice of therapy depends on the clinical presentation of the cancer.

■ CASE 16

A 57-year-old woman with a history of eczema presents to her primary care physician with a new rash near the nipple of her right breast. She tells her doctor that the rash first appeared 2 months ago, and that she had been treating it with the topical corticosteroid prescribed for her eczema. At first the rash improved somewhat, but over the past few weeks it has gotten worse and has expanded in size. Physical examination reveals a raw, scaly lesion around the nipple that is beginning to ulcerate. There is also a palpable mass in the affected breast, a few centimeters deep to the skin lesion.

What is the most likely diagnosis?

Paget disease of the breast, an eczematous skin lesion in the area of the nipple, is associated with underlying invasive or in situ breast carcinoma (Figure 13-8). In approximately 50% of cases, Paget disease is associated with a palpable breast mass. Paget disease is often mistaken for a benign skin lesion such as eczema.

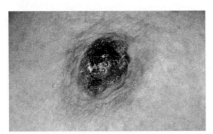

FIGURE 13-8. Paget disease of the breast. (Reproduced, with permission, from Wolff K et al. *Fitzpatrick's Color Atlas & Synopsis of Clinical Dermatology*, 5th ed. New York: McGraw-Hill, 2005: 495.)

What is the pathophysiology of this condition?

The skin lesion likely develops from underlying mammary adenocarcinoma cells that migrate through the ducts to the epidermis. However, an alternative theory suggests that epidermal keratinocytes transform into malignant cells independent of the underlying carcinoma.

What are the most likely findings on histology?

Histology often shows large cells with a halo of clear cytoplasm surrounding a prominent nucleolus. Additionally, the cytoplasm stains positive for mucin.

What are the most common sites of metastasis for breast carcinoma?

- Bone is the most common site for metastatic disease.
- Other common organ sites include liver and lung.
- Less common sites include bone marrow, brain, ovaries, spinal cord, and eye.

What is the lymphatic drainage of the breast?

Approximately 75% of lymphatic drainage of the breast is to the **axillary lymph nodes,** which include the pectoral (majority of drainage), apical, subscapular, lateral, and central node groups. The nipple drains to the pectoral group. The remaining lymph drains to the infraclavicular, supraclavicular, and parasternal (also known as the internal thoracic) nodes. To assess for lymph node metastasis in breast cancer, a sentinel lymph node biopsy is performed. To do this, a dye is injected into the tumor, and the first lymph node that the tumor drains into is dyed first. This lymph node is then biopsied to assess for lymphatic invasion.

Molecular analysis of a biopsy reveals that the cells express c-erbB-2 in high levels. What is the significance of this, and how does it affect treatment?

The human epithelial growth factor receptor (HER)-2/neu (also known as c-erbB-2) protein is a transmembrane growth factor receptor kinase. Overexpression of this molecule (present in 18%–20% of breast cancers) has been associated with a poorer prognosis. The drug trastuzumab is a humanized recombinant monoclonal antibody directed against this protein. The binding of trastuzumab to the extracellular portion of the molecule stimulates a cytotoxic immune response, leading to death of the cancer cells.

■ CASE 17

A 36-year-old African-American woman in week 34 of gestation presents to the emergency department with a 2-day history of headache, blurry vision, and sudden right upper quadrant (RUQ) pain. She reports that her husband has noticed increased swelling of her face since yesterday, and her rings are suddenly too tight. Physical examination is notable for hyperactive deep tendon reflexes and jugular venous distention. Her blood pressure at presentation is 165/110 mm Hg and 6 hours later is 170/110 mm Hg. Relevant laboratory findings are as follows:

Serum transaminase: 2 × normal
Serum creatinine: 1.5 mg/dL
Urinalysis: 3+ protein

What is the most likely diagnosis?

Preeclampsia and eclampsia are the two most common causes of pregnancy-induced hypertension (PIH). Preeclampsia can occur at 20+ weeks of gestation. Preeclampsia is characterized by proteinuria and blood pressure > 140/90 mm Hg. Eclampsia is preeclampsia associated with seizures and/or coma.

What signs and symptoms are commonly associated with this condition?

Mild preeclampsia is characterized by 1+ proteinuria and a blood pressure > 140/90 mm Hg. Common signs and symptoms include: headache, rapid weight gain, facial/hand edema, jugular venous distention, and hyperactive reflexes.

Severe preeclampsia is characterized by 3+ proteinuria and a blood pressure > 160/110 mm Hg. Common signs, symptoms, and laboratory results are visual changes, headache, somnolence, RUQ or epigastric pain, oligohydramnios, elevated liver enzyme levels, thrombocytopenia, renal failure, pulmonary edema/cyanosis, and intrauterine growth restriction.

Eclampsia is characterized by seizures or coma that develops in the setting of preeclampsia.

What is HELLP syndrome?

HELLP is a subcategory of preeclampsia that results in a high rate of stillbirth (10%–15%) and neonatal death (~ 25%). **HELLP** stands for Hemolysis, Elevated Liver enzymes, and Low Platelets.

What are the appropriate treatments for this condition?

If the baby is term, the fetal lungs are mature, or the case is severe, delivery is the best treatment. Mild preeclampsia is treated with bed rest, close monitoring, and blood pressure control with antihypertensive agents. In severe cases the mother should be hospitalized, and magnesium sulfate should be given for seizure prophylaxis (continued for 24 hours postpartum), in addition to antihypertensive agents. If severe, immediate delivery may be indicated to save the life of the mother.

■ CASE 18

A 17-year-old boy is awakened from his sleep by sudden, sharp scrotal pain. In the emergency department, the patient says he feels nauseous. He reports that the pain is mainly on the left side. On physical examination, he is afebrile, and there is evidence of swelling and reddening of the scrotum. He has a negative cremasteric reflex on the left. No transillumination of the scrotum is present.

What is the most likely diagnosis?

Testicular torsion. Testicular torsion is usually seen in adolescent males aged 16–18 years, although it can also occur in infancy. Approximately 50% of instances occur during sleep, but it can also occur at rest or with physical activity. Some patients have repeated episodes that spontaneously resolve (presumably because the testis is undergoing repeated torsion and detorsion).

What signs and symptoms are typically associated with this condition?

Symptoms of testicular torsion include the following:

- Sudden, acute onset of pain in the scrotum, often on one side.
- Swelling/reddening of the scrotum.
- Abdominal pain.
- Nausea/vomiting.

Signs of testicular torsion include the affected side's being higher than the other and horizontal in orientation as well as absent cremasteric reflex.

What conditions should be included in the differential diagnosis?

- **Epididymitis** should be considered but is not likely here given that signs of systemic infection (eg, fever) are not present nor is there epididymal tenderness or induration. Likewise, no history of sexually transmitted disease risk is noted. Notably, if scrotal elevation had relieved pain (Prehn sign), this would have indicated epididymitis in lieu of torsion.
- **Orchitis** should be considered but is also not likely in this patient given the lack of fever, lack of bilateral testicular involvement, and lack of other signs of mumps.
- **Trauma** should be considered but is not likely here given the lack of history consistent with this etiology.
- **Hydrocele** should be considered but again is not likely here because hydroceles rarely present with acute scrotal pain at night; however, when they are reactive hydroceles from other etiologies, pain may be present. Additionally, transillumination would be noted on exam.
- **Varicocele** should be considered but is unlikely in this case because the "bag of worms" sign would be noted on exam of the scrotum.
- **Hernia** should be considered but is also unlikely given that no mass was appreciated on exam.
- **Tumor** should be considered last, but is unlikely because no mass was noted on exam.

What complications are associated with this condition?

Testicular torsion results in the twisting of the spermatic cord, which contains the testicular artery, pampiniform plexus, and vas deferens. The main danger is the twisting of the testicular artery, which cuts off the blood supply to the testicle. If this is not reversed rapidly, it will result in **testicular atrophy and necrosis.** This is a true surgical emergency.

What is the appropriate treatment for this condition?

Manually untwisting the testis will produce immediate and dramatic pain relief if successful. The success of this method can be confirmed by evidence of return of blood flow to the testis on Doppler ultrasound. Even if successful, surgery should be performed to suture the testis in place to prevent repeated torsion. If manual detorsion does not work, emergent surgery must be performed. Treatment must be initiated within 6 hours of presentation to assure viability of the testicle. If it is not treated within 24 hours, there is little chance of the testicle's viability.

■ CASE 19

A 16-year-old girl is brought to her pediatrician because of an absence of menarche. She has short stature, a webbed neck, and a square chest. Physical examination reveals breast buds and female external genitalia. Her blood pressure is normal in both arms. CT scan reveals a small uterus and atretic, fatty ovaries. There is no known history of this condition in her family.

What is the most likely diagnosis?

Turner syndrome, characterized by gonadal dysgenesis secondary to the presence of a single X chromosome (XO) (Figure 13-9). This syndrome is the most common cause of primary amenorrhea. This genetic disorder affects 3% of all conceptions, but only 1:1000 45X embryos survives to term.

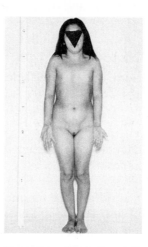

FIGURE 13-9. (Reproduced, with permission, from Le T, et al. *First Aid for the USMLE Step 1: 2008.* New York: McGraw-Hill, 2008: Color Image 109.)

What other conditions can cause primary amenorrhea?

Primary amenorrhea refers to the complete absence of menstruation by 16 years of age (compared with secondary amenorrhea, which is cessation of menstruation for more than 6 months after menarche). Other causes include the following:

- Absence of uterus, cervix, and/or vagina (**müllerian agenesis**).
- Hypothalamic hypogonadism (secondary to anorexia, exercise, stress, or gonadotropin-releasing hormone deficiency).
- Ovarian failure (gonadal dysgenesis, or polycystic ovarian syndrome).
- Pituitary disease.
- Transverse vaginal septum or imperforate hymen.

What diagnostic test is indicated based on the patient's clinical features?

Karyotype analysis should be performed.

What other conditions are associated with Turner syndrome?

- Coarctation of the aorta.
- Bicuspid aortic valve.
- Hypothyroidism.
- Sensorineural hearing loss.
- Renal abnormalities.
- Gastrointestinal telangiectasias.
- Osteoporosis.

What are the appropriate treatments for this condition?

Recombinant human growth hormone and hormone replacement therapy can initiate puberty and complete growth. Treatment of other associated conditions is also advised.

14

Respiratory

■ CASE 1

While working in a laboratory, a medical student accidentally opens a canister of highly corrosive gas and inhales a large quantity of the gas. He immediately goes to the emergency department for evaluation and treatment. Physical examination shows labored breathing and tachypnea as well as scattered crackles and tachycardia.

What conditions should be included in the differential diagnosis?

Given this patient's history, the differential diagnosis should include noncardiogenic pulmonary edema, acute pneumonitis, and acute respiratory distress syndrome. Onset of symptoms may take up to several days depending on the severity of the insult.

If protein-rich exudate is found in the alveoli, what diagnosis is likely and to what condition could it lead?

Protein-rich exudate in the alveoli suggests diffuse alveolar damage, which may lead to acute respiratory distress syndrome (ARDS). ARDS is a severe and potentially fatal lung disease in which acute inflammation and progressive parenchymal injury leads to hypoxemia. Typical histological presentation (Figure 14-1) involves diffuse alveolar damage and hyaline membrane formation in the alveolar walls.

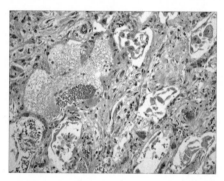

FIGURE 14-1. Histopathology of acute respiratory distress syndrome. (Reproduced, with permission, from USMLERx.com.)

What are the mechanisms of this condition?

Diffuse alveolar damage involves an increase in alveolar capillary permeability because of the damage caused by an inciting agent; in this case, the inciting agent is the corrosive gas and the body's response to it. Initial damage is due to neutrophilic substances that are toxic to tissue, oxygen-derived free radicals, and activation of the coagulation cascade. This insult leads to protein-rich exudates leaking into the lungs and the formation of an intra-alveolar hyaline membrane.

If this condition does not resolve, what complication can arise?

If the inflammation and hyaline membrane formation do not resolve, the damaged tissue can organize, resulting in **fibrosis**.

How are the other conditions in the differential diagnosis characterized?

- Noncardiogenic pulmonary edema is pulmonary edema caused by injury to the lung parenchyma (such as pulmonary contusion, aspiration, or inhalation of toxic gas).
- Acute interstitial pneumonitis is a severe lung disease that begins abruptly with cough, fever, and difficulty breathing and progresses to respiratory failure within days to weeks.

What is the most appropriate treatment for this condition?

Oxygenation is a cornerstone of treatment and usually involves some form of mechanical ventilation in the intensive care unit. Whenever ARDS develops, the underlying cause must be treated, and patients may also need medication to treat infection, reduce inflammation, and remove fluid from the lungs.

■ CASE 2

A 60-year-old man comes to his primary care physician because of dyspnea on exertion that has been worsening over the past several years. He also reports a nonproductive cough that he has had almost daily in the same period. On questioning, the man says he worked for 30 years stripping insulation on ships. On physical examination, chest expansion appears markedly restricted, and fine inspiratory crackles are heard that are most pronounced at the lung bases. The man also has multiple firm subcutaneous nodules on his hands.

What is the most likely diagnosis?

Asbestosis.

What other conditions should be considered in the differential diagnosis?

Interstitial lung diseases should also be considered, especially those caused by occupational exposure:

- **Silicosis** is caused by exposure to silica dust and characterized by fever, cough, shortness of breath, and cyanosis. X-ray of the chest will usually show multiple small nodules located primarily in the upper lung zones.
- **Coal worker's pneumoconiosis** is due to inhaled coal dust that accumulates in the lungs and, over time, causes inflammation and fibrosis. Symptoms are usually mild at first and include chronic cough and shortness of breath. X-ray of the chest often shows large masses of dense fibrosis in the upper lung zones.
- **Berylliosis** is classically associated with beryllium mining or exposure to fluorescent light bulbs. Patients develop small inflammatory nodules in their lungs (ie, granulomas) that ultimately progress to restrictive lung disease.

Conditions not related to occupational exposure, including idiopathic pulmonary fibrosis, should also be considered.

What is the pathophysiology of this condition?

The pathophysiologic process of asbestosis involves diffuse pulmonary interstitial fibrosis caused by inhaled asbestos fibers. Asbestos fibers penetrate bronchioles and lung tissue, where they are surrounded by macrophages and coated by a protein-iron complex **(ferruginous bodies)**; Figure 14-2 shows these phagocytosed bodies. Diffuse fibrosis around the bronchioles spreads to the alveoli, causing lung tissue to become rigid and airways distorted.

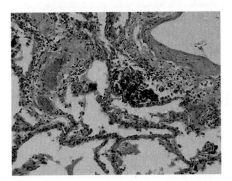

FIGURE 14-2. **Asbestos bodies.** (Reproduced, with permission, from USMLERx.com.)

What are the most likely x-ray of the chest findings?

In cases of minor exposure, the only findings may be pleural thickening or calcified pleural plaques. In cases of extensive pulmonary fibrosis, reticular or nodular opacities will be seen throughout the lung fields, most prominently at the bases.

▌CASE 3

A 7-year-old boy is brought to the emergency department (ED) after awakening in the middle of the night with difficulty breathing. He has a 2-day history of worsening productive cough and wheezing. The patient is found to have dyspnea, tachypnea, and a decreased inspiratory/expiratory ratio. Lung examination reveals diffuse rhonchi and expiratory wheezes in addition to pulsus paradoxus. He is afebrile and has no recent history of fever. This is the patient's second visit to the ED with these symptoms; his first visit was 2 years ago.

What is the most likely diagnosis?

Asthma exacerbation. Asthma is a form of obstructive lung disease.

What are other obstructive lung diseases, and how do they differ from this condition?

- **Bronchiectasis** is a disease state in which bronchi become inflamed and dilated, causing obstructed airflow and impaired clearance of secretions. It is often associated with AIDS, cystic fibrosis, and Kartagener syndrome.
- **Emphysema** is a long-term, progressive disease in which the small airways and alveoli (which maintain the lung's functional shape) are destroyed. This is usually the result of smoking.
- **Chronic bronchitis** is chronic inflammation of the bronchi that causes a persistent and productive cough that lasts for at least 3 months in 2 consecutive years. Smoking is almost always the cause.

Unlike these diseases, the airway obstruction seen in asthma is usually reversible.

What is the pathophysiology of this condition?

Acutely, **bronchial hyperresponsiveness** leads to episodic, reversible bronchoconstriction. Specifically, smooth muscle contraction in the airways leads to **expiratory airflow obstruction**. Chronically, **airway inflammation** leads to histologic changes in the bronchial tree.

What histologic findings in the lung are associated with this condition?

Histologic examination reveals smooth muscle hypertrophy, goblet cell hyperplasia, thickening of basement membranes, and increased eosinophil recruitment (in Figure 14-3 the arrow points to plate of cartilage, and the arrowhead points to infiltrate of inflammatory cells). Dilated bronchi are filled with neutrophils and may have mucous plugs.

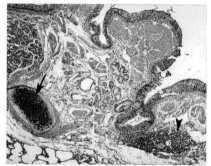

FIGURE 14-3. Histologic findings in asthma. (Reproduced, with permission, from Wilson FJ, et al. *Histology Image Review.* Norwalk, CT: Appleton & Lange, 1997: Figure 19-42.)

What are common triggers of this condition?

Triggers of asthma exacerbation include **stress, cold, exercise, dust and animal dander, mold,** and **viral upper respiratory tract infections.**

What is the appropriate treatment for this condition?

For acute episodes, albuterol, a β_2-agonist, helps relax bronchial smooth muscle and decrease airway obstruction. However, for long-term control of persistent symptoms, inhaled corticosteroids are the best treatment.

CASE 4

A pregnant woman suffering from markedly elevated blood pressure and thrombocytopenia suddenly starts having seizures. She is rushed to the delivery room, where she is determined to have eclampsia, and then immediately taken to the operating room for cesarean section. Her premature baby (< 32 weeks) is delivered and found to have increased work of breathing and an elevated heart rate. The baby is intubated, a drug is administered, and x-ray of the chest is taken (Figure 14-4).

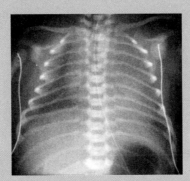

FIGURE 14-4. (Reproduced, with permission, from Tintinalli JE, et al. *Tintinalli's Emergency Medicine: A Comprehensive Study Guide,* 7th ed. New York: McGraw-Hill, 2008: Figure 4-0.1.)

What drug was most likely given to this baby to promote lung expansion?

Surfactant, normally produced late in fetal life (around week 28), can be given to the baby directly. Surfactant lowers the surface tension between alveoli, helping the lung to expand. Dexamethasone can be used antenatally to aid in surfactant production; it is given to women at risk for preterm delivery to reduce the risk of respiratory distress syndrome.

What is the most likely diagnosis?

The baby is suffering from neonatal respiratory distress syndrome, a disease in which parts of the baby's lungs are deficient in surfactant. This deficiency results in collapsed air spaces, incomplete expansion of the lungs (ie, atelectasis), hyaline membranes (Figure 14-4), and vascular congestion. Clinically, patients present with tachypnea, tachycardia, and cyanosis immediately after birth.

What are the primary types of atelectasis?

- **Adhesive atelectasis** occurs in patients with insufficient surfactant.
- **Obstructive atelectasis** involves obstruction of an airway, commonly at the level of the smaller bronchi, with collapse of the alveoli distal to the obstruction. A common cause for this type of atelectasis is secretions or exudates.
- **Cicatricial atelectasis** occurs in an area of scarred lung tissue.
- **Passive atelectasis** occurs because of poor ventilation (eg, after surgery).
- **Compressive atelectasis** is due to a space-occupying mass in the thorax that compresses a region of lung tissue.

How does obstructive atelectasis differ from compressive atelectasis?

In obstructive atelectasis, the mediastinum shifts toward the atelectasis due to loss of lung volume in that area. By contrast, the mediastinum shifts away from the atelectasis with compression.

During atelectasis, to what is the patient commonly predisposed?

Atelectasis results in mucus trapping and a decrease in ventilation, thereby predisposing the patient to infections.

CASE 5

A patient comes to his physician with a hacking cough and purulent sputum. His history is positive for a genetic birth defect called Kartagener syndrome in which ciliary motion is either abnormal or absent. The patient also claims to have a constantly runny nose, a prior diagnosis of chronic bronchitis, and numerous bouts of pneumonia. Before making a diagnosis, the physician orders a high-resolution CT scan of the patient's lungs (Figure 14-5).

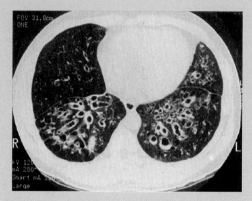

FIGURE 14-5. (Reproduced, with permission, from Fauci AS, Kasper DL, Braunwald E, Hauser SL, Longo DL, Jameson JL, Loscalzo J. *Harrison's Principles of Internal Medicine*, 17th Edition; Fig. 252-1.)

What is the most likely diagnosis?
Bronchiectasis.

What radiologic findings can help diagnose this condition?
In bronchiectasis, a "tree-in-bud" pattern is commonly seen on high-resolution CT scans. This represents the plugging of small airways with mucus and bronchiolar wall thickening.

What are the possible etiologies of this condition?
Etiologies include chronic bronchial necrotizing infections, cystic fibrosis, bronchial obstruction from granulomatous disease or neoplasms, α_1-antitrypsin deficiency, impaired host defense (eg, AIDS), and airway inflammation (eg, bronchiolitis obliterans). Additionally, tuberculosis and primary ciliary dyskinesia should be evaluated.

What complications are associated with this condition?
Complications of bronchiectasis include hemoptysis, hypoxemia, cor pulmonale, dyspnea, and amyloidosis.

What is the appropriate treatment for this condition?
If an infection is thought to be the cause, then antibiotics should be given. If the bronchiectasis is localized, surgery may be an option. For routine management, however, measures include postural drainage and chest percussion.

■ CASE 6

A 50-year-old woman visits a community health clinic because of a 1-month history of cough productive of yellow sputum. On questioning, she says she has had several periods of cough lasting 4–6 consecutive months each year for the past 5 years. She has smoked two packs of cigarettes per day for the past 30 years. On examination, the woman's breathing is shallow, and she exhales slowly with pursed lips. Her jugular venous pulse is visible to the jawline when she is reclined at an angle of 45°. Auscultation of the chest demonstrates wheezing and distant heart sounds. A positive hepatojugular reflux is demonstrated, as is 2+ pitting edema up to her knees. X-ray of the chest is shown in Figure 14-6.

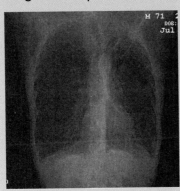

FIGURE 14-6. (Reproduced, with permission, from Tintinalli JE, et al. *Tintinalli's Emergency Medicine: A Comprehensive Study Guide*, 7th ed. New York: McGraw-Hill, 2011: Figure 73-2.)

What is the most likely diagnosis?
The history of productive cough for at least 3 consecutive months over 2 consecutive years accompanied by emphysema (suggested by pursed-lip breathing) indicates chronic obstructive pulmonary disease (COPD) with features of chronic bronchitis.

What radiologic findings can help diagnose this condition?
In patients with COPD, x-rays of the chest often reveal lung hyperinflation, flattening of the diaphragm, and decreased peripheral vascular markings.

What abnormalities would be expected on pulmonary function testing?
- In COPD, the forced expiratory volume in 1 second (FEV_1) is decreased, forced vital capacity (FVC) is normal or decreased, and the FEV_1/FVC ratio is < 70% of predicted.
- In restrictive lung disease, decreased vital capacity and total lung capacity result in a FEV_1/FVC ratio of > 80%.

How would this condition affect the patient's arterial blood gas levels (pH, PaO_2, $Paco_2$, and SaO_2)?
The pH decreases as a result of respiratory acidosis. Although pH may be normal in a patient with chronic compensated COPD, it is low in a patient with an acute exacerbation. Arterial oxygen tension (PaO_2) decreases, arterial carbon dioxide tension ($Paco_2$) increases, and oxygen saturation (SaO_2) decreases secondary to impaired gas exchange (from destruction of alveolar septae and pulmonary capillary bed).

Why is breathing with pursed lips adaptive in this condition?
Breathing with pursed lips maintains positive end-expiratory pressure (PEEP). PEEP prevents alveolar and small airway collapse, which is common in emphysema. Respiratory therapy often provides supplemental oxygen via a mask or nasal prongs. Positive airway pressure can be provided by continuous positive airway pressure, bilevel positive airway pressure, or intubation and ventilatory support.

What complication of this condition is suggested by the patient's enlarged neck veins, hepatomegaly, and edema?
Cor pulmonale. Right heart failure due to chronic pulmonary hypertension leads to systemic venous congestion, which presents with the symptoms mentioned here. This complication occurs only in patients with severe COPD who develop pulmonary hypertension.

■ CASE 7

A 67-year-old man comes to the emergency department complaining of a 3-day history of cough and fever and a 1-day history of shaking chills. He has smoked about half a pack of cigarettes per day for the past 45 years. For the past 9 months, the man has had an increasingly severe cough that has been productive of clear sputum. His cough now produces rusty sputum. On physical examination, he is found to have a respiratory rate of 24/min and a temperature of 37.8°C (100°F). An x-ray of the chest shows lung consolidation (Figure 14-7).

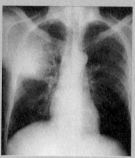

FIGURE 14-7. (Reproduced, with permission, from Le T, et al. *First Aid for the USMLE Step 1: 2011.* New York: McGraw-Hill, 2011: 514.)

What is the most likely diagnosis?

This patient presents with several classic findings of community-acquired pneumonia (CAP): a productive cough, fever, rigors (shaking chills), and tachypnea. His risk factors include an advanced age and a significant smoking history.

What are the likely lung examination findings?

Decreased breath sounds, crackles, dullness to percussion, and increased tactile fremitus are probable findings and can indicate areas of consolidation (ie, areas filled with fluid).

What are the most likely causative organisms?

- *Streptococcus pneumoniae* (20%–60%).
- *Haemophilus influenzae* (3%–10%).
- *Staphylococcus aureus* (3%–5%).
- *Legionella* (2%–8%).
- *Mycoplasma* (1%–6%).
- Viruses (2%–15%).

Gram stain of the sputum reveals gram-positive cocci in pairs and short chains. Additional testing reveals that the organism is optochin sensitive and the Quellung reaction is positive. What is the causative organism?

S pneumoniae is a gram-positive, encapsulated organism, hence the positive Quellung reaction, which is performed by adding anticapsular antisera that cause the capsule to swell. The organism is also catalase negative, α-hemolytic (partial hemolysis; the blood turns greenish), and optochin sensitive (which differentiates it from *Streptococcus viridans,* which is also α-hemolytic).

What are the appropriate treatments for this condition?

Penicillin V and amoxicillin are rarely used in clinical practice because resistance with these drugs is an increasing problem. The typical treatment is either a macrolide in combination with a cephalosporin or fluoroquinolone monotherapy.

What factors would indicate hospitalization for a patient with this condition?

Factors that increase the need for hospitalization include age older than 65 years, altered mental status, underlying chronic illness, elevated blood pressure, elevated temperature, and abnormally high kidney function tests (ie, creatinine and blood urea nitrogen).

■ CASE 8

A newborn boy has been diagnosed by prenatal ultrasound with a congenital cystic adenomatoid malformation (CCAM) in the right lower lobe of his lung. CCAMs are hamartomas of terminal bronchioles. Because of the risks of CCAM-associated complications, the boy undergoes a right lower lobe resection.

How many segments of lung will be resected if the entire right lower lobe is removed?

There are five segments in the right lower lobe (Figure 14-8): Medial, Anterior, Lateral, Posterior, and Superior (mnemonic: **MALPS**).

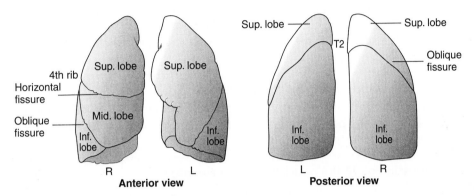

FIGURE 14-8. **Lobes of the lung.** (Reproduced, with permission, from Le T, et al. *First Aid for the USMLE Step 1: 2011.* New York: McGraw-Hill, 2011: 503.)

Which vessels supply arterial and venous branches to the lungs, and what paths do the branches follow to supply each lung segment?

The lung alveoli are supplied by branches of the pulmonary artery and vein. The bronchial tree also receives its arterial supply from the bronchial arteries (from the aorta) and venous drainage from bronchial veins that feed into the azygos and accessory hemiazygos veins. Pulmonary and bronchial arteries follow the airways into the periphery. Pulmonary veins course in the septa between adjacent lung segments.

When entering the thoracic cavity through an intercostal space, the surgeon preserves the intercostal nerves and vessels. What is the anatomic relationship between the intercostal nerves and vessels and the ribs?

The intercostal nerves and vessels lie in the costal groove inferior to each rib. They are positioned between the innermost intercostal and internal intercostal muscles for the length of those muscles.

During development, the pulmonary arteries arise from which aortic arch?

The sixth aortic arch produces the pulmonary arteries as well as to the ductus arteriosus.

During which week of gestation are the bronchial buds formed from the foregut?

Bronchial buds are formed in the fourth week of gestation. Depending on the histology and other associated anomalies, different types of CCAMs are suspected to result from insults at varying stages of development. For example, **type 2 CCAMs** are associated with anomalies such as esophageal fistulas and bilateral renal agenesis. Thus, type 2 CCAMs are thought to arise early in organogenesis, during the fourth week of gestation.

▮ CASE 9

A 15-year-old girl is brought to the emergency department in acute respiratory distress and is stabilized with treatment. On questioning, she reports an increasingly productive cough over the past few days. Her pulse oximetry shows 93% oxygen saturation on 2 L of oxygen, and she often gasps for air midsentence. Examination shows nostril flaring, subcostal retractions, and clubbing of the fingers. A birth history reveals she had a meconium ileus.

What genetically transmitted condition does this patient likely have?

The patient likely has cystic fibrosis (CF), which is caused by loss-of-function mutations in the cystic fibrosis transmembrane conductance regulator (CFTR) protein, a chloride channel found in all exocrine tissues. As a result of these mutations, secretions in the lung, intestine, pancreas, and reproductive tract are extremely viscous.

What test was likely conducted to confirm the diagnosis?

A genetic screen during the patient's infancy was most likely conducted. A sweat chloride test can also confirm the diagnosis, but it may be difficult to collect an adequate amount of sweat in a baby. Patients with CF have elevated sweat chloride levels.

What is the probable etiology of the patient's current symptoms?

The lungs in patients with CF are colonized at an early age with various bacteria not normally found in the lung. Therefore, patients suffer from repeated pulmonary bacterial infections (*Staphylococcus aureus*, *Haemophilus influenzae*, and *Pseudomonas aeruginosa* are the most common organisms), which increase production of viscous secretions. These increased secretions lead to increased cough and pulmonary obstruction, which can result in acute respiratory distress.

What vitamin supplements do patients with this condition usually require?

Patients with CF generally require the fat-soluble vitamins A, D, E, and K. The thick secretions block the release of pancreatic enzymes, resulting in pancreatic insufficiency.

What information can be provided if this patient asks for genetic counseling?

The frequency of CF in white people is 1: 2000; the carrier rate of CF in white people is 1:25. CF is an autosomal recessive disease, so all children of a patient with CF will at a minimum become carriers. Approximately 95% of males with CF are infertile because of defects in the transport of sperm. Infertility affects as many as 20% of women as a result of abnormally thick cervical mucus and amenorrhea from malnutrition.

What is the prognosis for patients with this condition?

- Prognosis for patients with CF is generally good.
- Most patients are able to survive into their 30s and lead relatively normal lives.

■ CASE 10

A 70-year-old woman with a 65-pack-year smoking history complains to her physician of worsening dyspnea. The dyspnea has now become so severe that she is experiencing shortness of breath at rest. She also admits that her cough is now occasionally productive of small amounts of thin sputum. Physical examination reveals a thin woman with an increased thoracic anteroposterior diameter. The physician notes that she breathes through pursed lips, has an increased expiratory phase, and is using her accessory muscles to breathe.

What is the most likely diagnosis?

- The most likely diagnosis is COPD with features of emphysema. Other obstructive lung diseases that should be on the differential include chronic bronchitis and asthma.
- By definition, a patient with chronic bronchitis experiences a cough with sputum production on most days for 3 months of a year for at least 2 consecutive years. Patients with chronic bronchitis also experience hypoxia that results in cyanosis of the skin and lips as well as fluid retention.
- Patients with asthma experience reversible and episodic airway obstruction, which is characterized by wheezing, coughing, and shortness of breath. Symptoms usually respond to treatment with an inhaled β_2-agonist and can often be prevented by avoiding triggers, such as allergens and irritants.

What is the pathophysiology of this condition?

Destruction of alveolar walls results in enlargement of air spaces. Compared with a normal lung (Figure 14-9A), the lung in emphysema (Figure 14-9B) shows destruction of lung parenchyma and marked dilatation of terminal air spaces. Destruction of lung parenchyma also decreases elastic recoil, which increases airway collapsibility, causing expiratory obstruction. As a result, patients with emphysema often find it easier to exhale through pursed lips (which maintains a high end-expiratory pressure, thereby stenting the alveoli open)—hence the term "pink puffers." Because of chronic hyperinflation, lungs are expanded close to total lung capacity with little inspiratory reserve, and diaphragms are flattened to a point of significant mechanical disadvantage.

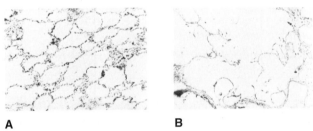

A　　　　　　　　　　　**B**

FIGURE 14-9. (A) Normal lung. (B) Lung in emphysema. (Reproduced, with permission, from Chandrasoma P, et al. *Concise Pathology*, 3rd ed. Norwalk, CT: Appleton & Lange, 1997: Figure 35-6.)

What findings are expected on lung and heart examination?

Air trapped in the lungs causes the chest to sound hyperresonant to percussion. Patients with COPD also have decreased breath sounds, wheezing, a prolonged expiratory phase, diminished heart sounds, and a PMI that may be displaced centrally.

What pattern of lung parenchymal destruction is likely to be found in this patient?

Smoking results in a destruction pattern termed **centrilobular emphysema**, which affects the respiratory bronchioles and central alveolar ducts. **Panacinar emphysema** is associated with α_1-antitrypsin deficiency and results in destruction throughout the acinus.

How do pulmonary function test results help distinguish this condition from other lung diseases?

In COPD, pulmonary test results are likely to be consistent with obstructive lung disease findings: dramatically reduced forced expiratory volume in 1 second (FEV_1) and reduced forced vital capacity (FVC), resulting in an FEV_1/FVC ratio of < 70%. By contrast, in restrictive lung diseases, both the FEV_1 and the FVC are reduced, resulting in a normal FEV_1/FVC.

■ CASE 11

A 4-year-old boy is brought to the emergency department by his mother because he is lethargic, drooling, and having difficulty breathing. Physical examination reveals an elevated temperature and a high-pitched upper airway wheeze. Further questioning of the patient's mother reveals that the child has not received any immunizations. A lateral x-ray of the neck shows soft tissue swelling.

What is the most likely diagnosis?

The stridor found on lung examination and the drooling—findings consistent with both tracheal and esophageal obstruction—suggest **acute epiglottitis**. The obstruction is due to swelling of the epiglottis caused by infection and is a **medical emergency**. The x-ray shows the classic "thumbprint" sign caused by the thickening and swelling of the epiglottis.

What is the likely source of this infection?

Given the child's unimmunized status, the most likely cause is type b *Haemophilus influenzae* infection. *H influenzae* is considered part of the normal flora of the nasopharynx. The organism may thus be spread by direct contact with respiratory secretions and by airborne droplet contamination. Epiglottitis may also represent a primary infection of the epiglottis rather than invasion from the nasopharynx.

What additional microorganisms can cause this presentation?

Epiglottitis can also be caused by *Pasteurella multocida*, which is often transmitted from dog or cat bites, and herpes simplex virus type 1.

What is the main virulence factor of the causative organism in this case?

The polysaccharide capsule is the major virulence factor of *H influenzae*, which has both encapsulated and nonencapsulated strains. The nonencapsulated forms are limited to local infections such as otitis media in children and mild respiratory infection in adults (Table 14-1). The encapsulated strains are significantly more virulent and can cause disseminated diseases such as meningitis, epiglottitis, and septic arthritis. There are six capsular types of *H influenzae*, designated a through f. The b-type capsule accounts for approximately 95% of serious *H influenzae* infections in children.

TABLE 14-1	Types of Infection Caused by *Haemophilus*			
	H INFLUENZAE		*H AEGYPTIUS*	*H DUCREYI*
	TYPE B	NONTYPEABLE		
Type of infection	Meningitis Epiglottitis Bacteremia Cellulitis Septic arthritis	Otitis media Sinusitis Tracheobronchitis Pneumonia	Conjunctivitis Purpuric fever (Brazilian)	Chancroid (painful ulcers of genitals, lymphadenitis)
Treatment	Ceftazidime Cefotaxime Ceftriaxone Gentamicin	Cephalosporin Fluoroquinolone Azithromycin	Rifampin	Azithromycin Cephalosporin Ciprofloxacin

How has the vaccine for this infection been redesigned to improve its efficacy?

The **Hib vaccine** consists of a purified b-type capsule conjugated to diphtheria toxin. The diphtheria toxin activates T lymphocytes, which are required for adequate antibody production against the capsular antigen. The original vaccine consisted only of b capsule and was not effective in eliciting an antibody response.

■ CASE 12

A 60-year-old man visits his doctor complaining of recurrent fever, chest pain, and difficulty breathing. He states that his symptoms wax and wane but never completely resolve. The patient's occupational history is significant for 30 years as a shipyard worker. Suspecting an occupational exposure to hazardous material, the physician orders a CT scan of the thorax (Figure 14-10).

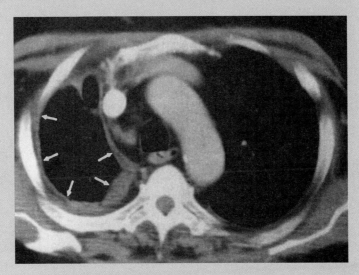

FIGURE 14-10. (Reproduced, with permission, from Chen MYM, et al. *Basic Radiology*. New York: McGraw-Hill, 2004: 101.)

What is the most likely diagnosis?

The pleural thickening (indicated by the arrows in Figure 14-10) in addition to a history of exposure to asbestos makes the diagnosis of **malignant mesothelioma** of high concern. Benign pleural plaques could also present similarly. As the malignant mesothelioma progresses, the lung is surrounded and compressed by a thick layer of tumor. Although mesotheliomas are rare, an exposure history greatly increases the risk. Common features of the disease include dyspnea, chest pain, and pleural effusions.

What occupations put patients at risk for exposure to the suspected agent?

Asbestos exposure is commonly seen in pipe fitters, shipyard workers, welders, plumbers, and construction workers. In addition to malignant mesothelioma, asbestos is associated with benign pleural plaques, interstitial lung disease, pleural effusions, and bronchogenic carcinoma. The diseases typically manifest several decades after asbestos exposure.

What are the typical findings on pulmonary function testing in this condition?

Pulmonary function testing reveals a **restrictive pattern**. Tumor growth decreases lung expansion and total lung capacity. Both forced expiratory volume in 1 second (FEV_1) and forced vital capacity (FVC) are decreased, but the FEV_1/FVC ratio is preserved.

What is the prognosis for patients with this condition?

Given only supportive care, the median survival for patients with malignant mesothelioma is approximately 6–12 months. With very aggressive therapies, such as extrapleural pneumonectomy plus chemotherapy and radiation, the median survival can be as high as 34 months.

■ CASE 13

A 70-year-old man with a history of laryngeal cancer presents to the emergency department with shortness of breath. He complains that for the past 3 days he has been unable to lie flat to sleep, and last night he woke up suddenly gasping for air. A decubitus x-ray of the chest shows layering of fluid (Figure 14-11; arrowhead points to the layer of fluid).

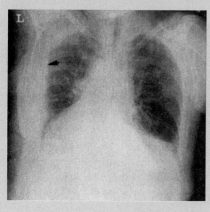

FIGURE 14-11. (Reproduced, with permission, from Tintinalli JE, et al. *Tintinalli's Emergency Medicine: A Comprehensive Study Guide,* 7th ed. New York: McGraw-Hill, 2011: Figure 56-3.)

What is the most likely diagnosis?

A **pleural effusion** consists of fluid accumulation in the pleural space (between the visceral pleura and the parietal pleura) of the lung. Normally, the pleural space is only a potential space, with a small amount of fluid.

How is this condition classified?

There are two types of pleural effusion:

- **Transudative pleural effusions** are caused by increased hydrostatic pressure of the pleural capillaries (as in congestive heart failure) or by a decrease in plasma oncotic pressure (as in disorders with decreased plasma albumin levels, such as renal and hepatic failure).
- **Exudative pleural effusions** are caused by a change in the permeability of the pleural surface (such as secondary to inflammatory or neoplastic changes). These effusions have a high protein content.

What are the common causes of this condition?

- Common causes of transudative pleural effusion include congestive heart failure, cirrhosis, constrictive pericarditis, nephrotic syndrome, and pulmonary embolism (PE).
- Common causes of exudative pleural effusion include infection (pneumonia, tuberculosis), malignancy (primary or metastatic lung cancer or mesothelioma), collagen vascular disease, and PE (note that PE can cause both transudative and exudative pleural effusions).

What are the typical laboratory findings in this condition?

Analysis of pleural effusion fluid includes measuring pH, total protein, lactate dehydrogenase (LDH), glucose, cell count, gram stain and culture. Cytology can also be performed to identify malignant causes. Meeting any one of the three **Light's criteria** qualifies the effusion as an exudate:

- Protein effusion/serum ratio > 0.5
- LDH effusion/serum ratio > 0.6
- Pleural LDH level greater than two-thirds the upper limit of serum LDH level.

What are the appropriate treatments for this condition?

Thoracentesis performed by needle insertion into the pleural space is both diagnostic and therapeutic. The needle is inserted through an intercostal space superior to the rib to avoid the intercostal nerve and vessels, which lie in the intercostal groove at the inferior border of the rib. Other treatments include **pleurodesis** (in which the pleura is made adherent and closed by chemicals such as talc or doxycycline or physical abrasion) and permanent catheter insertion into the pleural space for periodic fluid drainage.

■ CASE 14

An 18-year-old man comes to his physician complaining of a 3-week history of worsening dry and nonproductive cough. He also has a throbbing headache and a mild fever and complains of malaise and a sore throat. Treatment with penicillin has not relieved his symptoms.

What is the most likely diagnosis?

Mycoplasma pneumoniae, which causes primary atypical pneumonia (**"walking pneumonia"**), is the most common cause of pneumonia in teenagers (Table 14-2). This organism is the smallest free-living bacterium. It has no cell wall and its membrane is the only bacterial membrane containing cholesterol.

TABLE 14-2	Most Common Causes of Pneumonia According to Age		
6 WEEKS–18 YEARS	**18–40 YEARS**	**40–65 YEARS**	**> 65 YEARS**
Viral (respiratory syncytial virus)	M pneumoniae	S pneumoniae	S pneumoniae
Mycoplasma pneumoniae	C pneumoniae	Haemophilus influenzae	Viral
Chlamydia pneumoniae	S pneumoniae	Anaerobes	Anaerobes
Streptococcus pneumoniae		M pneumoniae	H influenzae

What diagnostic tests can help confirm the diagnosis?

A high titer of cold agglutinins (IgM) and growth on Eaton agar (which is specific for growing *M pneumoniae* and contains penicillin for selectivity) indicate *M pneumonia* infection.

What clinical findings are commonly associated with this condition?

Infection with *M pneumoniae* typically results in mild upper respiratory tract disease including low-grade fever, malaise, headache, and a dry, nonproductive cough. Symptoms gradually worsen over a few days and can last for more than 2 weeks. Less than 10% of patients develop more severe disease with lower respiratory tract symptoms. Classically, x-ray of the chest in these patients looks worse than would be predicted by their physical appearance.

What is the pathogenicity of this organism?

M pneumoniae is an extracellular organism that attaches to respiratory epithelium. As the superficial layer of respiratory epithelial cells is destroyed, the normal ability of the upper airways to clear themselves is lost. As a result, the lower respiratory tract becomes contaminated by microbes and is mechanically irritated. Close contact allows for spread of the organism.

What hematologic condition can develop secondary to this infection?

Autoimmune hemolytic anemia due to **cold agglutinins** (usually IgM autoantibodies that are able to agglutinate RBCs at temperatures below 35°C) can lead to lysis and mild anemia. Cold agglutinin production peaks during the third week of *M pneumoniae* infection and resolves spontaneously.

What are the appropriate treatments for this condition?

Azithromycin is most commonly prescribed to treat *Mycoplasma* infection. Tetracycline, clarithromycin, or erythromycin may be prescribed as well.

■ CASE 15

A 62-year-old woman presents to the emergency department with acute-onset shortness of breath. She also complains of "stabbing" pleuritic right-sided chest pain. The woman had a stroke 3 months ago but is otherwise healthy. Her temperature is 36.7°C (98.1°F), blood pressure is 90/60 mm Hg, heart rate is 110/min, respiratory rate is 40/min, and oxygen saturation is 80% on room air. Physical examination reveals jugular venous distention, and cardiovascular examination reveals a fast rate with regular rhythm and no murmurs. The woman's lungs are clear bilaterally with decreased breath sounds in the right middle lobe.

What is the most likely diagnosis?

This is a case of pulmonary embolism (also known as pulmonary thromboembolism, or PTE).

What other conditions should be included in the differential diagnosis?

The differential diagnosis includes the following:

- Cardiac: Myocardial infarction, unstable angina, pericarditis (all less likely to present with such a low oxygen saturation).
- Pulmonary: Pneumonia, pneumothorax (tension pneumothorax especially needs to be ruled out), exacerbation of chronic obstructive pulmonary disease.
- Musculoskeletal: Costochondritis (presents with point tenderness reproducible on physical exam).

What is the Virchow triad?

The Virchow triad refers to the three factors that increase the risk for venous thrombosis: local **injury** to the vessel wall, **hypercoagulability,** and **stasis.** It is believed that patients with PTE are predisposed to venous thrombosis; triggers include pregnancy, limb immobility, and surgery.

What test remains the gold standard for diagnosing this condition?

Pulmonary angiography remains the most specific test available for definitively diagnosing PTE. However, because of the invasiveness of angiography, CT of the chest with thin cuts is the most frequently used diagnostic test. A ventilation-perfusion lung scan is still often used. A lung scan showing normal perfusion virtually excludes PTE. An x-ray of the chest can show signs of PTE including Hampton hump (a wedge-shaped indicator of infarction in a region served by an occluded vessel) and Westermark sign (oligemia distal to a PTE) but neither sign is specific and additional imaging is necessary to confirm the diagnosis.

Plasma D-dimer levels have a negative predictive value in cases of low clinical suspicion but are elevated in more than 90% of patients with PTE. This assay is nonspecific and levels may also be elevated in conditions such as myocardial infarction or sepsis. The current strategy for diagnosing PTE and deep venous thrombosis is shown in Figure 14-12.

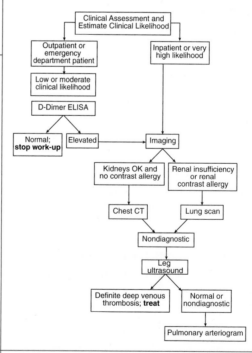

FIGURE 14-12. **Diagnosis of PTE.** (Adapted, with permission, from Kasper DL, et al. *Harrison's Principles of Internal Medicine,* 16th ed. New York: McGraw-Hill, 2005: 1563.)

What is the most likely finding on microscopic examination?

Under low-power magnification, characteristic lines of Zahn (alternating pale lines of platelets and fibrin with RBCs, indicating premortem clot formation) are visible in the thrombus.

What are the appropriate treatments for this condition?

PTE is treated with therapeutic levels of heparin for at least 5 days unless there is a contraindication to anticoagulation (eg, recent surgery). In most patients, warfarin and heparin may be started together and oral anticoagulation continued for at least 3 months. If there is a contraindication to anticoagulation or a high risk of recurrence of PTE, an inferior vena cava filter is recommended.

■ CASE 16

A 55-year-old woman with a history of chronic obstructive pulmonary disease (COPD) presents to the local hospital complaining of fatigue and weakness. On admission, she is found to have the following laboratory values:

Serum:
  Sodium: 144 mEq/L
  Chloride: 96 mEq/L
  Bicarbonate: 40 mEq/L
  Potassium: 4.2 mEq/L
  Blood urea nitrogen/creatinine ratio:
    18:1.0 mg/dL

Arterial blood gas values: pH of 7.32
Partial pressure of carbon dioxide (Pco_2):
  91 mm Hg

What is the most likely cause of these symptoms?

The patient has respiratory acidosis (pH < 7.4 and Pco_2 > 40 mm Hg) with compensatory metabolic alkalosis. Respiratory acidosis can be caused by COPD, airway obstruction, and hypoventilation.

What is the most likely diagnosis?

The patient has a chronic respiratory acidosis, as indicated by the large compensatory increase in bicarbonate to correct for an elevated Pco_2. It is most likely due to her underlying COPD since a patient with a more acute process would not be able to compensate as robustly.

In Figure 14-13, which area corresponds to respiratory acidosis, respiratory alkalosis, metabolic acidosis, and metabolic alkalosis?

Letter A in Figure 14-13 refers to respiratory acidosis, and letter B refers to metabolic acidosis. Letter C refers to respiratory alkalosis, and letter D refers to metabolic alkalosis.

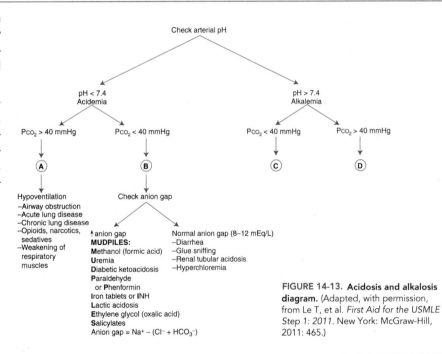

FIGURE 14-13. **Acidosis and alkalosis diagram.** (Adapted, with permission, from Le T, et al. *First Aid for the USMLE Step 1: 2011.* New York: McGraw-Hill, 2011: 465.)

How is this condition distinguished from metabolic acidosis?

In respiratory acidosis, the primary disturbance is an increase in Pco_2 to which the body responds by increasing renal bicarbonate reabsorption. In metabolic acidosis, the primary disturbance is a decrease in bicarbonate, which is compensated for by hyperventilation, resulting in a decreased Pco_2.

What is the anion gap, and what factors can increase the anion gap in this condition?

Anion gap is defined as [Na+] − ([Hco_3^-] + [Cl^-]). In this case it is [144] − ([40] + [96]) = 8, which is within the normal range (8–12). Causes of increased anion-gap metabolic acidosis include renal failure, diabetic ketoacidosis, lactic acidosis, and salicylate ingestion. Causes of normal anion-gap metabolic acidosis include diarrhea, renal tubular acidosis, and hyperchloremia.

■ CASE 17

A 35-year-old African-American man presents to his primary care physician with progressive dyspnea on exertion. He has no history of congestive heart failure or asthma and has had no known contact with any individuals known to have tuberculosis. His laboratory results reveal normal creatinine kinase (CK), CK-MB fraction, and troponin levels. An x-ray of the chest shows bilateral hilar lymphadenopathy and evidence of interstitial lung disease (ILD). A bronchoscopic lung biopsy reveals the presence of several small, noncaseating granulomas.

What is ILD and what are the common causes?

The term ILD is generically used to describe a collection of diseases that involve diffuse scarring and/or inflammation of lung tissue. Common causes of ILD are as follows:

- Prolonged exposure to occupationally inhaled inorganic agents such as silicone, coal, asbestos, talc, mica, aluminum, and beryllium.
- Idiopathic pulmonary fibrosis.
- Connective tissue disease (eg, Wegener granulomatosis, systemic lupus erythematosus, scleroderma, Sjögren disease).
- Sarcoidosis.
- Hypersensitivity pneumonitis, such as "farmer's lung" or "bird-breeder's lung," in which an immune reaction to an organic dust induces a type III or type IV hypersensitivity reaction.
- Radiation-induced disease.
- Antitumor drugs (eg, bleomycin).

What is the most likely cause of ILD in this patient?

Sarcoidosis is the most likely cause. This diagnosis is supported by the patient's race, the presence of **noncaseating granulomas** (discrete collections of tissue macrophages termed *histiocytes* often organized into multinucleated giant cells without central necrosis), and the bilateral hilar lymphadenopathy on x-ray of the chest.

What laboratory abnormalities may be found in this patient?

Vitamin D is secreted by the macrophages of the granulomas and is therefore elevated in serum. Angiotensin-converting enzyme is also secreted by the macrophages of the granulomas and is also elevated.

What pulmonary function testing findings are expected?

In ILD, lung compliance is decreased, reflecting increased stiffness from alveolar wall inflammation and fibrosis. Tidal volume and total lung capacity are typically decreased. Diffusion capacity is also decreased as a result of inflammatory destruction of the air-capillary interface. Unlike most ILDs, sarcoidosis has features of both obstruction and restriction.

What are some extrapulmonary manifestations of this patient's ILD?

Common extrapulmonary manifestations of sarcoidosis are in the eye (anterior uveitis) and skin (papules and erythema nodosum), but granulomas can also occur in the heart, brain, lung, and peripheral lymph nodes.

What is the appropriate treatment for this condition?

Corticosteroids.

■ CASE 18

A 56-year-old man presents to his physician complaining of generalized weakness, cough, and a 9.1-kg (20-lb) weight loss that has occurred over the past 8 weeks. His voice is hoarse and he is unable to keep up with his work as a construction worker. The patient has a 30-pack-year smoking history. Serum sodium is 119 mEq/L. The physician orders posteroanterior and lateral chest radiographs (Figure 14-14).

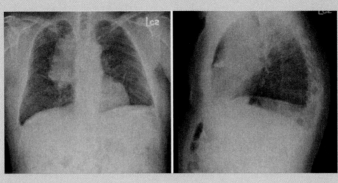

FIGURE 14-14. (Reproduced, with permission, from Kantarjian HM, et al. *MD Anderson Manual of Medical Oncology.* New York: McGraw-Hill, 2006: 239.)

What is this most likely diagnosis?

Small cell lung carcinoma is strongly suggested by the central, hilar nature of the lung mass; a significant weight loss; and a serum sodium of 119 mEq/L, as a result of syndrome of inappropriate antidiuretic hormone (SIADH) as part of the paraneoplastic process.

Which other paraneoplastic processes are associated with this condition?

Small cell lung carcinoma is known to cause hormonally mediated Cushing syndrome due to ectopic secretion of adrenocorticotropic hormone. In addition, up to 3% of patients with small cell lung carcinoma develop Lambert-Eaton myasthenic syndrome.

What additional symptoms can arise from an intrathoracic cancer?

Symptoms for tumors within the thoracic cavity derive from their location and the structures they displace or disrupt, and include superior vena cava obstruction, hoarseness of the voice due to recurrent laryngeal nerve compression, phrenic nerve palsy resulting in dyspnea, dysphagia from esophageal compression, and stridor due to tracheal compression.

To which areas does this condition commonly metastasize?

Small cell lung carcinoma is notable for its metastases to the central nervous system, liver, and bone. As a result, patients may present with bone pain, neurologic symptoms such as seizures or focal deficits, and pain in the right upper quadrant.

What is the prognosis for patients with this condition?

Untreated patients with this disease have a median survival of only 6–17 weeks. However, with combination chemotherapy, median survival may increase to up to 70 weeks. The prognosis largely depends on the tumor's reaction to chemotherapy; drugs include etoposide and cisplatin. Surgery is not an option in small cell carcinoma because of its early and highly aggressive metastasis.

CASE 19

A 55-year-old man comes to the emergency department after suddenly experiencing severe right-sided chest pain followed by profound difficulty breathing. He informs the physician that he has severe emphysema due to an extensive history of tobacco use. On physical examination, the patient is markedly tachypneic and tachycardic. His breath sounds are diminished at the right apex, and his chest wall is hyperresonant to percussion. No tactile fremitus is noted. Arterial blood gas analysis demonstrate a partial pressure of oxygen (PO_2) of 60 mm Hg and a partial pressure of carbon dioxide (Pco_2) of 50 mm Hg.

What is the most likely diagnosis?

Pneumothorax—more specifically, secondary spontaneous pneumothorax. Whereas primary spontaneous pneumothorax occurs in the absence of underlying lung disease, secondary spontaneous pneumothorax occurs in the setting of chronic lung parenchymal disruption.

What is the pathophysiology of this condition?

Spontaneous pneumothorax is most likely caused by rupture of a **subpleural bleb** (a pocket of air caused by destruction of lung parenchyma near the pleural surface), which allows air to escape into the pleural cavity. A tension pneumothorax ensues when a one-way valve is created, allowing air to progressively accumulate with each inspiration. This expanded and pressurized pleural compartment shifts and compresses other intrathoracic structures.

What diseases most often underlie this condition?

The most common underlying condition is chronic obstructive pulmonary disease. Additionally, patients with AIDS, *Pneumocystis jiroveci* (formerly *carinii*) pneumonia, cystic fibrosis, and tuberculosis are at higher risk for spontaneous pneumothorax.

What is the most common clinical presentation of this condition?

Dyspnea with pleuritic chest pain on the same side of the pneumothorax is a common presentation. Typical physical examination findings include diminished breath sounds, hyperresonance, and absent fremitus over the pneumothorax. Arterial blood gas testing typically shows hypoxia and hypercapnia.

What are the typical radiologic findings in this condition?

Partial collapse of the lung on the side of the pneumothorax with a thin line parallel to the chest wall is usually visible. In a **tension pneumothorax**, tracheal and mediastinal deviation can be present away from the pneumothorax. In a **nontension pneumothorax**, however, the trachea and mediastinum will remain unchanged or shift toward the side of the collapsed lung.

What is the appropriate treatment for this condition?

For a tension pneumothorax, needle decompression at the second intercostal space at the midclavicular line is the initial treatment. Then, as with other pneumothoraces, a chest tube (thoracotomy) is placed at the fifth intercostal space at the midaxillary line. Small pneumothoraces may be treated with high concentration oxygen to facilitate nitrogen resorption and followed clinically and radiographically. In the case of repetitive pneumothoraces, parenchymal sclerosing agents such as physical and chemical irritants are used to adhere to layers of the pleura to prevent future pneumothoraces by a process called pleurodesis.

APPENDIX

CASE INDEX

INDEX

ABOUT THE EDITORS

Tao Le, MD, MHS

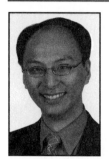

Tao has pursued the dream of better medical education for all for the past 20 years. As senior editor, he has led the expansion of *First Aid* into a global educational series. In addition, he is the founder of the *USMLERx* online test bank series as well as a cofounder of the *Underground Clinical Vignettes* series. As a medical student, he was editor-in-chief of the University of California, San Francisco *Synapse*, a university newspaper with a weekly circulation of 9000. Tao earned his medical degree from the University of California, San Francisco in 1996 and completed his residency training in internal medicine at Yale University and allergy and immunology fellowship training at Johns Hopkins University. At Yale, he was a regular guest lecturer on USMLE review courses and an adviser to the Yale University School of Medicine curriculum committee. Tao subsequently went on to cofound Medsn and served as its chief medical officer. He is currently pursuing research in asthma education at the University of Louisville.

James S. Yeh, MD

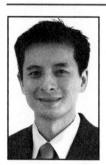

James is a resident physician at Cambridge Health Alliance and a clinical fellow in medicine at Harvard Medical School, where he received a teaching award in recognition of his work with medical students. He is a graduate of Boston University School of Medicine. While at Boston University School of Medicine, he was an Albert Schweitzer Fellow and was awarded the Henry J. Bakst Award in Community Medicine. He completed his undergraduate and graduate work at the University of California, Berkeley and at Harvard University. He looks forward toward a career in academic medicine with emphasis in medical education and evidence-based medicine. He has worked as author and editor on a number of projects in the *First Aid* series including *First Aid for the USMLE Step 1*, *First Aid for the Wards*, and the second edition of *First Aid for the Basic Sciences: General Principles*, as well as the *Step 1 Qmax* test bank. In his spare time, he enjoys traveling, cooking and eating with his wife, playing sports, the guitar, and riding his bike.

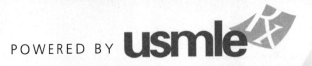
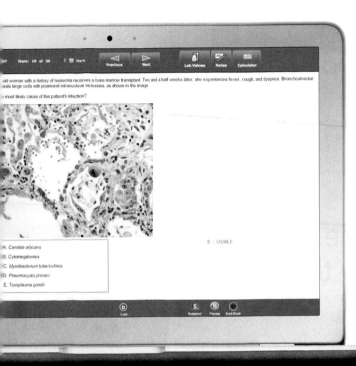
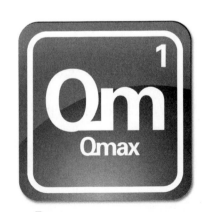

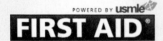

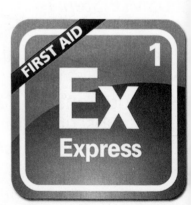